The Concepts of Psychiatry

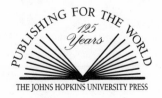

PUBLISHING FOR THE WORLD
125 Years
THE JOHNS HOPKINS UNIVERSITY PRESS

The Concepts of Psychiatry

A Pluralistic Approach to the
Mind and Mental Illness

S. Nassir Ghaemi, M.D.
Department of Psychiatry
Harvard Medical School
Boston, Massachusetts

The Johns Hopkins University Press
Baltimore and London

© 2003 The Johns Hopkins University Press
All rights reserved. Published 2003
Printed in the United States of America on acid-free paper
9 8 7 6 5 4 3 2 1

The Johns Hopkins University Press
2715 North Charles Street
Baltimore, Maryland 21218-4363
www.press.jhu.edu

Library of Congress Cataloging-in-Publication Data

Ghaemi, S. Nassir.
  The concepts of psychiatry: a pluralistic approach to the mind
and mental illness / S. Nassir Ghaemi.
    p.   cm.
  Includes bibliographical references and index.
  ISBN 0-8018-7377-0 (hardcover: alk. paper)
  1. Psychiatry.   2. Psychiatry—Philosophy.
  [DNLM: 1. Psychiatry—methods.   2. Mental Disorders—
therapy.   3. Psychological Theory.   4. Psychotherapy—
methods. WM 100 G411c 2003]
  I. Title.
  RC437.5 .G47 2003
  616.89—dc21   2002152164

A catalog record for this book is available from the British
Library.

For Heather, and for Valentine, and Zane too

[Psychiatry's] faults are, on the whole, much the same as the faults of philosophy—schematization without sufficient evidence, uncritical trust in the adequacy of language, and contention because the contenders do not agree about their axioms or fail to make them explicit.

—AUBREY LEWIS, 1967

Contents

Foreword

We read books from our own professional vantage points and with our own aims—if we're beginners, to learn; if we're practitioners, to refresh our knowledge; if we're investigators, to seek confirmation or refutation of opinions. Of late, I read psychiatric texts to help me see into the future. I want to know where we are going and how we might get there. In this pursuit, most recent books have disappointed me. They come in two varieties.

One group tries to reassure me. Books in this group recount how better off we psychiatrists are now that we have received a reliable classificatory system (DSM-III and IV), along with medications for use with the conditions DSM identifies and, some claim, along with a new understanding of the provocation of many of these mental disorders by "trauma" (present, past, remembered, or repressed). The future they prescribe for the discipline is: "more of the same."

Books in the other group try to dismay me. They bemoan the present neglect of individual psychotherapy. They note the frequent failures of pharmacological medications and wonder about the corrupting power over our thought and practice subtly brought to bear by pharmaceutical companies. They deplore the pervasive and constraining influence exerted on our profession and our patients' treatment by a health system dominated by profit-driven insurance and managed care companies. The future they prescribe for the discipline is: "back to the 1960s."

Truth abides in books in both these groups—admittedly, in some more than others. But I can cultivate feelings of satisfaction or dissatisfaction with the present status of psychiatry without reading them. I'm well aware how psychiatry has grown long on disorders, short on explanations, and vulnerable to accusations of mystification and invention. I'm looking for books that provide a coherent conceptual structure for psychiatry—ones that will permit us to advance rather than retreat, toward a future we can eagerly anticipate.

Dr. Ghaemi has written such a book. It provides what I seek and what I know students and leaders of this discipline need. He assesses the present form of our discipline—sometimes applauding, sometimes demurring to, its modes of thought and ways of practice. But then he provides a method-driven, comprehensive, and practical structure of thought to spur a discourse that is more critical than is customary today and can impel practice, teaching, and research forward. I hope his book will encourage others to continue along the same path and help resolve the impasse I sense from my reading elsewhere. He sets a high standard for all who would follow him.

Dr. Ghaemi first turns his attention to what might be called the "method school" of modern thought and its leaders. Beginning with a thoughtful discussion of Charles Sanders Peirce, he follows on with William James, Wilhelm Dilthey, and Max Weber and culminates with a comprehensive and critical assessment of the psychiatrist Karl Jaspers. Ghaemi points out just why Jaspers is the expert on psychiatric methods and just how his work clarifies the discipline. Armed by his reflections on Jaspers, Ghaemi then translates the clinical approaches of Sigmund Freud, Adolf Meyer, and Emil Kraepelin into the language of method so as to render their merits and their limits apparent to us. He moves then to the present by describing the contemporary synthesizers of information, such as Gerald Klerman, Edward Hundert, Robert Spitzer, and Eric Kandel, as they reflect on the past, imagine the future, and lead the conversation—sometimes forward and sometimes into conceptual cul-de-sacs. With all, he challenges views and prescriptions from a Jaspers-inspired base: one specifically emphasizing the methods employed and what those methods actually permit one to say.

On the basis of this extensive and thoughtful scholarship, Ghaemi champions what he and Dr. Leston Havens have referred to as "pluralism" in psychiatric thought and practice and what we at Johns Hopkins have referred to as "perspectivism." Pluralism, by any name, rests on three important but interrelated issues. (1) Psychiatry is a unique medical discipline attending to those disorders susceptible to diagnosis, prognosis, and treatment that emerge in personal consciousness—the domain of "mind" rather than the domain of "body." (2) Several different classes of mental disorder exist and demand distinct methods for their explanation (hence "pluralism"). (3) Each disorder disrupts some functional feature of human mental life and thus reveals, as a kind of experiment of nature, the natural role of this feature in health.

Ghaemi defines psychiatrists as practitioners who work with several methods, each relatively independent of the others even as they interrelate in any comprehensive description of the discipline. He demonstrates, with salient examples, how many commentators who would assess psychiatry and its place in medicine do not understand this idea.

And they should, because pluralism, by committing psychiatry to methodology (defined properly as the study of methods of psychiatric explanation so as to appreciate their applications, their elements, their strengths, and their limits), is the key to the future of the discipline. In particular, pluralism will advance a classificatory system that moves beyond the ever-expanding dictionary approach of DSM-IV. It will provide—by definition—the approaches to validity that the original authors of DSM-III said would have to come into play once psychiatric terminology became reliable.

Pluralism has an ecumenical stance, as it can eliminate the ongoing chaos of "camps" of therapists that bewilders onlookers to our discipline—and not a few of those who are seeking treatment. Thus, it transforms our conversation from one among adversaries with agendas—biologic, psychodynamic, biopsychosocial, etc.—to one among colleagues who see interesting and complicated clinical problems and want to bring about solutions.

Most important, with a methodological structure of reasoning on which to place factual information, the beginning student can engage teachers in a progressive and interactive conversation over what we know and how we know it—employing clinical experience then to advance rapidly in skill and comprehension. We all can hope that psychiatry will eventually join medicine in identifying how the disorders we recognize are not entities imposed from without on people but rather expressions of life under altered circumstances that we can work to correct. To achieve this goal, we need to grasp how we are both working with patients and thinking about their conditions.

Read here and see the future—not darkly and indistinctly hoping for inspiration, but face to face with the methods and practices that will bring the future to pass.

Paul R. McHugh, M.D.

Preface

Seymour Kety once told a parable that summarizes much of what I seek to do in this book. Kety was a biologically oriented psychiatric researcher, the first scientific director of the National Institute of Mental Health (NIMH), and a pioneer in establishing genetics research, particularly in schizophrenia, in the 1950s and 1960s. In 1960 Kety sought to highlight the limitations of all approaches in psychiatry, whether biological or not. His story, which he called "The True Nature of a Book," was along these lines:

> Let us imagine a community with inhabitants who are of high intelligence and quite civilized except that they have never seen a book and have developed other means for the transmission of knowledge. One day a million books appear in their midst, an event which arouses so much curiosity and consternation that they decide to establish a scientific institute to study them. They set up this institute by disciplines and establish a policy that each scientist may examine these objects only with the tools and techniques and concepts of his discipline.
>
> The first laboratory to be organized is the Laboratory of Anatomy. There the workers study these strange objects for a while and [conclude]: "The specimen is a roughly rectangular block of material, covered ventrally and dorsally with two coarse, fibrous, encapsulated laminae approximately three millimeters thick. Between these lie several hundred white lamellae a fraction of a millimeter thick, all fastened at one end and mobile at the other. On closer inspection, [it contains] a large number of black surface markings arranged in linear groupings in a highly complex manner."
>
> By that time the chemists have arrived on the scene. The first chemist to get hold of a specimen burns it, and satisfies himself that it obeys the law of the conservation of matter and is therefore in his province. . . . Next comes the analytical chemist, who discovers first its elementary composition but later breaks it down less completely into pure compounds; he also reports traces of elementary carbon, "which are probably impurities. . . ."

Then there are the biochemists, who slice the book and mince it and, best of all, homogenize it. . . . But all of these chemists have an uncomfortable feeling that though what they are doing is important, the real answers will come from the fellow down the hall who has just arrived and is still polishing his bright and expensive equipment—the molecular biologist.

With the self-confidence which comes from the adulation of the less fundamental sciences, he is anxious to begin work on the book he has selected because someone has told him that it is biased and distorted. Having hung a sign over his door which reads, "No twisted book without a twisted molecule," he proceeds to search for the molecule. By repeated extraction, centrifugation and ultracentrifugation, electrophoresis, hydrolysis, and repolymerization he finally isolates a pure substance, free of the carbon particles, and—what is even better—a macromolecule, and a twisted one at that . . . cellulose.

Simultaneously, the physiologists have been attacking the subject. Unlike the biochemists, they have read the report from the anatomists and proceed to study and speculate upon why and how the pages are attached on one another. They study the movement of the pages as the book is riffled and derive complex equations to describe it. Then a biophysicist discovers that in an appropriate electrostatic field the graphite deposits produce discontinuities in potential. Fine microelectrodes are developed to pick these up, and amplifiers and oscilloscopes to display them. . . . They develop thousands of tracings of these signals . . . [some of which] are reproducible but incomprehensible. . . . The pattern is fed into the . . . computers, which can generate and test thousands of hypotheses per minute. Finally, the electric typewriter begins to print; the meaning has been found in that complex pattern—it reads "THE."

By this time the behavioral scientists have been admitted to the institute and begin to study the problem. They are a strange lot. Some of them have read the reports of the anatomists, the chemists, and the physiologists, but many of them don't seem to care. Most will admit, if pressed, that the book is material in nature, that it obeys material laws, that it and its contents are nothing more than a highly specialized arrangement of chemical substances. But they don't slice the book, and they don't purify its chemical components—in fact, they seem to feel it is improper to do so. Instead, they ask questions peculiar to their disciplines and look in the book for the answers. The first one likes to count, so he counts the number of letters in the words and comes up with a frequency distribution of the words by their length. He finds a preponderance of four-letter words. . . . His colleagues . . . learn a great deal about classes of books, how they differ from one another, and what their effects are on the community. Although the behavioral scientist has learned much about the nature of books . . . his techniques falter in the area of the individual book, its characteristics, and his ability to make entirely reliable predictions about it. If it is important to learn something about the individual book, then there is need for a technique which can read it completely. Such a technique has not yet appeared, but some progress has been made in its development.

Finally, the book is brought in desperation to the psychoanalyst in the hope that he will be able to read it. That he does not do precisely, but instead asks the author to select portions and read them while he listens. Of course, the author is biased and reads what he wants to read, or, if there is "good transference," those passages which he thinks the analyst would like to hear. And the analyst himself doesn't always hear with equal acuity but, depending on his school or on his preconceived notions, is deaf to greater or lesser portions of the data.

Nonetheless, this anecdotal, biased, and selected patchwork may be the closest approximation which we have to the rich and almost inexhaustible fund of information which reposes in the individual human brain and, to a significant extent, determines individual behavior. (Kety 1960, 1867–69)

This story can be read in a number of ways. Kety was trying to convince his colleagues, both biologists and psychoanalysts, that they should be humble and open-minded—and that is an important message. But in addition, he seemed to mean his story as a pluralist object lesson. The headnote for the paper in which he told this parable is "Many disciplines contribute to understanding human behavior, each with peculiar virtues and limitations," which is a good definition of pluralism. Kety's own words are, "I have merely wanted to point out that we do not always get closer to the truth as we slice and homogenize and isolate—that what we gain in precision and in the rigorous control of variables we sometimes lose in relevance to normal function, and that, in the case of certain diseases or problems, the fundamental process may often be lost in the cutting" (Kety 1960).

But this is not a simple story of the limits of science and biology and the need for wholehearted plunging ahead into psychoanalytic or any other psychosocial orthodoxy (even the biopsychosocial model). By pluralism I do not mean something simple and uncontroversial. In fact, pluralism in psychiatry, as I understand it, is a difficult and demanding vocation. Many readers will find something unappealing in it. By pluralism I do not mean simple acceptance of different views. That is the eclectic error, which really represents the status quo in psychiatry. I feel the eclectic error is an obstacle to further progress, and I wrote this book partly to unmask this problem. Kety's fable is a pluralist tale that seeks to dethrone eclecticism as well as dogmatism. Kety's book could not be approached by any single approach available to the denizens of the planet where it appeared. Even the fanciest biological and the fanciest psychoanalytic approaches failed. But the answer is not to simply say that all approaches are equally valid, as in the eclectic error. There are two answers. The first answer is to try to find a single method that will allow you to solve the problem. At one level, the answer is simple: read the book. Don't grind it down into its biochemical constituents; don't psychoanalyze it; read it. And this does not mean that in other circumstances, biochemical analyses or even psychoanalysis might not be the best methods to use. In this circumstance, we need to find the best method to handle this problem. We need to simply read the book. Finding the right method for the right problem: that is the difficult task and the imperative of pluralism. This aspect of pluralism, a second definition of it, is different from Kety's first definition. One should not assume that the problem is intractable. Frequently, a single method does solve the problem. If one method proves clearly superior to others, then it is the preferred method. Not all methods are created equal. The eclectic error is to make this equality assumption beforehand and then not to carefully apply any method in its purity.

The first answer might be unavailable, however. It may be empirically demonstrable that no single method solves the problem, as in Kety's parable. And this is how Kety sets up his story. He tells us: "If it is important to learn something about the individual book, then there is need for a technique which can read it completely. Such a technique has not yet appeared." In that case, although every effort needs to be made to continue to develop such a technique, the second definition of pluralism holds: "A truer picture of the nervous system and of behavior will emerge only from its study by a variety of disciplines and techniques, each with its own virtues and its own peculiar limitations" (Kety 1960). This is the pluralism of Karl Jaspers, and of more recent thinkers, which I will explain in this book. This is not, however, the eclecticism of the biopsychosocial model, which mixes methods and techniques and disciplines, is supremely unaware of the strengths and limits of many of them, and is highly susceptible to the biases of the individuals who profess eclectic allegiances. When no single technique works well enough, pluralism means identifying the techniques that work best, knowing their limits, and also working on other techniques that may prove better. At the same time, multiple techniques from multiple approaches may provide a better overall picture of the matter at hand. However, each technique must be applied purely and carefully, not mixing it with others, but always recognizing its limits.

Most clinicians in psychiatry and allied fields have, in theory, given up dogmatism, the belief that one method is sufficient for all problems. And they profess eclecticism, which is a vague notion that all methods need to be used, simultaneously, mixed together; in practice, most clinicians are still dogmatists, though. This is worse in some ways than the past situation, because they no longer realize that they are dogmatists. Pluralism seeks to uproot dogmatism in practice and in theory, while allowing for the efficacy of a single method for some, though not all, problems. Pluralism is a complex, difficult approach to understanding the mind and mental illness. Most clinicians have never carefully thought about or understood it. Kety's parable reminds us how utterly important it is to progress in understanding pluralism in relation to human behavior.

My goal is to provide a context for these issues in our understanding of psychiatry and mental illness, as well as to try to map out a nondogmatic, noneclectic future for us all.

Though I will use the word *philosophy* in this book, I hope it does not scare away the reader. For those with a mild allergy to it, let me explain what I mean by philosophy. I do not mean metaphysical systems of thought that require much reading and produce much aching of the cranial musculature. One feels the shadow of Socrates hounding us with dialogues, of Plato's dreams of reasons, of Aristotle's lengthy discourses, not to mention the hefty speculations of Kant, Hegel, and the rest. The reader should read on. Though she might see these names in this book, they will not haunt her. The philosophy that I use here is not primarily of this type.

By philosophy, I simply mean thinking hard. I mean what William James meant when he said that philosophy consists of "an unusually stubborn effort to think clearly" (quoted in Lewis 1967). In fact, many nonphilosophers do not realize how far many contemporary philosophers have come from the old metaphysical days. Current academic philosophy might be divided into two major camps. The first, called analytic, is most prevalent in Anglo-American countries, and its leading thinkers have included Bertrand Russell and W. V. O. Quine. Analytic philosophers strongly oppose classical metaphysical systems in philosophy. They view the main task of philosophy to be the clarification of what we mean when we use certain words either in common speech or in complex philosophical argument. Further, analytic philosophers emphasize the importance of the logical form of an argument, not simply its content (perhaps they consider logic more important than content, since if a stream of thought is illogical, then its content becomes irrelevant). Hence, much of the work of modern analytic philosophy has focused on studies of logic (often mathematical) and language. These philosophers tend to be highly sympathetic to modern science, and this approach to philosophy is not at all antithetical to or irrelevant to a scientific approach to any field, including psychiatry.

The second group of philosophers today is often called the phenomenological school. They tend to be prevalent in continental Europe, especially France and Germany. Prominent leaders in this approach have included Edmund Husserl, Martin Heidegger, and Jean-Paul Sartre. These philosophers are not focused on language and logic, but rather on human experience, as understood through intuition and feelings. This group tends to engage in complex theories reminiscent of traditional metaphysics, but unlike their predecessors, these philosophers are likely to downplay reason and focus on emotions and intuition. This approach is often identified with varieties of existentialism and postmodernism, and it often expresses antipathy toward modern science and sympathy toward the humanities.

Most of my efforts in this book are in the analytic tradition. I focus on the logic of what we are doing in psychiatry and the meaning of the language we use. I also utilize some ideas derived from the phenomenological school, however, since, focusing on emotions and experience, this approach offers some insights that are useful for understanding mental illness and psychiatry. Yet in doing so, I am still applying an analytic method to those phenomenological ideas; I examine their logic and their meanings.

So for those who are wary of philosophy, I ask you to read on, since all I am trying to do is to engage in a stubborn effort to think clearly about mind, brain, and mental illness.

I wrote this book to encourage psychiatrists and other mental health professionals to think about what we do, and to help everyone else understand something more about what psychiatrists and other mental health clinicians do. Most clinicians are practical people: they do not theorize; they live in the world of the concrete. The individual patient, with all his idiosyncrasies, is their concern. The best of clinicians, especially when practicing psychotherapy, operate intuitively. When one asks them why they said a certain thing to a patient at a specific moment in therapy, or why they decided to do any particular thing in treatment, those excellent clinicians are rarely able to eloquently enunciate why they do what they do. They are obscure to even their most advanced students, much less their patients or the general public, mainly because they work by instinct.

This is all well and good. But instinct can be wrong as well as right. Ultimately, we need to be able to communicate with each other, with colleagues, students, patients, and the general public. What do we think and do in our understanding and treatment of mental illness, and why? These are the questions behind this book.

Consequently, my main purpose is to explore the conceptual basis of the understanding and treatment of mental illness. I engage in a certain kind of philosophizing, but only as a way to clarify concepts. This is not philosophy in the sense of grand schemes or theories. Since this book is about mental illness, much of it consists of practical matters: psychotherapy, psychopharmacology, treating patients, diagnosing illnesses. But it treats these practical matters from the standpoint of how we understand them conceptually. What do we *mean* when we say a person has such-and-such a diagnosis? *Why* do we treat that person with medications and another with psychotherapy? What do we *mean* when we say that an individual's self is affected in a certain manner?

This book reflects my own self-education as a psychiatrist also interested in philosophy. It is my attempt to understand what I am doing. I hope both psychiatrists and philosophers will find at least parts of it worthwhile.

I also hope that it will prove of interest to others: residents in psychiatry, psychologists and social work professionals and their students, students of medicine, and individuals diagnosed with mental illnesses and their families, many of whom I know to be yearning for guidance about a subject that to them is anything but academic. I hope that all these individuals will see this book as a way to organize their thinking about the mind and how we understand and treat it.

Part 1 is a section on theory; it engages most directly in a philosophical analysis of the concepts of psychiatry. I begin with a discussion of current theories in psychiatry and the mental health professions, which I describe as dogmatism, eclecticism, pluralism, and integrationism (chapter 1). I focus on the errors of eclecticism and the ideas of pluralism and integrationism. Next I turn to psychiatric reality: what kind of entities do mental health professionals interact with (chapter 2)? Then I discuss how we know anything about psychiatric reality; how can we know anything about someone's mind in the circumstances of mental illness (chapter 3)? This section seeks to provide a version of scientific method that is appropriate for psychiatric conditions (chapters 4–7). Last, I examine the ethics of the mental health professions: what kind of value judgments are inherent in our practice (chapters 8–9)?

Part 2 addresses the practice of psychiatry and allied mental health professions, attempting to understand what we are doing as practitioners. I examine controversies in psychiatric nosology (chapters 10–13: the nature of mental illness and diagnostic schemes), psychopathology (chapters 14–17: depression, mania, psychosis, insight), and treatment (chapters 18–22: the value and limits of psychotherapy and psychopharmacology).

In Part 3 I seek to summarize topics covered in the book. I also reexamine the weaknesses of eclecticism and suggest how we can better understand the diagnosis and treatment of mental illnesses pluralistically.

I can only echo Karl Jaspers in my hopes for how readers might approach this book:

> I would like my book to give the reader a wide education in psychopathology. It is indeed much simpler to learn up formulae and technical terms and appear to have the answer to everything. An educated attitude has to grow slowly from a grasp of limits within a framework of well-differentiated knowledge. It lies in the ability to think objectively in any direction. An educated attitude in psychiatry depends on our own experience and on the constant use of our power of observation—no book can give us that—but it also depends on the clarity of the concepts we use and the width and subtlety of our comprehension, and it is these which I hope my book will enhance. ([1913] 1997, 50)

Acknowledgments

This book is my education. It incorporates the topics that intrigued me as I came of age. Consequently, this project is a labor of many years and activities. Throughout the process of its writing, I realized how many people had helped me along the way, and I looked forward to publicly thanking and acknowledging them.

First and foremost, I credit my father, Kamal Ghaemi, M.D., a neurosurgeon and neurologist who is equally skilled in the humanities, for instilling a love of learning in me. This inheritance has become a guiding feature of my life. My father first showed me the mysteries of the mind and the brain, and the deep wonder of how we might understand these mysteries. He also taught me the importance of science as well as the relevance of philosophy. He instructed me, above all, not only in the science of life but also in the art of living. His knowledge and skills extend from his profession to a background in socialism and a deep knowledge of Islamic and Iranian literature. This work is a consequence of his efforts as much as mine. I also want to thank my mother, Guity Kamali Ghaemi, who did so much of the hard work of caring for our family and was able to teach me Persian poetry while she was washing the dishes. And I thank my grandfather, Mohammad Mehdi Kamali, who is, for me, a second father. In his deeply wise manner, he has handled quite difficult circumstances, running a company for six decades in a tumultuous country; in so many ways, he is for me a living embodiment of virtues in action.

When I first left my native state of Virginia, I found a new family of teachers in Boston. First among them without doubt is Leston Havens, who, both in his personal willingness to meet with me and in his written works, has been an invaluable source of guidance. He more than anyone else nurtured this book along within me and helped bring it to fruition directly. We met numerous times before its writing and in the process of its completion. I will never forget his wonderful advice when I was struggling with how to plan the manuscript: just start writing it, he said, and then we'll take it from there. Edward

Hundert served as a role model for me of a person who could seriously engage in both philosophy and psychiatry; I was privileged to be in touch with him as my assistant residency director, and thus I realized that I could actually pursue philosophy and psychiatry simultaneously. Daniel Dennett was the philosopher who welcomed me into his graduate school and showed me how open, creative, and fun modern philosophy could be. He and his colleagues at Tufts University, particularly Stephen White, George Smith, Mark Richard, Jody Azzouni, Jeff McConnell, and Norman Daniels, opened new doors of learning to me in modern analytic philosophy. They provided me with methodological tools that I did not possess, and I am deeply thankful for their instruction. I have found companionship and another set of tutors and colleagues in the Association for the Advancement of Philosophy and Psychiatry. Ever since they, too, welcomed me into their fold as a rather green psychiatric resident, these philosophers and psychiatrists have nurtured my interests and helped broaden my immersion in these important ideas. Foremost among them is Jennifer Radden, head of the Boston chapter and the overall president of the association. Michael Schwartz and John Sadler have also been quite supportive. I also must thank other members of the Boston chapter, whose monthly meetings have been enriching to me. I particularly thank Marshal Folstein, whose energy and clearheadedness I admire. The members of the Karl Jaspers Society of North America also accepted me and taught me more about this extremely important thinker in a way that has greatly altered my thinking about psychiatry. Among philosophers in this group, Gregory Walters has been an especially wonderful colleague, and Leonard Ehrlich and George Pepper have tutored me personally to my great benefit.

I also want to thank Frederick Goodwin, who has been an ideal psychiatric mentor for me. Fred has been the single deepest professional influence on me, and I owe him a great deal for helping nurture and promote my academic career. He also helped keep my interest in the conceptual aspects of psychiatry alive as we both engaged in psychopharmacological research. Ross Baldessarini has also more recently played an important role in showing me how important conceptual interests remain in modern psychiatry and psychopharmacology. His historical work on the Kraepelinian era has been quite enlightening for me. Paul McHugh's work has always been fascinating to me, and in various interviews over the years he also served as a role model of the modern psychiatrist who remains curious about the conceptual foundations of our field. He was especially helpful in convincing the Johns Hopkins University

Press to take a look at a first draft of this manuscript, and for that help I am grateful to him. I would also like to thank Wendy Harris at the Press for accepting the manuscript and helping me pull it together. My close friend and residency colleague Godehard Oepen has always been a wonderful companion in my philosophical-psychiatric interests; he helped revise chapters of this book, as did Jennifer Radden, Scott Waterman, and Leston Havens. I also thank Scott Waterman for inviting me to give a grand rounds at the University of Vermont near the end of the period of manuscript preparation, an experience that helped me clarify some issues regarding pluralism. My discussions with Scott were also helpful in providing another perspective from someone within psychiatry who has been struggling with many of the same topics. Paul Roazen also read parts of the manuscript and has helped me think about some of these ideas. I have greatly benefited from his intellectual companionship. David Healy has also been generous with his time in discussing some of his ideas, which I found quite stimulating. Joshua Shenk, who is at work on a book on Lincoln's melancholia, also traded fruitful thoughts about depression. My colleague David Brendel, a rare psychiatrist who is also a fully trained Ph.D. philosopher, cotaught a course with me on the concepts of psychiatry at the 2002 meeting of the American Psychiatric Association, which helped me hone aspects of this book. David Duncan also encouraged me and offered his experience as a writer in the early stages of my preparation for this work.

William Osler once remarked that a physician's teachers are like parents to him. Thus, I would be remiss if I did not thank and acknowledge my first psychiatric mentors at the Medical College of Virginia. John Gilliam was my first teacher in the wards, and Gustavo Corretjer, who treated substance abusers in the Veterans Administration hospital with philosophical group therapy, first showed me the clinical relevance of philosophy for psychiatry. Kenneth Kendler and Lyndon Eaves first introduced me to the wonders of psychiatric research, and their work has remained a prime example of principled scholarship for me. I actually learned to practice psychiatry during my residency at the hands of wonderful clinicians and supervisors at McLean Hospital outside Boston: Steven Sternbach, Jeffrey Gilbert, Walker Shields, Andrew Stoll, Harrison G. Pope Jr., Jonathan Cole, John Gunderson, Alexander Vuckovic, J. Alexander Bodkin, Roger Weiss, Mauricio Tohen, Philip Isenberg, Richard Schwartz. I thank each of them and feel very privileged to have learned about this complex field in the company of such a distinguished group of teachers. I also thank, in my fellowship years at Massachusetts General Hospital, Gary

Sachs, Andrew Nierenberg, and Maurizio Fava for taking me further into the fields of mood disorders and clinical research.

I also acknowledge and thank the chairman of the Department of Psychiatry at Cambridge Hospital, Jay Burke, who took a keen interest in my work and whose department supported me emotionally and practically during the final stages of preparing this book. I also thank my research assistants for the past three years, James Ko, Doug Hsu, and Klara Rosenquist, whose daily labors have allowed me to find the time to work on this project, and who also listened to many of my ideas as they developed.

I began this book shortly after marrying my wife, Heather, who has not only helped me think through some of these thoughts but also tolerated my immersion in it. It is no accident that I started and finished this work, which had been stewing within me for so long, only after she came into my life. Three years before this book was born, our daughter, Valentine, joined us, and she also deserves credit for living with her father's preoccupations. Sleeping by my side, or running down the hall, she too was a source of inspiration.

Parts of chapter 14 are derived from S. N. Ghaemi, "An Empirical Approach to Understanding Delusions," *Philosophy, Psychiatry, and Psychology* 6 (1999): 21–24. Parts of chapters 15 and 17 are derived from S. N. Ghaemi, "Depression: Insight, Illusion, and Psychopharmacological Calvinism," *Philosophy, Psychiatry, and Psychology* 6 (1999): 287–94. Parts of chapter 17 are also derived from S. N. Ghaemi, "Insight and Psychiatric Disorders: A Review of the Literature, with a Focus on Its Clinical Relevance for Bipolar Disorder," *Psychiatric Annals* 27 (1997): 782–90. Parts of chapter 19 are derived from S. N. Ghaemi, "All the Worse for the Fishes: Conceptual and Historical Background of Polypharmacy in Psychiatry," in *Polypharmacy in Psychiatry* (New York: Dekker, 2002). Parts of chapter 21 are derived from S. N. Ghaemi, "Rediscovering Existential Psychotherapy," *American Journal of Psychiatry* 55 (2001): 51–64.

The Concepts of Psychiatry

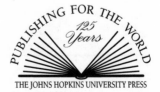

THE JOHNS HOPKINS UNIVERSITY PRESS

Part I / Theory

What Clinicians Think and Why

The psychiatrist has to ponder on the relation of mind to body, in resolving the clinical problems of every patient he sees; he must address himself to questions of value whenever he has to decide whether a patient has become healthy after he has been ill, or whether a particular disturbance of mental activity is a sign of illness; if he is at all reflective, he must examine the validity and limitations of human knowledge, gained through means upon which he relies for his understanding of himself and his patients, while at the same time recognizing how deceived those patients can be when they too rely upon such means of knowledge; and, finally, the problem of causation is thrust on his notice so insistently that even the most unsophisticated psychiatrist is aware that common sense will hardly serve his turn here. The psychiatrist then is confronted, whether he likes it or not, with many of the central issues of philosophy.

—AUBREY LEWIS, 1967

CHAPTER 1

The Status Quo

Dogmatism, the Biopsychosocial Model, and Alternatives

> These are the days when men of all social disciplines and all political
> faiths seek the comfortable and the accepted . . . in minor modification of
> the scriptural parable, the bland lead the bland.
> —JOHN KENNETH GALBRAITH, 1958

1.

What do we do in psychiatry and why? This is a question not asked often enough. Much is taken for granted. At a basic level, psychiatrists do one of two things. One activity is often subsumed under the heading of psychotherapy. Externally, psychotherapy consists of formal meetings, usually weekly, of an hour's duration, over an extended period of time (usually six months or longer). These external characteristics are important, because this prolonged regular contact allows for the development of much that happens in formal psychotherapy. The content of what happens involves, of course, listening and talking, but this listening and talking can be informed by certain methods or techniques (different psychoanalytic approaches, existential methods, cognitive-behavioral techniques, and so on). Importantly, the regular formal contact allows for this dialogue to lead to useful therapeutic outcomes. Of course, such an exchange, often informed by special techniques, can and does occur outside of the formal psychotherapy setting. In general medicine, it can be one component of a good "bedside manner." In general psychiatry, it is relevant to the optimal practice of psychopharmacology as well. Yet there is no doubt that formal psychotherapy represents one important aspect of psychiatry.

The other important part of psychiatry is psychopharmacology, the giving of medications. Psychopharmacology can be approached in various ways. It can be done aggressively, with many medications used for many purposes; and it can be done cautiously, with medications used less frequently. The psychopharmacologist might tend to be evidence-based, focusing on data from studies, or experience-based, focused on his own observations. He could be diagnosis-focused, using medications for diagnoses and syndromes, or he could be symptom-focused. He could view his activity as central to psychiatry, treating real diseases, or he could view it as peripheral, managing symptoms superficially, which are treated more radically through psychotherapy. Finally, in the age of managed care, the psychopharmacologist is also sometimes seen as simply performing *med checks*, a pejorative term that quite degrades his role. I am not sure how this term came about, or exactly what it means. But in practice it seems to imply that psychopharmacology is a simple process consisting of naming the medications, "checking" on their doses and side effects, "checking" on relevant symptoms, and making the relevant adjustments. In many managed care settings, only fifteen to twenty minutes are allotted for such "checks," as would seem to befit their rather superficial status. The work of psychotherapy is assumed to be definitely excluded from med checks.

This dichotomy has always existed in psychiatry, the split between a predominantly psychological approach and a predominantly biological approach, or, as it manifests itself today in practice, between psychotherapy and psychopharmacology. But this split has been exacerbated by the influence of managed care, and now it is reified into the performance of med checks by M.D. psychiatrists and psychotherapy by non-M.D. mental health professionals. Recent work has focused on this dichotomy as the status quo in contemporary psychiatry (Luhrmann 2000). I think most mental health professionals in practice are proponents of one or the other approach. In practice, I emphasize, because, as I stated, most psychiatrists and mental health clinicians do not often ask themselves what they are doing and why. They take for granted that their approach in practice, be it primarily biological or primarily psychosocial, is appropriate for their patients. In so doing, they are dogmatists, a label that is pejorative enough for everyone to deny it. But by *dogmatist* I only mean that these clinicians have an approach to psychiatry that is monistic, based on a belief that one approach to the field is more or less sufficient to explain most of what they observe and do. They are mistaken monists, which is what I mean by dogmatists, because they are not aware of the limits and partial nature of their approach.

When it is stated in this way, most everyone denies being a dogmatist. Some will avowedly defend their monism, such as some psychoanalysts who believe their views are essentially correct and others wrong, but most will deny that they hold monistic or dogmatic views. And when they deny dogmatism, most clinicians revert to a variety of eclecticism as their self-definition. By *eclecticism*, which I discuss in more detail later, they basically mean that they have no single view about what best explains psychiatry. Or they assert an *agnosticism*, meaning they claim that they do not know if any approach is better than any other. If pushed, most clinicians take refuge in the biopsychosocial model, by which they can mean many things, but which, I believe, usually reflects a vague eclecticism.

This back-and-forth between dogmatism and eclecticism is the underlying conceptual status quo of psychiatry today, I believe, more so than the more superficial dichotomy between biological and psychosocial approaches. The biopsychosocial model, as now used in psychiatry, is inadequate. And the status quo is unhealthy.

2.

The biopsychosocial model originates in two historical sources in psychiatry. The first is Adolf Meyer's "psychobiology" (Meyer 1948). Meyer, Swiss-born chair of the Johns Hopkins Department of Psychiatry for decades, was the dean of American psychiatry for most of the twentieth century, especially in the 1920s–1960s era. The DSM-II nosology published in 1968 essentially used Meyer's ideas as its primary basis. Meyer was heavily influenced by the American pragmatic school of thought. It is a little-recognized fact that for a time, when Meyer lived in New York, he lunched weekly with the pragmatic philosopher John Dewey (152). No doubt, the pragmatic ethos of American culture influenced Meyer's opposition to the Kraepelinian status quo of the early twentieth century in European psychiatry. As discussed in some detail in chapter 11, Meyer strongly opposed Kraepelin's biological approach to psychiatry. Meyer felt that Kraepelin was too biological, ignored psychosocial aspects in psychiatry, and was too pessimistic. A common complaint from Meyerians was that Kraepelin and his school only offered "therapeutic nihilism." If one believed that psychiatric illnesses were primarily biological, based on inheritance and other constitutional factors that could not be changed, then one seemed doomed to simply predict the future without any means of changing it. This was inadequate for Meyer. Even granting biological aspects of psychiatric illness, Meyer (1948) was mainly interested, on practical grounds, in those aspects, primarily psychosocial, that could be altered.

For the study of psychology we must adhere to the events as they occur; we study these for what they do, for the conditions under which they arise and for the ways in which we can modify them. . . . (144)

. . . Psychiatric experience has sadly suffered from veritable debauches in unwarranted systematization. . . . An orderly presentation of the facts alone is a real diagnosis. . . . The superstition about the value of a diagnosis of a disease prompts many to believe that a diagnosis once made puts them into a position to solve the queries about the case not with the facts presented by it and naturally considered in the light of principles based on experiment and on clinical experiences with concrete series of cases, but by a system of rules and deductions from the meaning of the newly defined disease entities, with their prognosis and autotoxic or other origin held out to the believer as sufficiently settled for practical purposes. . . . What we act on should be facts. If the facts do not constitute a diagnosis we must nevertheless act on the facts. (153–68)

Hence Meyer opposed the use of disease and syndrome concepts, like those of Kraepelin. Meyer proposed an approach based on viewing psychiatric conditions as "reactions" to life events and psychosocial circumstances. His psychobiology was meant to incorporate the prevalent belief at that time in the importance of biology in psychiatry, while at the same time essentially subordinating biology to being only a part of a broader view of psychiatry focused on the individual person.

We study behavior not merely as a function of the mind and of various parts of the body, but as a function of the individual, and by that we mean the living organism, not a mysteriously split entity. When we see somebody eating or drinking too much or too hurriedly, or overworking, with inadequate recreation, we want to know why and how this occurs, and we modify it not merely as a state of mind but as behavior. That is what we imply by psychobiological—undivided and direct attention to the person and to the function, health, and efficiency of the person as a living organism. . . .

. . . We study the facts (a fact is anything which makes a difference) for what they mean in actual life, and by that we mean the life of a "somebody." He is to us an organism with a life history, a biography. (1948, 434–36)

In all these ways, Meyer's psychobiology was rather hostile, in practice, toward biological approaches in psychiatry. Although Meyer himself kept psychoanalytic orthodoxy at arm's length, the eclectic approach to psychiatry that he fostered gave plenty of room for the psychoanalytic movement to expand its reach in the United States. By the 1950s, after Meyer's death, psychoanalytic dogmatism was paramount. The counterattack of the biologically oriented approach in the 1970s led to DSM-III, a major political success for the biological school. To preserve space for psychological approaches, the psychoanalytically oriented school then rediscovered some of Meyer's ideas in the biopsychosocial model, presented in a unique and attractive form by George Engel (1980).

3.

The biopsychosocial model was advanced most systematically by Engel in the 1970s. Engel held joint appointments in psychiatry and medicine from the 1940s onward, and with his colleague John Romano, he advocated greater emphasis on psychological components of mental illnesses. Engel also engaged in psychoanalytic training in Franz Alexander's institute, which was the center for the "psychosomatic" movement in the United States in the middle of the twentieth century. Alexander, a student of Freud, tried to introduce psychoanalytic ideas into general medicine. In his clinical work at the University of Rochester, where Engel spent most of his career, Engel mainly focused on what is now called "consultation-liaison" psychiatry, that is, the practice of assisting medical colleagues in treatment of psychiatric conditions. His main interests for a while included ulcerative colitis, psychogenic pain, and the psychological effects of gastrointestinal fistulae in children. Hence, Engel's work was primarily directed toward understanding the psychological aspects of medical conditions, rather than the biological aspects of psychiatric conditions. Although Engel and his colleagues had promoted their views for decades, his systematic exposition in the 1970s elicited great interest and became the standard model of psychiatry in the 1980s. It remains so today.

Engel apparently felt called to formulate the biopsychosocial model formally as opposed to "biomedical reductionism" because of the resurrection of biological psychiatry in the 1970s and the decline of psychoanalytic influences in psychiatry as well as in medicine. For many in psychiatry, the biopsychosocial model promised an end to the increasingly bloody conflict between the biological and psychoanalytic schools. Further, the biological school, though pushing forward a return to Kraepelinian nosology in DSM-III in 1980, was willing to back off on a commitment to a clear biological etiology for psychiatric disorders. The *neo* in *neo-Kraepelinian* stands, to a great extent, for this difference: Kraepelin strongly believed in an almost completely biological etiology and pathogenesis of major mental illnesses. Those who resurrected his nosology in the United States in the 1970s (see chapter 11) were willing to be "atheoretical" about this topic. They wanted to give up the Meyerian commitments of DSM-II, but they were also willing to avoid a biological commitment in etiologies. The biopsychosocial model filled this void, since it was consistent with all approaches. Engel's proposal quickly caught on in psychiatry, though not in general medicine as he had hoped. In fact, today, for a psychiatrist to pass her specialty boards, she needs to interview a patient and discuss that patient with board examiners who literally write down three categories— "bio," "psycho," and "social"—and the candidate is expected to cover material in each category. This is the case with practically every patient and every condition. Taken to such lengths, the biopsychosocial model has been exaggerated far beyond its origins in psychosomatic medicine (Brown 2000).

At least one benefit of the biopsychosocial model, in theory, is that it avoids dogmatism. If one takes it seriously, one cannot simply subscribe to biological reductionism or to psychoanalytic exclusivity. But this benefit is outweighed, it seems to me, by the model's drawbacks, which I now explain.

One of Engel's innovations was to link the biopsychosocial model to systems theory. Systems theory has a long and complicated history (originating with the biologist Ludwig von Bertanlaffy), but it is at one level consistent with what we discuss in chapter 2 as *emergence* in contemporary philosophy of mind. Systems theory views psychology as a different level of experience than biology, just as biology is different from chemistry and physics. Yet all these levels interact with each other. Complex systems consist of these interacting components, and such systems are viewed as a whole, rather than analyzed into their separately functioning parts. This approach returns to the holistic tradition in science and medicine, as opposed to the analytic tendencies of current scientific method in medicine. Presented as a discussion of *methods,* the biopsychosocial approach has some similarities to what I call pluralism, and I am not wholly critical of these views. However, in practice, the biopsychosocial model has evolved into a confusing set of assumptions about the *content* of psychiatric conditions. And here I think it has degenerated into a lazy eclecticism. As interpreted by most mental health professionals today, this model does little but assert that all illnesses have components that are, unsurprisingly, biological, psychological, and social (or interpersonal).

Thus, to take diabetes as an example, one possesses a genetic predisposition (biology), which produces the illness when coupled with excessive weight gain, which in turn has psychological (anxiety, depression) or social (availability of junk food, eating-out habits) roots. Engel's well-taken point is that one should not ignore psychosocial aspects of medical illness to focus only on the biological aspects, such as, with diabetes, simply recommending insulin, while ignoring the need to lose weight. It must have been clear to Engel and the early formulators of this theory that the biopsychosocial model applies better to some illnesses, like diabetes, than others, such as genetically transmitted diseases (e.g., Tay-Sachs disease). In Tay-Sachs, for instance, little can be said concerning the etiology of the illness beyond the bad luck of a random genetic transmission. This would seem to make the etiology purely biological. Nongenetic conditions that are purely biological are also common, like viral encephalitis, where the etiology simply seems to involve random viral infection and host immunological receptivity. Did Engel really mean to say that psychosocial factors are as important as biological factors in the etiology of such genetic and infectious diseases? I doubt it. In fact, biopsychosocial ideas have been incorporated into primary-care medicine with little controversy precisely because they are so commonsensical. The model, from one perspective, just underscores the well-known humanistic aspects of medicine, the need to pay attention to psychosocial factors when they are present, especially in certain illnesses in which they seem to play important roles.

Probably the first critique of the biopsychosocial model in psychiatry came from Paul McHugh and Philip Slavney (see below), who argue that the biopsychosocial model is excessively broad and provides no real guidance to clinicians or researchers. They compare the model to a list of ingredients, as opposed to a recipe. To cook a meal, it is not sufficient to simply know the list of ingredients. One also needs to know how much of each ingredient to use, and in which order. The biopsychosocial model only lists relevant aspects of psychiatry; it is silent as to how to understand those aspects under different conditions and in different circumstances. As a consequence, it becomes eclecticism, where the clinician essentially does whatever he wants to do (McLaren 1998).

Thus, in psychiatry, the biopsychosocial model has become a mantra, another ideology to replace (or perhaps hide?) the previous ones. Although Engel and the more nuanced biopsychosocial theorists surely did not so intend it, the model has become transformed into an excuse for intellectual laziness. All psychiatric conditions, from schizophrenia to stress-related anxiety, it seems, are held to be explainable biopsychosocially. Often, this means that while clinicians admit biological aspects to an illness, they insist on paying attention to the equally important psychosocial ones. So, if someone is depressed, one engages in extensive questioning regarding psychosocial stressors and pays little attention to basic phenomenological characteristics of illness (such as mania or hypomania); social histories are extensive, even when basic biologically relevant facts such as family history of illnesses often are less rigorously examined; mental status examinations are lengthy, but longitudinal histories of previous episodes (their onset, offset, years of occurrence, relationship to treatments) are left sketchy. I believe the biopsychosocial model in most cases seems to justify older psychological habits (concentration on the current mental status, psychological development, and childhood history) at the expense of progress in understanding the biological aspects of these conditions (careful pharmacological treatment history, detailed phenomenological history of mood or psychotic episodes, accurate genetic history). All this results in shoddy diagnosis and haphazard treatment success.

Another problem with the biopsychosocial model is that it not only confuses method and content, as described above, but also confuses cause and treatment. Hence it encourages sloppy thinking along the lines that if a condition is considered to have important psychological components, then psychological treatments should be preferred. If one truly holds that all psychiatric illnesses are biological, psychological, and social (especially if one believes that they are equally all three), then it would seem to follow that everyone should receive both biological and psychosocial treatments (treatments by both medication and psychotherapy). One hears this truism often, a false and faulty belief that stems directly from the biopsychosocial model (discussed further in chapter 24).

The superficial attraction of the biopsychosocial model is that it appears obviously true at one level. Any condition has all three aspects, it would seem, at least to some degree. Yet, if true, this is a trite interpretation. It has little meaning and provides minimal guidance to clinicians, researchers, or patients. Strongly ensconced in current psychiatric orthodoxy, a politically correct view that few have criticized, the biopsychosocial model is essentially sterile. To the extent that it is true, it is trite. And to the extent that it seeks to say anything, either it is better said with a principled pluralism, as I advocate later in this book, or it is simply asserting a problematic eclecticism.

Table 1.1 The Conceptual Status Quo in Psychiatry

1. Dogmatism
   a. Biological reductionism
   b. Psychoanalytic orthodoxy
2. Eclecticism
   a. Biopsychosocial model (Adolf Meyer, George Engel)
   b. Agnosticism (DSM-III onward)
3. Pluralism
   a. Karl Jaspers's methodological consciousness
   b. Leston Havens's approaches to the mind
   c. Paul McHugh and Philip Slavney's perspectives of psychiatry
4. Integrationism
   a. Edward Hundert's Hegelian neurobiology
   b. Eric Kandel's neuroplasticity

4.

What are the alternatives to dogmatisms (yesterday's orthodoxies) and eclecticism (today's orthodoxy)? I think the alternatives fall into two categories: pluralism and integrationism. Prominent proponents of pluralism are Leston Havens on the one hand, and Paul McHugh and Philip Slavney on the other. Proponents of integrationism are Edward Hundert and Eric Kandel. I will review their ideas here and return to them repeatedly throughout later chapters.

5.

In the early 1970s, before psychoanalysts were willing to accept it, the psychiatrist Leston Havens proposed an alternative to the hegemony of psychoanalytic theory in understanding the mind (Havens [1973] 1987). He also critiqued eclecticism, which has since become a synonym for the biopsychosocial model.

I will delay my comments on psychoanalytic hegemony until chapter 20, but mainstream psychiatry now holds that psychoanalytic theory has not delivered on many of its promises and that it is only one explanation of some mental phenomena, not the total explanation. Havens makes this point as part of his larger conceptual scheme. I think his most important critique is his discussion of eclecticism. It is sometimes assumed that eclecticism is the natural alternative to dogmatism. But in many ways, it is worse. At least supporters of psychoanalytic dogmas have certain beliefs. Eclectics eschew all theories, in theory. In practice, they either enact theories without being honest about it with themselves, or they do what seems right for the moment without any underlying rationale. The biopsychosocial model provides a cover for this idle eclecticism: everything is acceptable, and it can be justified by being labeled as biological or psychosocial as deemed necessary under the model's broad umbrella.

Havens's alternative is *pluralism*. He organizes differing approaches in psychiatry into four schools of thought. The key advantage of his work is that he divides the schools based on their methods, not on their content, which clears away many differences in theory that can obscure larger underlying agreements in methods. The four schools defined by Havens are the objective-descriptive, the psychoanalytic, the existential, and the interpersonal schools.

The objective-descriptive school is based on the traditional scientific method of empirical observation and statistical analysis. Its leader was Emil Kraepelin (1921), probably (other than Freud) the most prominent twentieth-century psychiatrist, who first clearly established the diagnoses of schizophrenia and manic-depressive illness.[1] This school of thought emphasizes the classical medical approach: obtain a list of symptoms and signs in the course of the psychiatric history and the mental status examination, relate these symptoms and signs to collections of syndromes, and then find the underlying diseases beneath those syndromes. The diseases would then be treated, as would any medical diseases, "somatically," that is, with medications or other physical treatments (e.g., surgery, electroconvulsive therapy). The causes of these diseases are mostly biological, such as viruses or brain abnormalities. Thus, Kraepelin's student Alois Alzheimer discovered the brain abnormalities underlying the dementia that now bears his name; also, many of the psychotic patients Kraepelin studied were discovered to suffer from syphilitic infection of the brain, a discovery that greatly influenced Kraepelin and others to pursue possible theories of underlying viral infections as the etiology of schizophrenia. The content of objective-descriptive theories can vary, but Havens makes the point that all the theories share one thing: the methodology of empirical observation and description as in the traditional medical model.

The second school is the psychoanalytic one, founded by Freud. Its basic method is free association, which is the use of "free-floating attention." The doctor or therapist is not pursuing the description of signs and symptoms, as above, but simply listening in a completely neutral way, without initially forming any judgments. By allowing the statements discussed to wander in whatever direction they take, Freud found that a certain logic imposed itself on the therapy which was not accessible to the objective-descriptive approach. That is, if the therapist tried to make sense of things, nothing made sense. Once the therapist stopped and simply let things go wherever they went, a sense of order grew up out of the apparently meandering associations produced. Havens's achievement in stripping the psychoanalytic school down to this bare essential is that his readers are less confused when faced with the myriad subschools produced by Freud's followers. Whether Adlerian or Jungian, Reichian or Kleinian—whatever the sect—they all subscribe to free association as their basic method. This is similar to the many biological theories in psychiatry (infectious disease models, hormone theories, neurotransmitter models, epilepsy analogies, and so on), whose theory content differs while their objective-descriptive methodologies remain the same. Freud's method especially helped its founder with a group of conditions (collectively called *hysteria*) that were poorly assessed and treated with the predominant objective-descriptive models of nineteenth-century Vienna (see chapter 20).

The third school is the existential school, and its leaders in psychiatry include Ludwig Binswanger (1963a), R. D. Laing (1969), and others.[2] The main method of this school is empathy, placing oneself in the position of the other person. As in the psychoanalytic school, from which some of the existentialists derived, the therapist begins with a neutral listening to the patient, but the existential therapist does not, as in psychoanalysis, later try to organize what is learned into a theory. The therapist's role is to simply understand the patient, not theorize about him. In fact, the patient-treater difference is annulled; the goal of treatment is a coming together wherein the patient (to use an objective-descriptive term) moves toward the therapist and the therapist moves toward the patient. The whole subject-object divide upon which the objective-descriptive school is based is thus erased in the existential school. Some of the most interesting work that has arisen from this school is research on the subjective experience of psychosis and the psychology of depression.

The fourth school is the interpersonal one, or what Havens also calls the social psychiatry school. One of its leaders is Harry Stack Sullivan, the only American among the founding leaders of these schools. Later proponents include Erich Fromm, Erik Erikson, Carol Gilligan, and others.[3] The methodology of this school, as derived from Sullivan, involves "clearing the interpersonal field." This refers to Sullivan's view that any interaction between two persons, such as a psychiatric interview between doctor and patient, involves interpersonal reactions that influence the psychological phenomena observed. These reactions frequently tend to distort the interpersonal field; this occurs not only in psychosis, where it may be due to the effect of paranoia, as described by Sullivan, but also in nonclinical interactions, such as communication between men and women (Tannen 1990). Before Sullivan, the orthodox psychoanalytic view was that such interpersonal phenomena, seen as "transference," were necessary stages toward gaining a deeper understanding of the patient's inner psychic life. Sullivan was unsatisfied with this approach, because—among other reasons—by focusing on the transference, psychoanalysis often seemed to only worsen the distortions produced. Sullivan's work largely consists of proposing methods to actively combat these transferential distortions (see chapter 22).

6.

Another pluralistic approach is based on Paul McHugh and Philip Slavney's *Perspectives of Psychiatry* (1998). Like Havens, they focused on identifying different methods underlying basic conceptual approaches in psychiatry. Unlike Havens, they did not focus on different schools of thought in psychotherapy, and they did not emphasize a historical approach of examining founders and followers among the different schools of thought. Instead, they described four different theoretical perspectives in psychiatry:

1. Disease: What the patient *has*. The goal of treatment according to this perspective is cure. This view agrees with Havens's objective-descriptive approach and consists of categorical knowledge: one either has or does not have the disease.

2. Dimension: What the patient *is*. The goal of treatment here is counseling, and this perspective is similar in parts to Havens's existential approach, where the focus is on the human being who may be suffering the illness, not the disease that underlies the illness. This involves continuous rather than categorical knowledge, since all human beings have certain characteristics, and what is relevant is how much of each characteristic someone has. Unlike diseases, which one either possesses or does not possess, the dimensional model applies to aspects of psychological functioning (such as personality traits) that everyone possesses but which may differ among individuals (who might have more or less of particular traits).

3. Behavior: What the patient *does*. McHugh relates treatment to a type of

reeducation in which the patient learns new methods of controlling or changing his actions. This is the underlying method behind popular behavioral approaches to treatment of depression and obsessive-compulsive disorder. Havens classifies this type of treatment under the objective-descriptive approach, since behavioral treatments subscribe to traditional methods of describing objective signs and symptoms.

4. Life story: What the patient *wants*. The goal of treatment is a kind of re-scripting of one's life goals. This perspective is future-oriented and takes an overtly hermeneutic approach in the sense that objective truth is not the goal one sets; this is similar to the major difference between the existential approach as described by Havens and all the other approaches (all of which seek to obtain objective accurate knowledge). Just as the existential approach simply seeks to understand things rather than explain them, the life story perspective is focused on understanding one's goals or one's ideals, what *might be* rather than what definitely will be or what has been.

7.

The basic viewpoint of pluralism is that multiple independent methods are necessary in the understanding and treatment of mental illness; no single method is sufficient. While all methods are partial or limited, they should be applied separately and purely—in this way pluralism differs from eclecticism (fig. 1.1).

It should be clear that there is a good deal of overlap between the theoretical structures advanced by Havens and by McHugh and Slavney. However, certain differences in emphasis and in content also stand out. Havens more clearly establishes a historical background for his theory, and he links the different methods to different historical schools of psychotherapy. McHugh and Slavney provide a better description of the cognitive-behavioral perspective in psychiatry, but Havens provides better descriptions of the unique methods of the psychoanalytic and the interpersonal schools of thought. The positions described by these authors can be put to some kind of empirical test. In particular, the distinction made by McHugh and Slavney between the categorical and dimensional forms of knowledge are liable to such empirical testing. I believe that the different perspectives of these two forms of knowledge apply to different psychiatric conditions and that this application is not arbitrary but the

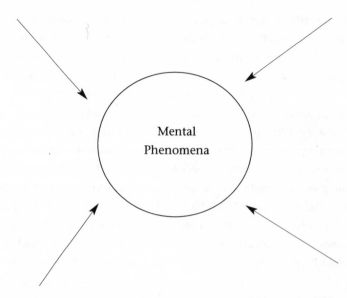

Fig. 1.1. A pluralist model of mind. The arrows represent either different perspectives (McHugh and Slavney), different schools of thought (Havens), or different modes of knowing (Jaspers), none of which is complete or sufficient, all of which are limited.

result of empirical studies of these conditions. We will return to these two pluralistic models repeatedly in the course of this book.

8.

What I call *integrationism* differs from pluralism in seeking to keep whole our understanding of the mind and mental illness. Integrationists are uncomfortable with the pluralist requirement to accept that no single method is sufficient and that all methods are limited. Yet integrationists are not reductionists, unlike dogmatists. Integrationists, like pluralists, can be thought to engage in *nonreductive materialism.*[4] I discuss this topic further in chapter 2 in relation to philosophy of mind. But for our purposes here, it is sufficient to point out that integrationists want to emphasize the interconnections of mind and brain, and they want to essentially remove the barrier between them. This is in contrast to the pluralists, whose position is most clearly exemplified by Karl Jaspers's views (see chapter 5). Pluralists are willing to allow for differences in understanding mental and brain phenomena and are not committed to seeking to integrate our understanding of mind and brain states. I return to these similarities and differences in the final chapter. Integrationism at least has the advantage of avoiding dogmatism while seeking to go beyond eclecticism.

The prominent integrationist views in psychiatry are those of Hundert and Kandel. I will comment on Hundert's model only briefly here, since I spell it out in more detail in chapter 3. I will treat Kandel, whose views have attained much recent attention, at more length here and again in chapter 23.

Edward Hundert is a psychiatrist who was heavily impressed by both Hegel's philosophy and the implications of neuroplasticity (Hundert 1989). He began with Hegel's view, explained further in chapter 3, that as human beings we shape what we know. Hegel tried to bridge the gap between subject and object, the constant problem for philosophy as well as for psychiatry. How can we get to know anyone else? How can we know what is going on with someone else? If there is a break between one person and another such that this gap cannot be breached, then many problems are introduced for psychiatry. In philosophy, the difficulties have centered around theory of knowledge and the mind-body problem. In psychiatry, these issues touch the core of what we do and what we can do. Dogmatists, recall, take one position or the other: either biology explains everything, or some psychological theory explains everything. Eclectics refuse to take a stand, simply asserting that it is all very complicated. Pluralists agree with dogmatists in claiming that specific methods need to be applied purely, but they agree with eclectics that no single method is sufficient. Integrationists like Hundert seek to describe a single approach that bridges the subject-object gap, but they are not limited to one approach, as in the various dogmatic schools.

Hundert begins with Hegel's philosophy. Hegel felt that the subject-object gap was bridged in human history. He held that as humans interacted with each other, they affected each other and changed each other, such that eventually they could know each other. Hegel focused on this process of change, rather than the apparent static opposition between a subject and an object. Hegel's view was highly influential for a time (e.g., among Marxists), but it fell into disrepute in many philosophical circles in the twentieth century, especially since it was rather abstruse and speculative. Hundert felt that modern neurobiology supported Hegel's views. It was Hundert's contention that the discovery of neuroplasticity was a key finding for philosophy and psychiatry. Previous neurobiological theory held that neurons could not regenerate; once dead, they could not recover. Thus, over a lifetime, one only lost neurons. Once formed, neurons were viewed as static entities. Eric Kandel and others discovered that neurons could in fact alter their shape throughout life and that indeed they could regenerate as well as decay in adulthood. Furthermore, other studies showed that environmental influences affected the size, shape, and connections of neurons. This is neuroplasticity. In other words, the environment literally shapes the brain. And humans, using their brains, obviously alter the environment. Here, Hundert seemed to be saying, was Hegel's philosophy confirmed in modern biological research. If we take this view seriously, then at some level the interface between brain and environment becomes so fuzzy that there no longer would appear to be a distinct break. The subject-object gap would be bridged, and integration would be achieved.

Hundert did not draw the conclusion that psychological phenomena could then be reduced to biological phenomena. Integrationism is not reductionist. It is a nonreductive materialism. The brain is central and necessary to understanding mental phenomena, but it is not sufficient. Mental phenomena also impact the brain. The interactions go in both directions, though without brain, there would be no mind. The brain is influenced by the environment such that our brains evolve so as to accurately represent the environment that impinges upon them. This is the Hegelian neurobiology that Hundert proposes. It is primarily an epistemological argument, as I point out in chapter 3, but in this chapter I want to emphasize its underlying views regarding mind and brain. Its basic view is that mind and brain interact and influence each other and that at some level the two entities can be integrated.

Hundert later went on to support the biopsychosocial model, as Engel had proposed it; and indeed a strictly methodological approach to the biopsychosocial model, as I mentioned, shorn of its vaguer eclectic adornments, is not entirely inconsistent with integrationism. However, the integrationism proposed by Hundert is at odds with both Meyer's pragmatic disinterest in such issues and Engel's systems theory–based views.

9.

In 2000 Eric Kandel became the first psychiatrist to win the Nobel Prize since Julius von Wagner-Jaurregg in 1929.[5] The awarding of the prize to Wagner-Jaurregg proved so controversial that it is perhaps not surprising that the Nobel committee shied away from psychiatric awardees for seven decades (Valenstein 1986). Wagner-Jaurregg won the prize for the use of malaria therapy to treat psychosis. Of course, as one committee member noted, it was not entirely obvious that a Nobel was a just reward for replacing one illness with another.[6]

Yet, at the time, malaria therapy was the only treatment that had cured any psychotic patients. So little of lasting significance seemed to have been achieved in psychiatry that the Nobel committee was gun-shy for decades. Prizes were awarded to neurophysiologists, like Julius Axelrod, who worked on the mechanisms of psychotropic drugs, but no individuals who had been trained as psychiatrists again received Nobel recognition. Until Kandel. He trained in psychiatry at the Massachusetts Mental Health Center in Boston in the 1960s, an era in which psychoanalytic ideas reigned supreme. Kandel was influenced by such views and has always retained a deep respect for and interest in psychoanalysis. He said in his Nobel autobiography: "It is difficult to recapture now the extraordinary fascination that psychoanalysis held for young people in 1950. During the first half of the 20th century psychoanalysis provided a remarkable set of insights into the mind—insights about unconscious mental processes, psychic determinism, and perhaps most interesting, the irrationality of human motivation. As a result, in 1950, psychoanalysis outlined by far the most coherent, interesting, and nuanced view of the human mind[—more] than did any other school of psychology" (2000).

In medical school Kandel became interested in the biological basis of the mind and, in particular, the possibility of a biological basis for psychoanalysis. So he turned to basic science research on neurophysiology, eventually focusing on the cellular mechanisms of learning and memory; he felt these investigations were the most relevant to psychiatry and psychoanalysis. Kandel eventually found that neurons themselves were not the source of memory, but rather the connections between neurons, and the nature of those connections, seemed to be the relevant features.

> We realized that the cellular properties of hippocampal neurons were not sufficiently different from those of spinal neurons to explain the ability of the hippocampus to store memory. Thus, it dawned on us what in retrospect is quite obvious: that the neuronal mechanisms of learning and memory probably did not reside in the properties of the neurons themselves. Rather, because the signaling properties of neurons are quite alike, we began to think that what must matter is how neurons are functionally connected. The basis of learning must reside in the modification of interconnections by appropriate sensory signals. (Kandel 2000)

His work focused on how memory was encoded in the brain. Kandel applied behaviorist ideas about learning to neurophysiological experiments with a simple invertebrate model of learning, the snail *Aplysia*.

We found that all three simple forms of learning—habituation, sensitization, and classical conditioning—lead to changes in the synaptic strength of specific sensory pathways, and that these changes parallel the time course of the memory process. These findings, which had been fully anticipated by our earlier studies of analogs of learning, gave rise to one of the major themes in our thinking about the molecular mechanisms of memory storage. Even though the anatomical connections between neurons develop according to a definite plan, the strength and effectiveness of those connections is not fully determined developmentally and can be altered by experience. (Kandel 2000)

He and his colleagues then showed that such synaptic changes involved effects on second messenger systems within cells. The details of this aspect of his work are not relevant to our needs here, but they are mentioned to give a sense of how Kandel went from a clinical interest in psychoanalysis and the importance of memory and learning, to a study of neuronal connections, and then to the molecular biology of the changes observed in neuronal connections that were associated with learning and memory.

In this process, Kandel practiced integration of mind and brain experimentally. And he was interested in what his findings meant for our understanding of psychiatry. In all, Kandel was central in demonstrating the process of neuroplasticity, especially as it applied to memory. As mentioned, neuroplasticity was a revolutionary idea that overturned a century of belief about neurons and had major implications for neurology and psychiatry. In 2000 Kandel won the Nobel Prize with Arvid Carlsson and Paul Greengard "for their discoveries regarding signal transduction in the nervous system." The award was for neurobiological work, but as stated, Kandel had long taken seriously the implications of these discoveries for our understanding of mind, brain, and the work of psychiatry.

As early as 1979, in his article "Psychotherapy and the Single Synapse", Kandel applied some of these implications to the mind-brain problem and to our basic understanding of psychiatry. Before Hundert, he alluded to the relevance of neuroplasticity for psychiatric practice. He speculated that psychotherapy could be an environmental influence that altered the brain, thus opposing the one-way direction of influence from brain to mind that is assumed in traditional reductive materialism. Kandel's speculation was confirmed by later research with Positron Emission Topography (PET) scanning, in which changes in blood flow and glucose metabolism could be shown to occur in different parts of the brain after treatment with behavioral psychotherapy as opposed to no such treatment for anxiety disorders (Baer 1996). Whereas the research on this topic usually involves cognitive-behavioral therapy for anxiety disorders, Kandel's interest was in psychoanalysis. No such empirical studies have been conducted with psychoanalysis, but, in principle, it would seem logical that any psychotherapy could have neuronal effects.

In a recent article (discussed in more detail in chapter 23), Kandel has followed up on his earlier speculations and now states with more certainty that psychotherapies influence the brain and that further research should seek to provide a neurobiological basis for psychoanalysis (1998). Some philosophers and cognitive psychologists are taking these ideas very seriously and are trying to demonstrate that psychological phenomena, broken down into simple subsets, can be "translated" at a fine-grain level of analysis into neurobiological terms. The neurobiological terms closest to the psychological phenomena would be complex, involving connections between neurons and physiological relationships such as sensitization. These neurobiological phenomena could then be broken down into smaller entities, eventually moving from cells to genes. Hence, although complex mental states cannot be reduced to minute molecular states, nonetheless there exists an unbroken chain from genes and cell proteins, through neuronal circuits and connections, to simple psychological states, to more complex psychological phenomena. This represents a kind of integrationism that is not at the same time reductionist on a general level.

Figure 1.2 is my attempt to summarize or simplify some of Kandel's ideas, as well as some similar ideas proposed by others, as they are relevant to our topic.[7]

10.

In summary, then, the conceptual status quo in psychiatry can be divided into dogmatic, eclectic, pluralist, and integrationist approaches. Most clinicians are dogmatists in practice and claim to be eclectic in theory. Either approach is highly problematic, in my opinion. The biopsychosocial model in particular has become the mainstream schema of current psychiatry, yet it suffers from a vagueness that makes it nothing but a cease-fire in the conflict between differing approaches in the field. The pluralist and integrationist approaches are the two most promising new concepts of psychiatry. The pluralist approach is in fact old, dating back to Karl Jaspers, whom I discuss in later chapters, and it has been represented recently by McHugh and Slavney and Havens. The inte-

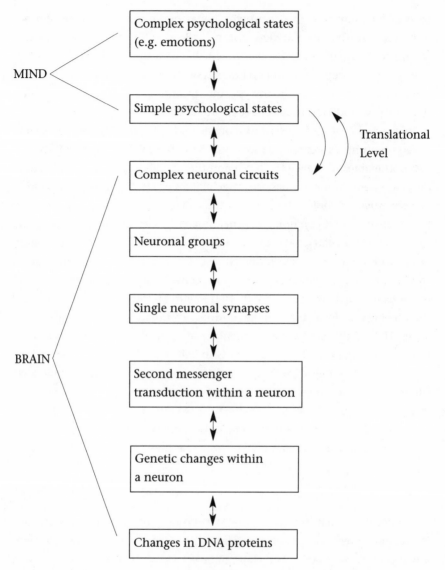

Fig. 1.2. An integrationist approach to mind and brain

grationist approach is often identified with Kandel, and it has also been promoted by Hundert. In subsequent chapters I return to all these models, particularly the errors of eclecticism and the meaning of pluralism. At the end of the book, I revisit these themes and, with the discussions that have transpired as background, discuss the relative merits of these approaches in more detail.

11.

When these concepts of psychiatry are laid out, I often find that clinicians lean toward one view or another almost reflexively. When I examine why my colleagues hold certain views, I often find that their opinions are based on underlying theories regarding the nature of mind and brain. In other words, to understand the current conceptual status quo in psychiatry, we need to examine philosophy of mind, and we need to think about what philosophies of mind are held by mental health professionals.

CHAPTER 2

What There Is

Of Mind and Brain

My first year in college, I read Descartes' *Meditations* and was hooked on
the mind-body problem. Now here was a mystery. How on earth could
my thoughts and feelings fit in the same world with the nerve cells and
molecules that made up my brain? —DANIEL DENNETT, 1991

1.

A common view in modern analytic philosophy is that the purpose of philosophy is the logical analysis of conceptual arguments. This perspective has
little in common with other versions of the goals of philosophy, such as building metaphysical systems of thought (Hegel), seeking epistemological certainty
(Descartes), or providing support for ethical (Kant) or religious (Aquinas) systems.
Understood this way, we can make sense of Karl Jaspers's statement that the study
of psychiatry requires an understanding of philosophy (Jaspers [1913] 1997).
This is so because otherwise psychiatry, like any other scientific discipline, would
operate with uninvestigated assumptions and logically immature arguments.
Psychiatry in particular runs this risk because its subject matter, the mind, is culturally imbued with many assumptions and beliefs, some of which may be
false. For instance, many persons believe mental phenomena are separate from
the body, and they thus might be inclined toward psychotherapy, as opposed
to biological, treatments for various conditions. Such persons might in fact deny
that psychiatric illnesses are medical diseases. Others, who believe that the brain
is sufficient to explain all mental phenomena, hold opposite views. These differing perspectives are based on varied philosophies of mind and dissimilar assumptions about the nature of the mind, rather than on either reasoned discourse about that subject or careful investigation of the nature of the mind.

If this is the reason why any student of the mind should have an awareness of philosophy, is there anything useful to be learned for psychiatry in the work of philosophers who specialize in the subject area of philosophy of mind?

2.

One of the first things that strikes a psychiatrist, used to interviewing patients and faced with the concrete anxieties and moods of the clinical treatment setting, is an initial sense of a certain lack of relevance in some current philosophical controversies. However, these controversies do have useful connections to our clinical experiences. For instance, one of the main topics of controversy in philosophy of mind has been the dilemma of color (Jackson 1982).[1] The prototypical problem is this: Suppose Mary is a color scientist, and she knows everything there is to know about color (its physical basis, an understanding of light and the spectrum of color, knowledge of brain pathways of color vision and the neurobiology underlying them), but she has one problem. She is in a black and white room. She has never left it, and she has never actually seen anything with color in it. The question is, Would she know what it is like to see color?

There are variations on this theme. Do we know what pain is if we understand everything about the neurobiology of pain but never experience it? Is the neurobiology of pain the same thing as the pain itself? If not, what is there that is added to neurobiology to account for the phenomenon of pain (Flanagan 1991)?[2] Another version reminds us that bats do not see; they navigate by their sense of hearing and by using electromagnetic waves. Do we, as humans, have any idea what it is like to be a bat? We can understand everything about the bat's physiology, but will that allow us to understand what it is to be a bat (Nagel 1974)?

These questions all share one essential core: is there something different about experiencing a thing (color, pain, being a bat) above and beyond our scientific understanding of the mechanisms of that thing (the neurobiology of color, pain, being a bat)? In other words, returning to older philosophical language, is there something subjective about mental experiences that is different from the objective bases of those experiences? And is this subjective aspect ineffable? That is, is it by definition nonunderstandable in an objective scientific manner? Or is there some version of subjective knowledge to which it is amenable?

3.

These issues hopefully give the reader a flavor for certain issues in contemporary philosophy of mind. The reader might note that we have here a series of questions, but few answers. The current consensus in philosophy appears to be that these questions are too difficult to answer if one adheres to a strict "psychophysical identity" theory. This view, which likely is held by many physicians, is that the there is no difference between the experience of something and the understanding of its neurobiological basis. Thus, the experience of color is the understanding of its neurobiology; and Mary would be able to understand color fully even if she had never seen anything with color. Pain would be identified with the firing of specific neurons in the central nervous system; no level of subjective phenomena would need to be added to understand pain. This perspective does not appear to hold up to careful scrutiny. The philosophical "thought experiments" described above support the intuition that mental experiences are not reducible to their physical bases. It does seem insufficiently accurate to reduce the complex phenomenon of pain to its neurophysiology.

At the other extreme, a number of philosophers hold the view that the subjective aspects of mental phenomena are ineffable, that they are purely nonobjective and unreachable by human understanding. These ineffable subjective qualities, called *qualia*, are beyond our mental reach. Although the thought experiments can lead to the conclusion that mental phenomena are not identical with brain phenomena, it is not clear why one must therefore conclude that mental phenomena are ineffable and nonobjective. They are simply different from, not identical to, the neurophysiology of the brain.

4.

It is my view that the most fruitful approaches in modern philosophy of mind fall in the middle perspectives on the above thought experiments. These can be categorized as *functionalism* (Daniel Dennett and others), *eliminative materialism* (Patricia and Paul Churchland), and *emergence theory.*

Daniel Dennett has published a prominent theory of mind in his book *Consciousness Explained* (1991). Because he seeks to have an empirical basis for his theory, he intends that many of the predictions of his theory should be liable to confirmation or falsification. Thus Dennett's approach can be tied into current knowledge and research in neuroscience and clinical neuropsychiatry.[3]

Philosophically, Dennett rejects the view that mind and brain are unrelated and that there is something special about mind that is ineffable or not explainable based on objective science. He also rejects traditional "identity" materialism, however; that is the view that mind and brain are identical, and thus for every "mind phenomenon" (like a thought), there is an identifiable "brain phenomenon" (like a neuronal action) to which the former can be reduced. The middle road, which one might say modern mainstream American philosophy has taken, is functionalism.

This is the view that mind is dependent on brain but not reducible to brain. This dependence is not identity; mind cannot be explained by simple reference to brain-related statements (one cannot replace "I am hungry" with "Neurons x and y are firing in my hypothalamus"). Mental phenomena possess their own unique symbolic language, analogous to the language of computers, which involves symbols that are arranged in a systematic manner to produce the results desired. Thus, although the mind is dependent on the brain, the mind possesses its own language and its own rules. Functionalism defines thoughts by the function they serve in between other thoughts (inputs and outputs) or actions.

Dennett's variation on functionalism is to assert that the mind's symbolic language is tied into neurobiology in certain ways. Some have criticized functionalism for ignoring neurobiology; it admits a dependence on the brain, but functionalism then ignores the brain and focuses entirely on understanding symbolic functions of mental phenomena. Dennett insists that neurobiology is relevant; for instance, we cannot understand the blind spot in the visual field, which influences visual mental phenomena, unless we understand the neurophysiology of the retina and its connections in the occipital cortex. In general, Dennett views mental phenomena as representing a kind of functional software program growing out of the "hard-wiring" of the brain. More originally, he holds that this software program is serial (mental phenomena are sequential in time; A follows B, which follows C), whereas the hardware program is parallel (neurons are structured in multiple parallel pathways). As a result, there is no direct one-to-one relationship between serial mental phenomena and their multiple underlying parallel brain connections. This is why the materialist identity theory fails. But there do exist empirical relationships between brain neurophysiology and the ability to experience various mental phenomena. So the antimaterialist approach fails as well.

Dennett tries to offer a theory of mind that is consistent with what we know about brain neurophysiology and what we know about the mind and human psychology. Interested readers should consult his work for details of this important discussion. Since my task here is not primarily to write a treatise on philosophy of mind, I cannot do justice to this complex topic in this chapter. But I will return to some of Dennett's ideas in later chapters, where I relate them to important psychiatric topics.

5.

What is the connection between the parallel network of brain physiology and the serial process of psychological experience? At a conceptual level, the connection may lie in the concept of *emergence*. By this, philosophers mean to say, basically, that the whole is more than the sum of its parts. That is, sometimes two things (call them A and B) combine to form a third thing (call it C). The concept of emergence holds that this relationship is not arithmetic: C is more than A + B. This is so because combining A and B produces something completely different, with certain properties that do not exist in either A or B by themselves. With this synergy, new properties "emerge" in the combination that were not present in the component parts. Applying this concept to the mind-brain connection, neuronal activities of certain types (pathway A plus pathway B), when combined and occurring at a certain place in the brain, produce the subjective psychological phenomenon of some state—perhaps pain, or perhaps rage. Although these psychological phenomena exist at a different level of description from that of their neurophysiological bases, psychological states nonetheless cannot exist without neurons, whereas neurons can exist without psychological states. It is in this sense that the materialists were right: brain comes before mind. But the nature of these relationships allows for a unique psychological description, not only a neurophysiological description.

6.

Emergence theory, alternatively labeled *supervenience,* has roots reaching back to the 1930s and 1940s, when figures such as Lloyd Morgan and others in Britain proposed this approach to understanding mental states.[4] It also has analogies to gestalt psychology and theories of holistic science advanced by German scientists in the late nineteenth and early twentieth centuries.

The concept of supervenience or emergence rejects mind-brain identity; a mental state is not identical to a brain state, although it depends on and derives from a brain state. Something extra happens when brain states lead to a mental state; the mental state "supervenes upon" or "emerges from" the constellation of brain states that underlies it. This may be analogous to the way biological states supervene upon or emerge from their underlying physical and chemical states. Hence, biology cannot be reduced to physics or chemistry, although biological life-forms depend on physical and chemical laws and properties to exist. Similarly, mental life has its own laws and is not reducible to brain states.

Emergence theory seems plausible and appealing on the face of it. But critics argue that this relationship of supervenience or emergence is vague; it is not clear what exactly happens when something supervenes upon or emerges from another thing.

Stanley Cobb, a neuropsychiatrist of the early to mid–twentieth century, wrote about the mind in a manner quite consistent with emergence theory: "The lines between physiology, neurology, psychology, and psychiatry are entirely arbitrary. They are purely academic and of administrative interest only. They have no biological significance. Psychology is the department that studies the 'higher' and more complicated levels of integration. It takes over physiology when it becomes too complex for the physiologist." It is "intellectually sinful," Cobb concluded, to separate mind and brain; but he did not reduce mind to brain, either (1943, 120, 157).[5]

What exactly are the characteristics of the process of emergence? This is another complex topic in philosophy of mind with potentially major implications for psychiatry. Here I can only point out the importance of this subject and again direct interested readers to relevant texts for more intensive study.[6]

Emergence theory at least has the advantage that it would allow one to adhere to a materialist theory of brain and mind, while still allowing for the utility of psychology as a separate science from neuroscience.

7.

Another approach, which goes in the opposite direction from emergence theory, would eliminate all talk of psychology in favor of neuroscience. Most concretely spelled out in Patricia Churchland's book *Neurophilosophy* (1986), this view emphasizes the identity hypothesis that brain activity is directly linked to the psychological phenomena it produces.[7] For instance, it can be predicted that certain parts of the brain produce certain psychological phenomena. The neurosurgeon Wilder Penfield famously demonstrated this fact almost a half century ago, when he directly elicited psychological states such as fear or déja vu feelings by electrical stimulation during surgery on certain parts of the temporal lobe of the brain (Penfield 1958, 1975, 1977; Penfield and Jasper 1954).[8]

Lesions of certain regions of the brain predictably produce certain mental phenomena: damage to the frontal lobe alters one's personality, making one often docile and uninterested in things; lesions of the thalamus can produce manic episodes, and lesions of certain parts of the left frontal lobe produce depression; stimulation of the occipital lobe can produce visual experiences or hallucinations; and activity of certain parts of the temporal lobe are associated with the experience of hearing voices. All of these mental phenomena, whether abnormal or normally occurring, are directly related to their neurological causes. It appears that more complex mental phenomena, such as my thoughts right now as I write these words or your thoughts as you read them, involve much more complex neuronal connections of different parts of the brain that are difficult to detect and describe.

A view that is often ascribed to the philosophers Paul and Patricia Churchland is that once this level of neuroscientific detail is known, many of our current psychological concepts will be deemed unnecessary or wrong. The classic example used is how progress in chemistry and physics rendered useless the old notion of the existence of a material called "phlogiston," the purpose of which was to explain fire. Once fire was explained through the chemistry of oxygen, the notion of phlogiston fell away. Similarly, our current notions of psychology will fall away once neuroscience advances, according to the Churchlands. They hold that, with scientific progress, our current psychological concepts (called "folk psychology" because they are based on "commonsense" intuitions regarding human nature that are culturally accepted) will be rendered as useless as phlogiston or alchemy. This *eliminative materialism* can be exaggerated, and a nuanced view can be that proponents of this theory do not mean to propose that all of our current psychological concepts are baseless, only that some will be shown to be so with advances in neuroscience. They also uphold a healthy skepticism toward pronouncing certain things, such as knowledge of mental phenomena, unknowable in principle by scientific methods. One has to wait and see how science progresses; if history is a guide, many things that seem unknowable will be understood quite well. Dennett subscribes to a similar epistemological optimism, which I share. I would add that besides advances in neuroscience, we can hope to benefit from progress in the scientific study of psychology and psychiatry themselves, as we update and hone our folk psychology.

8.

Psychiatry has yet to establish what we might call its own *ontology*. Much of the ontology of psychiatry comes down to the mind-brain problem. What is the relationship between the two? Are they totally separate and unrelated, as pure dualists would argue? Are they exactly the same, as identity theorists claim? Will we eventually eliminate the differentiation? Does one emerge from the other? Should we speak of mental function by analogy with computer software, while the brain provides the hardware? Will artificial intelligence research provide answers? Is there any use for psychological concepts, and folk psychology in particular?

The mind-brain problem is also implicated in what counts as an explanation, or cause, for psychopathological symptoms. If one takes, for instance, a strict identity theory view, then one would seek to explain psychiatric symptoms solely in terms of brain neurophysiology. If one were to take a pure qualia view, one might seek to explain those symptoms solely in terms of other psychological phenomena (e.g., childhood events and family environment).

Philosophers certainly have not answered these questions. But it is important for psychiatrists to at least begin to listen to the discussion going on among philosophers on these matters.[9] This is so at one level because philosophies of mind can explain a great deal about what we do in psychiatry and what we should or should not be doing. As just mentioned, I believe that many clinicians have extreme philosophical assumptions about the mind (whether extreme materialism or extreme antimaterialism) and enact these assumptions in their beliefs about the nature of psychiatric conditions (are they diseases, or simply psychological reactions to stress?) and treatments (medications or psychotherapy?). I believe that if one takes the functionalist or emergence theory approach, for instance, one would be inclined toward pluralistic or integrationist models of psychiatry, rather than dogmatism or eclecticism (see chapters 23 and 24).

At another level, the clinical experiences of psychiatrists may inform the competing philosophies of mind with facts relevant to choosing among them. This is already the case with neurology; interesting cases and findings, such as split brain experiments, have triggered important and fascinating discussions among philosophers of mind. Many psychiatric phenomena should prove relevant to understanding the nature of mind and its relation to the brain. For example, what does the phenomenon of impaired insight teach us about human self-consciousness (discussed in chapter 17)?

The question of *what* there is connects to the problem of *how* we know what there is (ontology leads to epistemology), which takes us to the next chapter.[10]

CHAPTER 3

How We Know
Understanding the Mind

> Research methods define their objects by the methods chosen. . . . Every
> advance in factual knowledge means an advance in method.
>
> —KARL JASPERS, 1913

1.

For a psychiatrist to understand a patient, to grasp the contents of her mind, seems fraught with so many difficulties. Karl Jaspers's clinical experiences convinced him of this. He saw the problem of one human, as subject, trying to understand another human, as object, to be nearly impossible to understand. Jaspers did not devise a theory that would get him out of this dilemma. In fact, he was antitheory in philosophy, believing that complex systems of thought, with the philosopher Hegel's system as the prime example, did too much violence to the reality of human concepts and human life (Ehrlich, Ehrlich, and Pepper 1994).[1]

Therefore, as he often repeated, Jaspers engaged in "philosophizing" about human life and experience, rather than engaging in "philosophy" with theories and systems to explain nature and humanity. If we simply accept facts as they are, if we accept in psychiatry that we have this patient before us and we, as strangers to her, wish to understand her, then we are faced, Jaspers held, with this dilemma: no single way of approaching the patient is sufficient to understand her. No matter what we do, that gap between us and her remains. We can try the traditional medical approach (what Havens calls the objective-descriptive approach) and elicit her signs and symptoms, trying to correlate these with objective events in her life and our knowledge of syndromes of diseases. But that does not suffice. We can try to understand her as a human being by discussing her feelings and how they relate to people in her life, such as her parents in childhood. But that does not suffice. We can apply specific techniques, for example Freud's method to assess her unconscious feelings, or the ideas of behaviorism, looking for the conditioning effects of her life experiences. But none of that suffices. We can even try understanding her individually and almost spiritually, attempting to put ourselves in her place, thinking like her, imagining living like her, trying as hard as possible to empathize with her, becoming existentially the same as her. But ultimately we know that we are not her and that a space, however small, will always separate us from her. This is the dilemma of the epistemology of psychiatry. How can we ever really know someone? How can we ever get inside someone's head?

2.

Jaspers would hold that we cannot. And Havens would add that this is a good thing, for it is the ultimate protection against totalitarianism that individual human beings are separated from each other at least mentally. Only cults and totalitarian regimes try to violate this separateness. This psychological separateness is the guarantee of political freedom, we might say, more so than Adam Smith's "invisible hand," or the wisdom of the Founding Fathers. But however useful politically this may be, it poses a huge problem for psychiatry.

3.

The conceptual basis of psychiatry rests on theories about mind and brain, as just discussed. Also, it is closely related to epistemology, or our theories regarding how we can know anything about the human mind. One of the few modern psychiatrists who have analyzed the underlying epistemology of psychiatry is Edward Hundert (1989). He suggests that the strongest basis of knowledge in psychiatry rests on an integration of psychological knowledge with progress in neuroscience. Drawing on ideas derived from the philosophy of Hegel, he asserts that advances in neuroscience provide support for accurate knowledge in psychology and psychiatry.

Hundert's integration of neuroscience with an epistemology of psychiatry is an important effort, which deserves a careful critique. In the course of the following examination, I will suggest that he may be correct in general terms, but there are many questions that remain to be answered.

4.

Hundert begins with a naturalistic interpretation of Immanuel Kant's philosophy (Kant [1781] 1998). Kant held that knowledge is not simply an accurate description of external reality, such as might occur by the direct influence of sense impressions on the tabula rasa of the mind (as attributed to the philosopher David Hume). Rather, Kant proposed that the mind was an active organ, which influenced sense impressions by its own cognitive activities. Kant labeled these psychological activities *categories,* and Hundert interprets them as aspects of psychological analysis and the thinking process. So Hundert suggests that, if one reinterprets Kant naturalistically, we can begin to make sense of Kant's epistemology in modern terms relevant to psychiatry.

At the very least, Kant's theory of knowledge suggests that there is no pure "objectivity" such that the world's sense impressions are the only relevant facts of knowledge. And there is no pure "subjectivity" either: the mind's psychological categories do not by themselves produce knowledge.

The problem with Kant's theories, as formulated by the philosopher himself, is that they imply that no truly accurate knowledge of objective reality can be obtained, since the mind's psychological categories necessarily interpret external reality in some way. In some sense, the sense impressions are distorted by the mind, and thus the external reality that produced them can never be known in its purity. These *things-in-themselves,* as Kant called them, are a logjam in Kantian philosophy. If Kant's views are accepted, then further work is needed to show how knowledge can be accurate and reliable. Hegel hoped to provide this philosophical contribution.

Hegel's view was that we should not try to separate an objective reality "out there" from the subjective viewer inside each of us, "in here." He tried to bridge the subject-object divide.

5.

In his *Phenomenology of Mind,* Hegel describes a way of thinking about subject and object that might bridge this gap completely. He begins with a view of a situation where the subject and object are two human beings, say, a master and a slave. For the master, the slave is an object. But the slave is also a subject, who views the master as, among other things, an object. As the two interact, they develop a complex matrix of subjects and objects whereby eventually the line between subject and object becomes blurred. Ultimately, for the slave, the creation of things in the world as a result of his labor leads to a situation where these objects, created by the slave, are essentially dependent on the slave for their existence. In this way, through "labor," the objects the slave creates are part of the subject, the slave, himself, and cannot exist without the subject. In this abstract form, Hegel eventually leads to the notion that human history provides a different perspective on the subject-object divide than natural history does. Meditating on nature, Kant could not bridge the divide. Things just seemed to exist as objects in the world outside of the subjective existence of human beings. But Hegel meditated on history, where individuals are dealing with each other rather than nature. And one person is an object to another person but also a subject to himself. Ultimately, through the creations of civilization, in human history, humans surround themselves with objects that are part of themselves, that are created by the subject, the human being himself. Marx took this argument one step further, stating that the alienation of human beings from some of the objects around them is not an abstract stage in the philosophical development of the world's Spirit, as Hegel later argued in his more theologically oriented work, but rather a historical stage in the economic development of human society. With further economic development, namely communism, this alienation would disappear. In Marx's ideal world, Hegel's philosophical abrogation of the subject-object divide would become a historical reality. People would live that way: from each according to his abilities, to each according to his needs (in Marx's famous dictum)!

In any case, Hegel, in focusing on human relations, pointed a way out of Kant's dilemma, at least in terms of knowledge outside of the bounds of natural science. Such knowledge would seem to encompass human psychology. And this is part of what Hundert builds on.

Hundert wants to say that with the creation of a world around them, humans, as subjects, can have a complete knowledge of that world. This is because the subject-object gap is not absolute; the objects depend on the subjects for their existence. The concepts of the mind are conditioned by the world in which the human being grows up. These concepts then seek to understand that world. Since the subject, the human being with those concepts, is influenced by the surrounding world, the concepts are in a way molded to that world.

Our concepts correspond to the world and truly reflect it. This correspondence is actively achieved, based on the literal impact of the environment on the actual anatomy and chemistry of the brain. The process of neuroplasticity becomes the scientific underpinning for Hegel's metaphysics.

6.

If we accept this view, then we can happily proceed with our empirical research in psychiatry and seek to understand ourselves with little skepticism about what we are doing. A few cautions suggest themselves, though: what about aspects of the world that may not have influenced our minds? Are we just unable to understand those parts of the universe? Some prominent philosophers believe that there are such inherent limits to the capacity for human understanding (McGinn 1990).

But Hundert takes things one step further. He calls on neuroscience to provide a more empirical backing for his philosophical application of Hegelian ideas to psychiatry. He describes much of the scientific literature on synaptic neuroplasticity. This is the notion that the brain is an adaptable organ, never completely whole or unchanging.

This is obvious in children: the brain grows in size, and the different parts of it develop in different ways. The process is reflected intellectually in children's ability at certain ages to perform tasks they could not perform earlier: spelling, higher mathematics, reading skills, and so on. Similar psychological skills also develop with age, and some have even suggested that moral skills develop with age as the child becomes an adult (Kohlberg 1981).

This plasticity of the brain reflects the influence of the environment. If primates are placed in environments with limited stimulation, their brains develop differently than in more stimulating environments. These small-size adaptations of the brain, which are now known to go on throughout life (though less markedly in adulthood than in childhood), are the neuronal equivalent, in a way, to the Hegelian interaction between subject and object. The brain is influenced by the environment in its very structure and connections, and the ideas that spring from the brain in turn are adapted to that environment. Certain molecules, like GAP-43, seem to be essential to this process, and Hundert spends a good deal of time discussing their significance.

Although the details of this story are likely to change, Hundert probably has the outlines right. In a way, neuroscience provides biological evidence in support of Hegel's theory of truth. The internal standard of truth, that the subject and the object are in many ways the same, is not simply an abstract notion; it is concrete and is reflected in the environment's influence on neuronal development. The brain provides an external justification for Hegel's criterion. The truth of subject-object knowledge is not simply abstract and philosophical; it reflects the natural and human world around us.

7.

No longer can we simply "compare" thoughts and things to determine the truth of our knowledge, for the wheel of knowledge is always turning. No longer is our brain, or our mind, a simple "mechanism" for experiencing external objects, but instead must be understood as a tool, an instrument with which we search for truth. But, unlike Hegel's dialectic, which was grounded in a search for truth within his own self-conscious experience, ours has been grounded in the experiences of human subjects interacting with their environment, in cognitive mechanisms which by definition apply equally to all members of the species. Reason (and the laws of logic) are thus not "relative" to just any reality, but physical reality as it actually evolved in all its biological wonder. It is this biological world of things which has been implicated in our thoughts, even in the a priori form of those thoughts. (Hundert 1989, 280–81)

In other words, there are two functions of the brain, "as a mechanism for experiencing" and "as a tool for knowing." As a mechanism for experiencing, the brain is a passive receptacle, as in Kant's model. Kant's mistake was to extend this cognitive property of brain function to philosophical truth. As a tool for knowing, the brain is an active creator, created by that which it creates, Nature, and thus able to comprehend Nature. Hundert's most original idea, a neuroscientific version of what Marx did politically, is just this: "The mind not only 'contains' its knowledge, but it actively participates in achieving its knowledge. But more than this, our biological, social world also actively participates in the mind, as we accommodate even our 'formal concepts' through the plasticity of the brain we use to 'know things'" (1989, 299).

8.

All this appeals to me. Hegel got something right, if his ideas can be incorporated relatively easily into evolutionary theory and research findings in neuroscience. However, I think pluralism offers a more parsimonious alternative to eclecticism than does a Hegelian integrationism. I expand on this critique in chapters 23 and 24. A simple skeptical objection to Hundert's approach, which I do not share, would be to object to the attempt to fit new empirical findings to any philosophy. This is a mistaken attitude. As Karl Jaspers so presciently foretold in the introduction to his *General Psychopathology,* where he expected the same criticism, everyone has a theory, whether the person knows it or not.

No one is so perfect as to be able to operate in a complete unbiased fashion. We all have certain theories or ways of thinking that underlie our actions or, in science, our research hypotheses. This is, when thought about, an unexceptional idea to which almost everyone who considers it seriously gives assent. It is a truism among philosophers of science. Scientists who have not thought of it are the only ones who might hesitate to accept it. So, if we all have theories that influence us, ignoring those theories puts us at the peril of accepting biased ones. This was Jaspers's argument for engaging in conceptual and even philosophical discourse in every science. He tried to do so in psychiatry. It is to Jaspers we must now turn in our search for an epistemology for psychiatry.

9.

It is probably not an exaggeration to say that Karl Jaspers thought more seriously about the problems of limits on human understanding as it applies to the human mind than any other philosopher or psychiatrist. Hundert's meditation on Hegel seems to suggest a way out. But long before Hundert's work, Jaspers suggested another approach: pluralism.

The source—what is Jaspers's most important contribution to psychiatry— is his *General Psychopathology (GP)* ([1913] 1997).[2] This is a theoretical work on the philosophical bases of psychiatry. He became famous for it, and yet he never practiced in the field. He had a chronic illness that kept him from engaging in the "rigors" of clinical work, as he recounts it in his autobiography.[3] Thus, at the end of his residency training, he persuaded his chairman to allow him to conduct a library project, an investigation into the theoretical bases of contemporary psychiatry. This became his *GP,* which he revised three decades later and which remains, in my view, the premier theoretical work in the field. Freud's originality and Kraepelin's empirical rigor notwithstanding, no one has thought longer and harder than Jaspers about what it is that psychiatrists are doing.

Jaspers's key insight in the *GP* is the following: since no single method or technique in psychiatry is sufficient to completely understand a patient, we must use them all separately, with a clear knowledge of when they are most useful, based on their strengths, and when they are inaccurate guides, based on their weaknesses.

Jaspers essentially upheld a methodological pluralism that is principled and remains usable today. It picks up where Hundert did, but instead of suggesting an alternative theoretical epistemology that might allow us to be certain of our knowledge in psychiatry, Jaspers accepts our uncertainties as they are and simply upholds methodological pluralism and skepticism about any one method of obtaining true knowledge. No method in psychiatry was so sufficient as to be completely true. Kraepelin's empirical skills only took him so far. Freud's brilliant theorizing only captured certain things. Jung's take on things, or Adler's—they were all partial truths. Even all together, there still seemed to be something about a human being—her freedom (dare we use the word?), her soul—something transcendent that failed to be comprehended in any clinical or intellectual description.

Jaspers felt that strict positivistic scientific method needed to be modified in psychiatry because each individual human being is unique. To flesh out Jaspers's contribution, which is extremely important, I will need to review the *GP* (on account of its age and length, it is sadly unfamiliar to many clinicians). I will do so in chapters 5 and 6, but before delving deeper into Jaspers's work, I think it is important to touch on some basic ideas in modern philosophy of science. Then I will go into a reading of the *GP* and an analysis of Jaspers's attempt to devise a scientific method for psychiatry.

CHAPTER 4

What Is Scientific Method?

It is wrong, always and everywhere, and for anyone, to believe anything on insufficient evidence.

—W. K. CLIFFORD

In the late nineteenth century, when some believed that Darwinism had undermined religious faith, the English mathematician W. K. Clifford made the above startling pronouncement, adding, "It is sinful" to hold such beliefs. In one pithy statement, he captured the spirit of the new age: he turned the concept of sin against religion. It was now literally sinful to believe, rather than to disbelieve. This was a challenge to the faithful, and a response came from an eccentric source: one who did not plainly believe in a religion, but one who wanted to have the freedom to believe what Clifford's ascetic scientific faith proscribed. This person was the psychologist and philosopher William James, and he made his comments in his classic essay "The Will to Believe" (James [1897] 1956).

This nineteenth-century controversy sheds light on some of the conceptual tangle in psychiatry today about what it means to assert that something is or is not scientific. What is scientific method, and what is it in particular when applied to psychiatry?

Clifford had an extreme view of science, what philosophers term *positivism*. James wanted to oppose this with a more nuanced understanding of the scope of scientific method. James began by asserting that one cannot avoid belief. Even not believing is a belief. As Jaspers argued, if one does not examine one's theoretical assumptions, one will simply operate with them unconsciously. Everyone has theories and beliefs, and only the simplest matters in life can be decided based on facts alone. This is because there are rarely enough facts to go around; we never have 100 percent proof or data on anything. So James's first point is that we all have beliefs. The question is, Are we justified in those beliefs?

Clifford held that we are never justified unless we have sufficient evidence. James argued that this makes sense only for those beliefs for which sufficient evidence is available. Suppose I believe the world is flat. James would agree that I should give up that belief because there is sufficient evidence that the world is round. I merely need to inform myself of that evidence; then I will no longer be justified in thinking the world flat.

But, James wondered, do we always have sufficient evidence? Of course not, but Clifford might reply that we then simply need to gather the evidence. We still can avoid believing anything; we simply abstain from any belief until sufficient evidence is available. James perceived, however, that there might be some circumstances in which this agnostic strategy would fail.

1.

Are there times when there simply cannot be sufficient evidence? Are certain questions beyond the pale of that standard?

James answered yes, and he focused on the question, Does God exist?

This question, which has belabored thinkers for centuries, is one that many individuals would agree is not open to proof or disproof. One cannot prove that God exists or does not exist. Most would agree—neither science nor logic appears capable of definitively solving this question.

I would add that there is a whole class of questions that fall in this category of problems that cannot be answered by sufficient evidence. These include, Is life worth living? Should I marry?

In many cases, individuals who are ill commit suicide; they are suffering from depression, usually. In some cases, persons seriously consider suicide, and there is no way to prove or disprove the merits of living. One cannot guarantee to such a person that future life will be limited in sorrow; calculations of pleasure and pain may argue for suicide in some circumstances.

James touched on another example: marriage. A young person must decide to marry or not. There is no third option. To pretend not to decide, or to avoid deciding, is equivalent to choosing not to marry.

In all these cases, people decide one way or the other, because they must. One has no choice. One either chooses to kill oneself or not. One either chooses to believe in God or not. James takes away the option of indifference, agnostics notwithstanding. The posture of abstention from belief is equivalent to disbelieving when there is no true choice. I would grant James's main point.

There obviously are some junctures in life where a decision needs to be made and not deciding is in itself a decision. If skeptics object to the examples drawn from James, here is another.

Suppose you were a German living outside a concentration camp in 1943. A Jewish prisoner escaped and fled to your door. You had a choice. Either you would hide the prisoner or not. You could not refuse to decide. Suppose you told the prisoner: "I will not decide in either direction; I will not hide you, nor will I send you away." That would be equivalent to not helping the prisoner; left alone at your door, the prisoner would be captured, just the same as if you turned him in. Thus, not deciding would be the same as deciding against helping the prisoner.

James makes the point that there are many issues in life of that ilk.

Let us give the name of *hypothesis* to anything that may be proposed to our belief . . . let us speak of any hypothesis as either *live* or *dead*. A live hypothesis is one which appeals as a real possibility to him to whom it is proposed. If I ask you to believe in the Mahdi, the idea makes no electric connection with your nature,— it refuses to scintillate with any credibility at all. As an hypothesis it is completely dead. To an Arab, however, (even if he be not of the Mahdi's followers), the hypothesis is among the mind's possibilities: it is alive. This shows that deadness and liveness in an hypothesis are not intrinsic properties, but relations to the individual thinker. They are measured by his willingness to act. The maximum of liveness in an hypothesis means willingness to act irrevocably. Practically, that means belief; but there is some believing tendency wherever there is willingness to act at all.

Next, let us call the decision between two hypotheses an *option*. Options may be of several kinds. They may be—1, *living* or *dead;* 2, *forced* or *avoidable;* 3, *momentous* or *trivial;* and for our purposes we may call an option a genuine option when it is of the forced, living, and momentous kind. (James [1897] 1956, 2–3)

In these cases, what James terms "forced momentous options," one has to choose. Yet there is also insufficient evidence to decide the case. Thus, one must choose a position based on insufficient evidence, exactly what Clifford says must not be done. Not deciding to choose owing to insufficient evidence is the same as not choosing. "He who refuses to embrace a unique opportunity loses the prize as surely as if he tried and failed" (James [1897] 1956, 4).

In sum, then, James grants Clifford's point for many decisions and matters, but not for certain essential aspects of life.[1]

2.

This controversy teaches us a lesson: we must get away from the oversimplified version of scientific method, the positivistic assumption that we can avoid any kind of belief and that we can know everything completely on the basis of data and facts alone. This is not the case in life, and not even the case in specific sciences, since all sciences have certain conceptual assumptions. But for a field that deals with life, like psychiatry, it is even less the case.

Yet this does not argue against scientific method in psychiatry; rather, we have to examine more closely what we mean by the term *scientific*. Modern philosophy of science has gone places, in this regard, where researchers and clinicians in psychiatry have little followed.

One of the transitions away from positivistic views of science began with Thomas Kuhn, who in the early 1960s published his powerful work *The Structure of Scientific Revolutions* (1962). The positivistic myth had been that science was an orderly affair. From fact built on fact, new theories were proven. But Kuhn examined nodal points in history when revolutionary scientific ideas appeared to overthrow older ones. These did not follow the orderly positivist pattern.

Take Galileo, excommunicated and hounded for his work. Or Darwin, the center of heated controversy. Or Freud, passionately rejected by mainstream medicine. Or Einstein, spinning his unusual theories from the periphery of mainstream physics, alone in his Swiss patent office. None of these founders of radical new scientific theories built unobtrusively on previous work. None of them were accepted in a friendly manner by their scientific colleagues.

Kuhn created his famous concept of a *paradigm shift* to explain these discontinuities. He argued that there were two phases to scientific research: "normal" science and "revolutionary" science. In periods of normal science, scientists operate within an existing paradigm, asking questions and providing evidence regarding details, as it were, within the accepted scientific framework. This normal science is uncontroversial and involves the gradual addition of pieces of knowledge. This is essentially the positivistic view, but circumscribed to a certain phase of research. However, when data that challenge accepted theories begin to accumulate, researchers question their basic axioms, and the result is a paradigm shift. If enough such evidence accrues, some researchers, and then others, replace earlier theories with new ones. And then a new process of normal science begins again. Sometimes the challenging evidence, although present for a long time, had been ignored in favor of traditional theories. Under social and cultural influences, paradigm shifts could occur as a result, allowing reinterpretations of previous data.

Kuhn's theory has been exaggerated by some to imply that science is completely socially and culturally determined, as opposed to dealing with "reality." In point of fact, Kuhn's view need not be seen so extremely. I find his concepts useful to psychiatry in keeping us aware of the need to recognize that certain facts that may seem unusual today may lead to important theories tomorrow. Further, it is relevant to recognize the strictly nonobjective, social-cultural factors that influence what we accept as our prevailing theories.

3.

Even though we accept that our science does not occur in a social and cultural vacuum, and that progress in science is fitful rather than smooth, we still are faced with thinking about what it means to speak of science in general, and psychiatry in particular.

There are two standard approaches in the philosophy of science. The first approach, identified with the nineteenth-century American philosopher Charles Sanders Peirce ([1905] 1958), is the inductive approach. Peirce is a fascinating and still underappreciated figure in philosophy and certainly in psychiatry. He is one of those philosophers—like Locke, James, and Jaspers—who came to philosophy from the sciences. Peirce's highest degree was a master's in chemistry, and his main employment for over three decades was as a physicist and astronomer for the U.S. Coast and Geodetic Survey. His only academic position was a brief stint as a professor of logic, owing to his mathematical background, at Johns Hopkins University. His influence on philosophy was mainly mediated by his younger colleagues William James and John Dewey. Peirce lived, much like Socrates, underemployed and unpaid, a man outside the academic mainstream who stimulated a whole new way of thinking in younger colleagues. He was a philosophic gadfly and, like Socrates, he died a painful death, though for Peirce it was penury and poverty that dogged him in the final decade of his life.

Peirce, like Jaspers, demands to be rediscovered by all those interested in the mind. Peirce, rather like the positivists, argued that science proceeds through the gradual accumulation of facts. These facts involve evidence confirmatory of a particular theory. However, David Hume ([1777] 1988) had shown a century earlier that such confirmatory inductive evidence could never be definitive. In discussing causation, Hume argued that one could never be absolutely certain that one event caused another in nature, because the future can always, even with minuscule probability, be different. Thus, we say that the sun will rise tomorrow because it has risen every morning that we have been alive. But that does not guarantee that it will always rise; perhaps some morning, for whatever reason, it will not. Hume emphasized that our experience of "constant conjunctions" does not translate into an ironclad, immortal law of nature. Peirce took this argument and tried to determine how science might know that something is true, or real, despite the limitations of such inductive experience. Eventually, he concluded that inductive data could approximate the truth very closely, in such a manner that they would be trivially doubtable. Peirce thought that we could be more sure of such truths if they were agreed upon by a community of objective scientists.

Since Peirce's perspective is of central importance to much of my discussion in this book, I will let him speak for himself as he develops his argument in a key essay, "The Fixation of Belief."

The object of reasoning is to find out, from the consideration of what we already know, something else which we do not know. . . . We are, doubtless, in the main logical animals, but we are not perfectly so. Most of us, for example, are naturally more sanguine and hopeful than logic would justify. . . . That which determines us, from given premises, to draw one inference rather than another is some habit of mind, whether it be constitutional or acquired. . . .

We generally know when we wish to ask a question and when we wish to pronounce a judgment, for there is a dissimilarity between the sensation of doubting and that of believing.

But this is not all which distinguishes doubt from belief. There is a practical difference. Our beliefs guide our desires and shape our actions. The Assassins, or followers of the Old Man of the Mountain, used to rush into death at his least command, because they believed that obedience to him would insure everlasting felicity. Had they doubted this, they would not have acted as they did. So it is with every belief, according to its degree. The feeling of believing is a more or less sure indication of there being established in our nature some habit which will determine our actions. Doubt never has such effect.

Nor must we overlook a third point of difference. Doubt is an uneasy and dissatisfied state from which we struggle to free ourselves and pass into the state of belief; while the latter is a calm and satisfactory state which we do not wish to avoid. . . .

Thus, both doubt and belief have positive effects upon us, though very different ones. Belief does not make us act at once, but puts us into such a condition that we shall behave in a certain way, when the occasion arises. Doubt has not the least effect of this sort, but stimulates us to action until it is destroyed. . . .

The irritation of doubt causes a struggle to attain a state of belief. I shall term this struggle *inquiry*. . . . Hence, the sole object of inquiry is the settlement of opinion. (1958, 95–100)

Peirce goes on to identify four methods of inquiry, the last and most satisfactory of which is science, while at the same time he proposes a pluralist tolerance for the strengths and limits of all four methods:

[One type of] man feels that if he only holds to his belief without wavering, it will be entirely satisfactory. . . . [The first] method of fixing belief . . . may be called the method of tenacity. . . . [The second] method has, from the earliest times, been one of the chief methods of upholding correct theological and political doctrines. . . . In judging this method of fixing belief, which may be called the method of authority, we must, in the first place, allow its immeasurable mental and moral superiority to the method of tenacity. Its success is proportionally greater. . . . For the mass of mankind, there is perhaps no better method than this. . . . But no institution can undertake to regulate opinions upon every subject. . . . [The third] method [called the a priori method] is to be found in the history of metaphysical philosophy. Systems of this sort . . . have been chiefly adopted because their fundamental propositions seemed "agreeable to reason." . . . This method is far more intellectual and respectable from the point of view of reason than either of the others which we have noticed. But its failure has been the most manifest. . . .

To satisfy our doubts, therefore, it is necessary that a method should be found by which our beliefs may be caused by nothing human, but by some external permanency—by something upon which our thinking has no effect. . . . Such is the method of science. Its fundamental hypothesis . . . is this: There are real things, whose characters are entirely independent of our opinions about them; those realities affect our senses according to regular laws, and, though our sensations are as different as our relations to the objects, yet, by taking advantage of the laws of perception, we can ascertain by reasoning how things really are, and any man, if he have sufficient experience and reason enough about it, will be led to the one true conclusion. The new conception involved here is that of reality. It may be asked how I know that there are any realities. If this hypothesis is the sole support of my method of inquiry, my method of inquiry must not be used to support my hypothesis. The reply is this: (1) If investigation cannot be regarded as proving that there are real things, it at least does not lead to a contrary conclusion; but the method and the conception on which it is based remain ever in harmony. No doubts of the method, therefore, necessarily arise from its practice, as is the case with all the others. (2) The feeling which gives rise to any method of fixing belief is a dissatisfaction at two repugnant propositions. But here already is a vague concession that there is some one thing to which a proposition would conform. Nobody, therefore, can really doubt that there are realities, or, if he did, doubt would not be a source of dissatisfaction. The hypothesis, therefore, is one which every mind admits. . . . (3) Everybody uses the scientific method about a great many things, and only ceases to use it when he does not know how to apply it. (4) Experience of the method has not led us to doubt it, but, on the contrary, scientific investigation has had the most wonderful triumphs in the way of settling opinion. These afford the explanation of my not doubting the method or the hypothesis which it supposes; and not having any doubt, nor believing that nobody else whom I could influence has, it would be the merest babble for me to say more about it. If there be anybody with a living doubt upon the subject, let him consider it. . . .

It is not to be supposed that the first three methods of settling opinion present no advantage whatever over the scientific method. On the contrary, each has some peculiar convenience of its own. . . . Yes, the other methods do have their merits: a clear logical conscience does cost something—just as any virtue, just as all that we cherish, costs us dear. But we should not desire it to be otherwise. The genius of a man's logical method should be loved and reverenced as his bride, whom he has chosen from all the world. He need not condemn the others; on the contrary, he may honor them deeply, and in so doing he only honors her the more. But she is the one he has chosen, and he knows that he was right in making that choice. And having made it, he will work and fight for her, and he will not complain that there are blows to take. (1958, 102–12)

In sum, Peirce begins with the opposition of doubt and belief. He argues, as against Popper's later view (see below), that doubt is not sufficient. It is not sufficient to falsify arguments; doubt is only an irritant that gives us impetus to attain belief. We always believe, as James pointed out; the only issue is whether we are sufficiently justified in our beliefs. Peirce identifies four such justifications, methods for what he calls "fixing belief." The first is essentially an intuitionist perspective, which we shall review in chapter 9 in the setting of Eastern/Islamic views. Peirce rejects this view as solipsistic; he wants an external criterion for belief that goes beyond any individual. The methods of authority (religion, ideologies) and philosophy (reasoning) are dismissed as insufficiently universal; there are still too many differences of opinion and no obvious way of settling those differences. The scientific method is his solution, resting on inductive observation and reasoning about external reality, agreed upon by most or all investigators, with fruitful consequence, and open to the confirmation or refutation of any investigator.

This interpretation of science is not much different from the intuitions of the average scientist. In fact, Peirce, who was a trained physicist, argues that his entire philosophy of pragmatism stems from the attempt to expand the way of thinking of the laboratory scientist to all areas of human thought. There always seems to be at least slight room for doubt with any amount of evidence. But if numerous investigators, in good faith, hit upon similar findings, more and more reliance can be put upon those results. I see this approach as, in many ways, very similar to the methods of evidential inquiry in the legal profession. In the law, it is recognized that human matters rarely if ever avail themselves of absolute certainty. Thus, different levels of evidence are required for different types of judgments. Some evidence needs to be held "beyond a reasonable doubt," which means something like 99 percent likelihood, the kind of near-certainty Peirce had in mind. Other judgments are based on much looser standards, such as the "preponderance of the evidence," meaning more than 50 percent likelihood. And still others involve a middle level of certainty, in between those two.

For some, this kind of probabilistic knowledge is insufficient. It seems to them that some facts just are more certain, and that science should be more firmly based than the law. Karl Popper sought to explain how science might be more certain by using a *deductive,* rather than an inductive, philosophy of scientific method (1959). Popper's intuition was based on his comparison of the acceptance of Einstein's revolutionary theories with the controversies swirling around Marx's and Freud's revolutionary ideas. Popper argued, like Hume and Peirce, that confirmatory evidence was always probabilistic. He therefore hypothesized that *disconfirmatory* evidence would be absolute. Many pieces of evidence supporting a theory may be disproved by just one clear refutation. If a theory is refuted by some data, then it is absolutely false. Thus, Popper emphasized that a scientific theory is scientific insofar as it is falsifiable.

If it can be disproved, then it can be shown to be false; theories should seek to provide predictions that can be disproved. Only by doing this, by opening themselves to falsification, can they be scientific. Popper saw Einstein as having done just this. Einstein made predictions based on his theories; these predictions were falsifiable, but they were not falsified; thus, he convinced the world of his theories. Conversely, Marx and Freud produced doctrines that were not falsifiable and in fact were infinitely malleable, twisting inconvenient facts into their theoretical matrix. This was the hallmark, for Popper, of their nonscientific nature.

Popper was quite taken with physics, and that is the main drawback of his theory. It does not apply to many activities in science. For instance, Darwin's theories were based on masses of induction, rather than attempts at falsification, and some have even argued that evolutionary theory is not scientific because it is not falsifiable. Certainly in psychiatry, if Popper's dicta are to be taken literally, many aspects of empirical research would have to be demoted to the realm of the nonscientific.

It is not uncommon these days to hear talk of paradigm shifts and falsifiability among scientists and nonscientists alike. But these references usually are perfunctory. Paradigm shifts do not mean that suddenly we change our minds about our theories, and reliance on falsifiability does not mean that we denigrate any inductive confirmatory evidence as unimportant. The tension between induction and deduction, between Peirce and Popper, lives in psychiatry today.

4.

Some would argue that we should stop discussing what scientific method is in theory; we should simply observe what scientists do in practice. The problem is that scientists themselves often define what they are doing as science based on their assumptions about scientific method in theory. Thus, in the positivistic era, science was seen as simply equivalent to unbiased induction. Today, where Popperian views are popular, science is often viewed as a cautious search for falsifiable hypotheses.

An important issue here is to distinguish between science as a body of knowledge and science as a method of knowledge. Francis Bacon first made this distinction, and Peirce emphasized it:

Lord Bacon remarks that "the sciences, as we now have them, are nothing but certain orderly arrangements of things previously discovered; not methods of discovery, or schemes for obtaining new results." This is a first anticipation of the contrast between the way in which an active science appears to any devotee of it and to one who has a general reader's . . . interest. . . . The latter person . . . will insist upon defining science as an "organized body of knowledge"; while for the former, science is a mode of life, like the profession of priest, or practicing physician, or active politician; and that which distinguishes the life of science, in the eyes of the scientific man, is not the attainment of knowledge, but a single-minded absorption in the search for it for its own sake—a single-mindedness that forgets every theory the moment the facts of observation appear against it. (Peirce 1958, 227–28)

In this sense, Popper's insistence on falsifiability has a place even in Peirce's own writings—not as the primary criterion of identifying what is to be accepted as scientific knowledge, but rather as an important attitude, the doubting attitude, which is an indispensable aspect of science viewed as a method, rather than a body of knowledge. We also see in this comment by Peirce another expression of the underlying theme of this book, the pluralistic-pragmatic injunction to focus on method rather than content in our understanding of the mind and psychiatry.

5.

Consequently, the perspectives of Popper and Peirce on scientific method, though covering most of this important territory, do not give us a complete map of it. Darwin's methods in particular also deserve careful scrutiny. In fact, in psychiatry, Darwin's methods are much more relevant than those of Einstein, and, I would suggest, Peirce's views on science are correspondingly more relevant than those of Popper. The evolutionary biologist Ernst Mayr makes this point indirectly when he discusses Darwin's scientific method:

Darwin's method was actually the time-honored method of the best naturalists. They observe numerous phenomena and always try to understand the how and why of their observations. When something does not at once fall into place, they make a conjecture and test it by additional observations, leading either to a refutation or strengthening of the original assumption. This procedure does not fit well into the classical prescriptions of the philosophy of science, because it consists of continually going back and forth between making observations, posing questions, establishing hypotheses or models, testing them by making further observations, and so forth. Darwin's speculation was a well-disciplined process, used by him, as by every modern scientist, to give direction to the planning of experiments and to the collecting of further observations. I know of no forerunner of Darwin who used this method as consistently and with as much success. (Mayr 1991, 9–10)

I will return to other aspects of Darwin's method in chapter 7. But for our purposes here, I want to emphasize that the greatest advances in the fields most relevant to psychiatry, such as Darwinism in biology, have proceeded along the lines of a philosophy of science that is similar to that propounded by Peirce but less consistent with the views of Popper. Yet, many assume that Popper's view is the most accurate, which has, in my opinion, unwelcome consequences for understanding the mind and mental illness.

6.

The psychiatrist and geneticist Kenneth Kendler, in an article on psychiatric diagnosis, gave a succinct description of scientific method: "The essence of the scientific method is hypothesis generation and hypothesis testing" (1990, 970). Both Popper and Peirce focus on the aspect of hypothesis testing, Popper emphasizing the need for refutation and Peirce the importance of consensual confirmation. I have emphasized that the modern climate of opinion utilizes Popperian ideas, whereas science generally continues, as it should, on a Peircean model. Kendler adds the importance of the first aspect, the framing of hypotheses: "The critical initial step . . . is to form empirically testable hypotheses" (970). This is the feature that limits the utility of so many nonempirical schools in psychiatry, such as the psychoanalytic school. They do not formulate their ideas in ways that are, even in principle, empirically testable, positively or negatively. If they fail to do so in either way, then they cannot be considered scientific either on Popperian or Peircean grounds. However, empirical testability does not necessarily mean definitive testability; parts of a theory might be testable, and, in some ways, one might argue that the concept of defense mechanisms is a part of psychoanalytic theory that is testable and has been tested. Darwinian theory is another notion that is not simply testable as a whole, yet it is an important part of the scientific canon of biology.

Hence, there is the question of whether empiricism is an essential aspect of science. By this we mean that no matter what scientific method one employs, the evidence one utilizes ultimately involves observation and experience in the spatiotemporal world of nature. And such observations and experiences need to be of a certain character to be empirical and scientific: they must be external, replicable, and quantifiable. Most science proceeds on those assumptions. Internal subjective experiences, such as those that occur when one is day-dreaming, are not seen as the type of data on which scientific principles can operate.

But this leads us to another dilemma, beyond the induction-deduction dilemma. If psychiatry has to do with mental states, then it runs across the problem of empiricism, of subjective states that are not easily amenable to observation. So where will we find a scientific method for psychiatry? Again, I think that we can begin with the work of Karl Jaspers, who, in his *General Psychopathology*, tried to trace such a method for psychiatry.

Since I view Jaspers's work as the most comprehensive attempt to conceptually understand psychiatry, I will devote the next chapter to a careful reading and commentary on Jaspers's text. I will follow with another chapter specifically relating Jaspers's ideas to the understanding of scientific method for psychiatry.

CHAPTER 5

Reading Karl Jaspers's
General Psychopathology

To sum up: If anyone thinks he can exclude philosophy and leave it aside
as useless he will eventually be defeated by it in some obscure form
or other. —KARL JASPERS, 1913

Certain books, such as Karl Marx's *Capital,* Charles Darwin's *Origin of Species,*
or Freud's *Interpretation of Dreams,* are often discussed and rarely read. There
must be a reason for this. Length, outdated language, the seepage of ideas from
great books into the general culture—all these no doubt play a part. But there
is a danger in relying on discussions about great books without having read
them: each discussion introduces an often tiny, perhaps imperceptible, change
in the original thought, until, after many such ripples of misinterpretation,
later concepts hardly approximate the views of their originator. It was not without reason that Marx famously remarked (in French, for added effect): "Moi, je
ne suis pas Marxiste."

I wish to avoid that fate with Karl Jaspers. I already have referred to him
many times and will continue to do so. Since his original work is little read
these days, I will take some space to allow him to express his thoughts directly,
based on his prime psychiatric work, the *General Psychopathology* (hereafter
GP).[1] I also am entering into his ideas in great detail because my own views
set forth in this book relate most closely to his. Readers who are familiar with
his ideas, or who have limited interest in the details of the *GP,* may wish to skip
this chapter altogether and proceed to the next, where I analyze Jaspers's two
main contributions to psychiatry. But I hope this chapter can serve as a detailed
description and commentary on Jaspers's thought for those new to him and
stimulate a wider audience for the *GP.*

1.

Until the age of thirty, Jaspers did not study or teach philosophy. He was first a medical student and then a resident in psychiatry at the University of Heidelberg. It is noteworthy that the philosopher John Locke was a trained physician, and one might call Aristotle a proto-physician, since that was his father's profession and he closely observed and followed its practitioners. But the philosophical personality closest to Jaspers, especially in terms of his background in medicine and psychiatry, might be William James, who also trained in medicine and then studied and taught experimental psychology, before turning to philosophy. It was James who made the comment that the first philosophy course he ever attended was the first one he taught! There are, interestingly, many similarities between James and Jaspers (a pluralistic theory, a strong interest in science, a respect for religious faith, a mistrust of philosophical systems, a devoted coterie of students, political liberalism). All of this leads up to the point of this introduction: Jaspers believed strongly that the way into philosophy passed through the fields of science. And in his case, the particular science he experienced was the medical science of psychiatry. As a result, his first major work, the psychiatric tome entitled the *General Psychopathology,* was, for Jaspers, not simply a psychiatric book but a compendium of thinking that marked his transition to philosophy. For the field of psychiatry, Jaspers's work was more than an introduction to his philosophical career, however; it was an uncommon achievement in itself that has continued to influence this branch of medicine for almost a century. "Here . . . was a rare bonus for psychiatry," commented the psychiatrist Michael Shepherd. "One of the foremost thinkers of the day, a trained physician, had spent a long enough period in the practice of the subject to write a major volume on its foundations" (1982).[2]

2.

Jaspers wrote the *GP* when he was just shy of age thirty. He appeared to suffer from a chronic illness, perhaps the lung condition bronchiectasis, which impeded him from engaging in the physically taxing work of a medical resident. He proposed an idea to his departmental chairman, Franz Nissl (most famous in medicine for developing a special staining technique for neuronal cells): let me spend the final year of residency in the library, working on a dissertation on the theoretical basis of psychiatry. Nissl was at first skeptical, but, convinced by Jaspers that there was much methodological confusion and conceptual drift in the field, Nissl relented. This is how Jaspers describes the setting:

Stagnation of scientific research and treatment was widely felt in German psychiatric hospitals. . . . In view of their own infinitesimal knowledge and skill, intelligent but intellectually sterile psychiatrists took refuge in skepticism and in the elegantly phrased hauteur of men of the world. In Nissl's hospital, too, therapy was unambitious. At bottom, we were therapeutically hopeless but kind. . . . All this I found when I came. Fascinated by each fact and method, I tried to absorb everything. . . . Often the same thing was said in other words, usually vague ones. Several schools had terminologies of their own. They seemed to be speaking different languages, and the divergencies extended to the jargon of each individual hospital. . . . At our regular staff meetings and demonstrations I sometimes felt we were constantly starting all over. One cause of this intellectual jumble seemed to me to lie in the nature of the case. For the subject matter of psychiatry was man, not just his body. . . . Our subject was also that of the Geisteswissenschaften [the human sciences]. They had developed the same concepts, only far more subtly and distinctly. One day we were taking down utterances made in states of confusion or paranoid talk, and I told Nissl, "We must learn from the philologists." I started looking for what philosophy and psychology might have to offer us. ([1957] 1986, 5)

The result was the book *General Psychopathology.*

3.

After writing the *GP,* Jaspers turned his complete attention to philosophy and spent the rest of his years as a professor in that field. However, the book has had a long and storied life. And Jaspers himself returned to it again and again in numerous revisions. It ran to nine editions. The second came out in 1920, and the third was an expanded version. Jaspers rewrote the book with detailed changes for the fourth edition in 1941–42, when he was in an enforced period of inactivity because of his opposition to the Nazi regime in Germany. Later editions exist in Germany, but the English translation is based on the fourth edition.

Although Jaspers has always had an influence on psychiatry and philosophy in his native Germany, the extension of his impact to other nations required adequate translation into English. This has proved difficult, and observers in psychiatry have considered this problem chief among the reasons for Jaspers's relative obscurity among rank-and-file practitioners. "It is not an easy work to read," noted the British psychiatrist Michael Shepherd, "concentrated in argument and diffuse in form, difficult enough in the original German and often understandably opaque in another language despite the heroic efforts of the translators" (1982). Even after enough of the translation could be understood for readers to realize that something of importance was being said, the actual content of the book eluded easy summary. The British psychiatrist Paul Harrison commented, "There is an apocryphal saying that in order to pass the membership examination of the Royal College of Psychiatrists, Jaspers' name should be invoked at some stage, preferably being followed by a comment as to the great significance of his *General Psychopathology* and of how much is lost in translation" (1991).

Professor Leonard Ehrlich and his colleagues have done much in the last decades to provide new and more accurate translations of Jaspers's philosophical work (Ehrlich, Ehrlich, and Pepper 1994). But the daunting task of retranslating the *GP* remains undone. Another task has succeeded, however. Since the English edition of 1963 was long out of print until recently, readers had to search used bookstores or rely on luck to find a copy of the book. In 1997, the Johns Hopkins University Press published a new version of the English translation, with a wonderful foreword by Paul McHugh, chairman of the Johns Hopkins Department of Psychiatry. As noted previously, McHugh's work is a prime living example of Jaspersian psychiatry today. His department, as a result, has long explicitly seen Jaspers's work as an important part of psychiatric training, and the field owes a great debt to the Johns Hopkins group for providing easier access to the new edition of Jaspers's *GP*.

4.

Thus, today the *GP* again is easily found, although the translation remains a difficult read. There is another factor, however, which has complicated the reception of this book, one that Shepherd (1982) first noted: "Perhaps the principal difficulty posed by the book for the reader is that of fitting it into a recognizable and familiar mould. *General Psychopathology* cannot be classified as a textbook. Rather it should be regarded as an intellectual map, a guide to a series of separate but related areas of knowledge." As a result, the *GP* is not the kind of book that one should begin on page 1, with hopes of smoothly passing from chapter to chapter to a satisfying conclusion. The *GP* is not a novel. Nor is it a psychiatric textbook. One cannot easily skim the table of contents and move to interesting sections, or look up specific matters in the index and read a few pages of neatly summarized material. Not a medical text, it fails also as a book of philosophy; the bulk of it consists of descriptions of psychopathological states, rather than conceptual arguments or exercises in logic. The *GP* is not any one of these things—but a bit of them all. Shepherd's phrase, "an intellectual map," probably best captures its nature. Jaspers rather clearly identified its purpose: to understand the conceptual basis of what we do in psychiatry.

> I would like my book to give the reader a wide education in psychopathology. It is indeed much simpler to learn up formulae and technical terms and appear to have the answer to everything. An educated attitude has to grow slowly from a grasp of limits within a framework of well-differentiated knowledge. It lies in the ability to think objectively in any direction. An educated attitude in psychiatry depends on our own experience and on the constant use of our power of observation—no book can give us that—but it also depends on the clarity of the concepts we use and the width and subtlety of our comprehension, and it is these which I hope my book will enhance. (50)

Shepherd (1982) again best captures the spirit in which the *GP* should be approached for the first time, after noting the above quote by Jaspers:

> The attainment of this objective depends primarily on the clarification of a host of concepts which are traditionally either ignored or over-simplified in the psychiatric literature. To do justice to such themes as the mind-body relationship, the role of scientific inquiry, the principles of classification, personality, the subjective-objective dichotomy, or the notions of health and disease calls for a familiarity with the history of ideas in other disciplines. It is here that Jaspers comes into his own, bringing a massive tradition of philosophy and social theory to bear on these perennial problems in relation to psychopathology.

Paul McHugh presents his view in the foreword to the Hopkins edition (1997, vii):

> Jaspers sensed that psychiatry inhabited a middle ground between science, where laws of nature are discerned, and history, where fateful events are conceived as emerging from human choices and actions. . . . He believed and emphasized in

his phenomenological studies that the individual human being—even afflicted by mental disorder—was always more than we can know. In essence, Jaspers' object was to show psychiatrists exactly what they know, how they know it, and what they do not know and cannot claim. He wrote this book with these aims in mind. . . . I call this book indispensable even though it was written eighty-four years ago—before the discovery of the EEG, DNA, or norepinephrine. . . . We have more information than Jaspers found crowding the shelves of Heidelberg, but we still disagree about how best to order this information so as to encourage its steady progress and to read its fundamental messages.

5.

Jaspers would argue that all this can be summed up by saying that the *GP* was not a psychiatric text or a philosophical book, but a book on psychopathology, a field that stands in a middle relation to both psychiatry and philosophy. This is what makes the *GP* of interest to professionals in both fields. In fact, since Jaspers explicitly discusses the nature and goals of the *GP* in its introduction, it is perhaps best to let him speak for himself:

> General psychopathology is not called upon to collect individual discoveries but to create a context for them. Its achievement should be to clarify, systematise, and shape. It should *clarify* our knowledge of the fundamental facts and the numerous methods used; it should *systematise* this knowledge into comprehensible form and finally shape it so that it *enriches the self-understanding of mankind*. It thus specifically assumes the function of furthering knowledge, a function which far exceeds the simple process of fact-finding. (38–39)
>
> *Conscious critique of methods in place of dogmatism:* Instead of forcing the subject-matter into a strait-jacket of systematic theory, I try to discriminate between the different research methods, points of view and various approaches, so as to bring them into clearer focus and show the diversity of psychopathological studies. No theory or viewpoint is ignored. I try to grasp each different view of the whole and give it place according to its significance and limitations. (41)
>
> *Classification according to methods:* . . . We obtain our facts only by using a particular method. Between fact and method no sharp line can be drawn. The one exists through the other. Therefore a classification *according to the method used* is also a *factual classification* of what is, as it is for us. (43)

> *Overlapping of chapters:* . . . In each chapter there is only one method that is paramount, and the reader's gaze is directed to all that it reveals. . . . but [each method] has some relation to other subject-matter which is duly comprehended by other methods. (47)

6.   Reading the *General Psychopathology*

The *GP* consists of two volumes and six parts. The first part is a section on phenomenology, where Jaspers carefully describes various psychopathological states. The second part consists of a discussion of those phenomena using the method of understanding *(Verstehen)*, and the third part does the same using the method of causal explanation *(Erklaren)*. These are the two ways of knowing that Jaspers introduces into psychiatry, and the fourth part (conception of the psyche as a whole) seeks to connect the two, doing so most interestingly in discussions of nosology and personality. The fifth part touches on social and historical factors affecting psychiatry, factors often ignored among the biologically oriented. The sixth and final part (the human being as a whole) discusses the connection between philosophy and psychiatry in more detail and introduces Jaspers's philosophical ideas. This last step makes sequential sense to Jaspers since he sees his entry to philosophy as occasioned by recognizing the limits of what he could know through science (specifically psychopathology). The introduction and the appendix both function as largely general reviews of the major topics discussed in the text, particularly the understanding–causal explanation distinction and the importance of methodological pluralism. Thus, to avoid getting bogged down in apparently unconnected theory, I would suggest that the introduction be initially skimmed. Then, unlike previous commentators, I recommend a sequential reading of the two volumes, with focus on the sections I highlight below. At the end, the appendix will flow easily, and finally I recommend a rereading of the introduction, which will tie everything together.

7.   The Introduction

Here Jaspers provides the conceptual background for the book and outlines the general theory that he seeks to detail in the book. This general concept, as will be discussed further, is that any science utilizes specific methods and that these methods both allow the science to discover certain things and limit the ability of that science to know about other things. One needs to know one's methods, consciously and clearly, to adequately apply one's science and comprehend its object. In the case of psychopathology, the *GP* intends to apply just this "methodological consciousness." The introduction should lead to recognition that this is the method and the ultimate outcome of the whole endeavor of the *GP.* Jaspers lays out this central core of his thinking in sections 3 and 4 ("Prejudice and Presupposition" and "Methods," pp. 16–37) of the introduction. In my opinion, if a reader had to choose just one section of the *GP* to read, these nineteen pages would be it. Hence I will quote extensively from what Jaspers writes there:

> [There] were periods in which philosophy tried to create from "above" what only experience could bring from "below." Nowadays we seem to have abandoned this orientation but it reappears here and there in the form of abstruse theories. Behind our accepted systems of general psychopathology the old spirit hovers and can be identified. Our rejection of purely deductive and barren philosophical theorising is justified but it is often linked regrettably with the opposite misconception, that the only useful approach is to go on with the collection of particular experiences. It is thought better to amass data blindly than sit down and think. From this follows a contempt for the activity of thinking, which alone gives a place to facts, a plan to work to, a standpoint for observation and the passionate drive for rewarding scientific goals. (16)

> Reality is constantly seen through the spectacles of one theory or another. We have, therefore, to make a continual effort to *discount* the theoretical prejudices ever present in our minds and train ourselves to *pure appreciation of the facts.* We can only appreciate these latter in terms of category and method, and we have therefore to be fully aware of the presuppositions lying in every discovery according to the nature of its subject-matter—"theory lurks in every fact." (17)

> The investigator, however, is more than a vessel into which knowledge can be poured. He is a living being and as such an indispensable instrument of his own research. The *presuppositions* without which his enquiry will remain sterile are contained within his own person. Clarification may free us from prejudice, but presuppositions are a necessary part of understanding. They appear as tentative ideas which we then take as experimental hypotheses. . . . Presuppositions provide guiding ideas, and form the mental life of those engaged in research; they need to be

strengthened and cultivated and they should be acknowledged. They do not prove the correctness of an insight but are the source of any truth or relevance it attains. (21)

Prejudices (that are false) are rigid, circumscribed presuppositions which are wrongly taken as absolutes. . . . *Presuppositions (that are true)* are rooted in the investigator himself and are the ground of his ability to see and understand. Once elucidated, they will be well and truly grasped. (21)

In psychiatric literature, there is much discussion of mere possibilities and a great deal of subjective and speculative comment that lacks the substance of authentic experience. . . . It is a pity to waste time on tortuous, meaningless argument or on imaginary models, however much they clamor for attention. If we are to apperceive essentials with certainty, our guide should be a clearly grasped methodology. (22)

Every advance in factual knowledge means an advance in method. (23)

A clear definition of *the original data* is of decisive importance. If it is not unequivocally defined and identifiable by any other research worker at any time, calculation becomes meaningless. Exact method based on inexact data can lead to the most remarkable mistakes. (24)

The main problem is to find those methods that will extract some definite realities from the endless and confusing flood of life. . . . Discovery of a way to make certain facts comprehensible, so that they can be re-identified by others, is the beginning of all research. (25)

Some scientists tend to deny the validity of any psychological source of scientific knowledge. They only accept what can be perceived objectively by the senses, not what can be meaningfully understood through the senses. Their viewpoint cannot be refuted since there is not proof of the validity of any ultimate source of knowledge. But at least we might look for consistency. Such scientists should abstain from talking of the psyche or even thinking in terms of psychic events. They should give up psychopathology and confine themselves to the study of cerebral processes and general physiology. . . . This seems a sterile nihilism shown by people who would persuade themselves that their incompetence is due to their subject-matter, not to themselves. (28)

Jaspers warns against certain particular methodological errors in psychiatry, such as "unlimited ad hoc hypotheses":

> We need working hypotheses for the interpretation of our fact. . . . [But frequently] we keep on making more and more far-reaching concepts, develop our theoretical constructions and employ one concept after another simply for the sake of concept-building. . . . We must, therefore, ask of every method whether it increases our knowledge and gives it depth and shape, and whether it makes it more possible to identify phenomena as they arise. Does it widen our experience and increase skill? Or does it lead to a void of abstractions and so entangle us with ideas and paper-schemes that we suddenly find ourselves in a world remote from what we see or do, and ourselves moving from one vacuum into another? (33)

> According to Kant expert opinion in the courts on mental states should fall within the competence of the philosophical faculty. . . . In practice of course it will not do. . . . Kant's dictum stands, however, in that the psychiatrist's competence is really commensurate with how far his education and knowledge would qualify him to belong to the philosophic faculty. This goal is not served where (as has occurred in the history of psychiatry) he learns a certain philosophical system by heart and applies it automatically. This is worse than if he had learnt nothing at all. But he should acquire some of the viewpoints and methods that belong to the world of the Humanities and Social Studies. (36)

8.   Part 1, "Individual Psychic Phenomena"

Once the introduction is finished, the reader begins the book itself. In part 1, Jaspers engages in his classic detailed descriptions of psychopathological states. In this section he is engaging in *phenomenology,* the school of thought in existential philosophy with which he would be most associated. This approach, derived from the philosopher Edmund Husserl, sought to know the phenomena of the world without presuppositions of any kind. Thus, Jaspers seeks to describe varied psychopathological states without reference to any theory or any concepts regarding their etiologies. He wants to be as unbiased as possible, merely observing and describing.

The simple separation of observation and value-judgment is something that must
be required from every psychopathologist in his work, not so that all human values must be relinquished but that, on the contrary, we shall possess truer, clearer,
and profounder values the more we observe before we judge. What is needed is a
quiet absorption into the facts of psychic life without the adoption of any specific
attitude to them. Human beings have to be approached in an unbiased fashion
with lively interest and without any kind of appraisal. (17)

This part in itself has exerted an immense influence on psychiatry; it forced
the field to notice certain phenomena that were often ignored owing to biological or psychoanalytic biases. Part 1 may be less interesting to philosophers,
except those interested in abnormal psychology for specific purposes, since, as
the phenomenological method entails, Jaspers avoided explicit philosophical
discussion. However, psychiatrists have found important ideas in section 1, titled "Experience of Space and Time" (pp. 79–88), where Jaspers first discusses
the concept that the experience of time is slowed down in clinical depression
and speeded up in mania. Here also Jaspers provides an initial discussion of
delusions, which has sparked a great deal of research that continues to this day
and in which Jaspers's ideas continue to play a central role (see chapter 14).

9.   Part 2, "Meaningful Psychic Connections"

In parts 2 and 3, Jaspers seeks to comprehend psychopathology by the two
methods of *Verstehen* (understanding, meaningful connections) and *Erklaren*
(causal explanation). This distinction is another crucial aspect of Jaspers's work,
which he lays out most explicitly in the introduction to part 2 (pp. 302–3). It
derives from previous thinking in Germany in the disciplines of history and
sociology, as is discussed further below.

In natural sciences, we find causal connections only but in psychology our bent
for knowledge is satisfied with the comprehension of quite a different sort of connection. Psychic events "emerge" out of each other in a way which we understand.
Attacked people become angry and spring to the defence, cheated persons grow
suspicious. (302)

The evidence for genetic understanding is something ultimate. When Nietzsche
shows how an awareness of one's weakness, wretchedness and suffering gives rise
to moral demands and religions of redemption, because in this roundabout way

the psyche can gratify its will to power in spite of its weakness, we experience the force of his argument and are convinced. . . . Such conviction is gained *on the occasion* of confronting human personality; it is not acquired inductively *through repetition of experience.* (303)

In any given case the judgment of whether a meaningful connection is real does not rest on its self-evident character alone. It depends primarily *on the tangible facts* (that is, on the verbal contents, cultural factors, people's acts, ways of life, and expressive gestures) in terms of which the connection is understood, and which provide the objective data. All such objective data, however, are always incomplete and our understanding of *any particular, real event* has to remain more or less an *interpretation* which in only a few cases reaches any relatively high degree of complete and convincing objectivity. (303)

Psychological understanding only serves psychopathology in so far as it makes something visible to our experience and fosters our observation. As I understand, I find myself asking what are these facts I am looking at and what am I indicating? When do I reach the limit of my understanding? (312)

In sum, Jaspers used this distinction to explore two different ways of comprehending psychopathological states. In part 2, "Meaningful Psychic Connections," the meaning of such states, in terms of subjective understanding, is pursued. In part 3 the causal explanation of such states, based on biological and empirical research, is intended.

Part 2 is the more interesting, in my opinion, for time has not faded its impact, as Jaspers seeks to empathize with the experiences of psychiatric patients. This section should be of interest to psychiatrists and philosophers. Jaspers again expands on his use of the method of understanding in the fifth segment of chapter 5, "The Basic Laws of Psychological Understanding and Meaningfulness" (pp. 355–63), including an initial discussion of Freudian psychoanalysis as a type of psychology of meaningful connections. Jaspers faults Freudian theory for seeking to provide one theory for all psychology and for not respecting the inherent freedom of human beings, an unpredictability that puts a limit on the ability of understanding to interpret human existence:

The limits of every psychology of meaningful connections must necessarily remain the same for psychoanalysis in so far as the latter is meaningful. Understanding halts first before the reality of the *innateness of empirical characteristics.* . . .

> Secondly, understanding halts before the reality of *organic illness and psychosis,* be-
> fore the elementary nature of these facts. . . . Thirdly, understanding halts before
> the reality of *Existence itself,* that which the individual really is in himself. The il-
> lumination of psychoanalysis proves here to be a pseudo-illumination. . . . Psy-
> choanalysis has always shut its eyes to these limitations and has *wanted to under-*
> *stand everything.* (363)

Of particular note is chapter 7, "The Patient's Attitude to His Illness" (pp.
414–27), where Jaspers lays out for the first time in psychiatry a clear discussion of the concept of *insight,* or awareness of illness. Jaspers discusses how insight is lacking in many psychiatric conditions, as patients are unaware of their
psychopathology. This is analogous to the concept of *anosognosia,* a neurological stroke syndrome associated with lack of awareness that one is paralyzed.
Philosophers have taken careful note of the phenomenon of anosognosia,
since it shows (in a way that Freudian theory of the unconscious does only at
the speculative level) that one can be subjectively unaware of important aspects of one's psychic and physical reality. It is noteworthy that Jaspers made
the same clinical point in terms of unawareness of psychopathology in 1913,
and recognition of the importance of lack of insight in psychiatry has grown
with time.

> Psychic illness looks different to the medical observer from what it looks like to
> the patient reflecting on himself. Thus it happens that someone, who regards him-
> self as quite healthy, may be analysed as mentally ill or that someone may con-
> sider himself to be ill in a way that has no objective validity and is in itself a mor-
> bid symptom, or that someone through his contriving may influence morbid
> processes for good or bad. (414)

> In psychosis, there is no lasting or complete insight. Where insight persists we
> do not speak of psychosis but personality disorder (psychopathy). Individual phe-
> nomena may be judged correctly, but, apart from that, the innumerable manifes-
> tations of the illness are not recognised as such and inversely there are morbid
> feelings where the content is a false one and is itself a symptom. (421)

10. Part 3, "The Causal Connections of Psychic Life"

Part 3, though conceptually relevant, will likely seem quaintly outdated to
psychiatrists and opaque to philosophers. Empirical scientific research requires

a background of terminology and method that makes it difficult to follow for nonscientists. That is part of the problem. Another part is that most empirical research is out of date within a decade, much less nearly a century. It is commendable that Jaspers sought, in the 1941 revision, to update this section with footnotes referring, for example, to neuroanatomical studies, but such work is generally of minimal relevance compared to more recent research. The point of part 3, in any event, is to detail this approach to psychopathology, the empirical biological approach. The general concept is what is relevant today rather than the actual research studies reviewed. In the introduction to part 3, Jaspers provides a useful theoretical review of the strength and limitations of the causal explanatory method in psychiatry (451–62). For instance, he discusses the view that psychiatric conditions are basically brain disorders in a manner that could have been written in a contemporary philosophical article on the mind-body problem:

[The view has been held that] *"mental illness is cerebral illness."* . . . This declaration is as dogmatic as its negation would be. Let us clarify the situation once more. In some cases we find connections between physical and psychic changes taking place in such a way that the psychic events can be regarded with certainty as consequences. Further, we know that in general no psychic event exists without the precondition of some physical basis. There are no "ghosts." But we do not know of a single physical event in the brain which could be considered the identical counterpart of any morbid psychic event. We only know conditioning factors for the psychic life; we never know *the* cause of the psychic event, only *a* cause. So this famous statement, if measured against the actual possibilities of research and the actual findings, may perhaps be a possible, though infinitely remote, goal for research, but it can never provide a real object for investigation. To discuss statements of this sort and try to solve the problem in principle indicates a lack of critical methodology. Such statements will vanish from psychiatry all the more quickly in proportion as philosophic speculations vanish from psychopathology and give place to a philosophical maturity in the psychopathologist. (459)

All categories and methods have their specific meaning. It is nonsense to play off one against the other. Each can realise itself fruitfully if it preserves its independence, accords with its facts and observes its limitations. . . . But if we turn it into an absolute, this will end every time in empty claims, ineffective discussion and attitudes which destroy any free approach to the facts. In relation to causal events in particular, it is a basic impulse of knowledge to advance constantly in the direction of more profound compelling causality. Hope may lend wings but the goal is difficult and calls for patience. But however far our causal knowledge goes, we shall never be able to know the event simply in itself and as a whole, and so be able to manipulate it. Causal knowledge is always faced by something which no matter how we operate it implies that in the end all the well-being of man is still dependent on something decisive in himself, which is only approachable if we understand. (462)

Jaspers expands on these introductory comments in chapter 11, "Explanatory Theories—Their Meaning and Value" (pp. 530–55). There he specifically critiques the errors that can occur with an exclusively empirical approach to psychiatry, which his contemporary the neuroanatomist Carl Wernicke claimed to take, or with the claim that one is following an empirical approach when in fact a meaning-oriented approach is utilized, as was true of Freud. Wernicke's work in neuroanatomy and in psychopathology is appraised as important and fruitful, especially since he tends to avoid too much speculation, but he is faulted for his view that considering mental illness to be cerebral illness would provide a comprehensive and complete understanding of psychiatric conditions. This critique would apply equally to contemporary empirical-biological psychiatry. The commentary on Freud, which is strewn throughout the *GP,* is continued here. Since Freud's views are the other main competitor to those of Jaspers in terms of "understanding" psychology, it is worth quoting:

> Freud's new attempt at psychological understanding was epoch-making for psychiatry. . . . A critique of Freud's teaching might resolve itself into the following theses. . . : 1. Freud is actually concerned with the *psychology of meaningful connections* and not with causal explanation as he himself believed. 2. Freud teaches us in a most convincing way to recognise many particular meaningful connections. We understand how complexes repressed into unconsciousness reappear in symbolic form. . . . To some extent here Freud fills out in detail the teachings of Nietzsche. . . . 3. The falseness of the Freudian claim lies in the mistaking of meaningful connections for causal connections. The claim is that *everything* in the psychic life, every psychic event, is *meaningful.* . . . 4. In a great number of cases Freud is concerned neither with understanding the meaning of unnoticed connections nor with the bringing of them into consciousness but with a *"hypothetical understanding"* of extra-conscious connections . . . [such as] Jung thought he had discovered in the case of dementia praecox [schizophrenia]. 5. One lapse in

Freud's teaching consists in the increasing *naivete of understanding* which goes with the transformation of meaningful connections into theory. Theories call for a certain simplicity whereas the understanding of meaning uncovers an infinite manifold. As it is Freud believed that practically everything psychic could be traced back to sexuality in a broad sense as if it were the sole and primary power. In particular the writings of many of his followers are intolerably boring by reason of this very naivete. One knows beforehand that the same thing will be found in each one of them. The psychology of meaningful connections cannot make any progress here. (539–40)

Jaspers goes on to link the errors of the two extremes, Wernicke's totalistic biological psychiatry and Freud's totalistic meaningful psychology, which, as discussed below, foretold that seesaw of psychiatry in the next century between the two dogmatisms:

Wernicke started with his theory from the "outside," with the brain. Freud on the other hand started his theory from the inside, with what is psychically understandable. Both review a whole field of facts and both generalise what has only a circumscribed validity and apply it over the whole realm of psychopathology and psychology; both end in abstract constructions. They are complete opposites as regards the content of their study and interests . . . yet their modes of thought are structurally related. They are indeed opposites but on the same plane and with the same limitations and restrictions on their thinking. (546)

11. Part 4, "Conception of Psychic Life as a Whole"

Jaspers seeks to connect the two approaches of understanding and explanation in part 4. The most influential segment of this part is the initial chapter (chapter 12, "The Synthesis of Disease Entities—Nosology," pp. 564–616). Here again Jaspers inaugurates a discussion, touched on earlier in the chapter on personality, that has continued to this day. Jaspers directly addresses the perspective of the empirical-biological school, led in his age by Emil Kraepelin. This discussion remains relevant today, especially as mainstream psychiatry has returned to the basic nosology established by Kraepelin (now termed *neo-Kraepelinian*). This nosology is purely empirical and has been criticized, in the spirit of Jaspers, for not allowing for meaning-oriented approaches in psychiatry. Further, the Kraepelinian nosology held that psychiatric diagnoses could be delineated by careful clinical observation, and that eventually the underlying brain pathology for these diagnoses would be discovered. This is still the mainstream view in psychiatry today. Kraepelin's opponents in 1913 held the "unitary psychosis" model, the view that psychiatric diagnoses could not be accurately separated from a single general psychotic condition. A few prominent psychiatrists continue to hold this view, and some even argue that there are no psychiatric diagnoses or diseases at all, but that mental conditions are defined by social and legal deviations from the norm of human behavior. Jaspers came out against the concept that psychiatric illnesses could be reduced to diseases of the brain, but he also recognized the utility of the clinical empirical approach:

> There has been *no fulfilment* of the hope that clinical observation of psychic phenomena, of the life-history and of the outcome might yield *characteristic groupings* which would *subsequently be confirmed in the cerebral findings*, and thus pave the way for the brain-anatomists. . . . The original question: are there only *stages and variants* of one unitary psychosis or is there *a series of disease-entities* which we can delineate, now finds its answer: *there are neither*. The latter view is right in so far that the idea of disease-entities has become a fruitful orientation for the investigations of special psychiatry. The former view is right in so far that no actual disease-entities exist in scientific psychiatry. (568–70)

Earlier, in the introduction, Jaspers also had added:

> In the psychiatric assessment of a case . . . except in the case of well-known cerebral changes, diagnosis is the least relevant factor. If it is made the main issue, it will prejudge what ideally should emerge from the investigation. What matters is the process of analysis. The chaos of phenomena should not be blotted out with some diagnostic label but bring illumination through the way it is systematically ordered and related. Psychiatric diagnosis is too often a sterile running round in circles so that only a few phenomena are brought into the orbit of conscious knowledge. (20)

But here in part 4, Jaspers explains why a classification scheme is important in psychiatry, and he provides one that is remarkably similar to the current nosology in psychiatry, arrived at in 1980 with the major changes enacted in DSM-III in the United States.

> We have detailed knowledge of particular phenomena, of causal connections and meaningful connections, etc., but complex disease entities remain an endless, in-

extricable web. The individual configurations of disease are not like plants which we can classify in a herbarium. Rather it is just what is a "plant"—an illness—that is most uncertain. *What* do we diagnose? . . . Diagnosis is expected to characterise in a comprehensive manner the whole morbid occurrence which has assailed the person and which stands as a well-defined entity among others. . . . But however we devise [a diagnostic schema] we realise that it cannot work; that we can only make temporary and arbitrary classifications; that there are a number of different possibilities which account for the fact that different workers construct entirely different schemata; and that classification is always contradictory in theory and never quite squares with the facts.

Why then do we keep on making this vain attempt? In the first place we want to see properly what this idea of disease-entity has *achieved* in respect of the *overall picture* of existing psychic disorders, and particularly where we have failed because it is the basic and radical failure which makes us aware of the actual state of our knowledge. In the second place every *presentation of special psychiatry* requires some classification of psychosis at its base. Without some such schema it cannot order its material. In the third place we need a classification in order *to make statistical investigations* of a large case material. (604)

Jaspers goes on to provide his proposed diagnostic schema:

An ideal schema would have to satisfy the following requirements: It must be such that any given case would have only one place within it and every case should have a place. The whole plan must have a compelling objectivity so that different observers can classify cases in the same way. . . . We abandon the idea of disease-entity and once more have to bear in mind continually the various points of view (as to causes, psychological structure, anatomical findings, course of illness and outcome) and in face of the facts we have to draw the line where none exists. Such classification therefore has only a provisional value. It is a fiction which will discharge its function if it proves to be the most apt for the time. There is no "natural" schema which would accommodate every case. (605)

With those caveats, Jaspers proposes a nosology quite similar to the big shift in 1980 with DSM-III in modern U.S. psychiatry. He proposes dividing psychiatric conditions into three main groups: Group I, "Known Somatic Illnesses with Psychic Disturbances" (such as cerebral tumors, meningitis), coincides with DSM's Axis III, which describes psychiatric conditions secondary to known medical illnesses. Group II, "The Three Major Psychoses" ("genuine epilepsy," schizophrenia, and manic-depressive illness), would correspond with the major mood and psychotic disorders on DSM's Axis I, primary psychiatric conditions (with epilepsy now moved to Axis III since a cerebral basis has been established for it). Group III is the "Personality Disorders," which corresponds to DSM's Axis II, also defined as personality disorders. Heuristically, with the caveats given previously, Jaspers goes on to accept Kraepelin's definition of the distinction between schizophrenia and manic-depressive illness based on the outcome criterion as the main factor, that is, invariably poor outcome with schizophrenia and frequent recovery with manic-depressive illness. This too is a distinction that mainstream psychiatry dropped for many years in favor of psychoanalytic theories, but to which the field returned in 1980 with the neo-Kraepelinian nosology of DSM-III (see chapter 11).

Jaspers's acceptance of an affective disorder–schizophrenia distinction in the nosology debate was based on the distinction between conditions with which one could empathize, those in whom meaningful connections could be made, and those which were not understandable. He felt that this distinction would provide one of the few organizing principles for nosology:

> The most profound distinction in psychic life seems to be that between what is meaningful and allows empathy and what in its particular way is ununderstandable, "mad" in the literal sense, schizophrenic psychic life (even though there may be no delusions). Pathological psychic life of the first kind we can comprehend vividly enough as an exaggeration or diminution of known phenomena and as an appearance of such phenomena without the usual causes or motives. Pathological psychic life of the second kind we cannot adequately comprehend in this way. Instead we find changes of the most general kind for which we have no empathy but which in some way we try to make comprehensible from an external point of view. . . . The affective illnesses appear to us to be open to empathy and natural but the various types of "madness" do not seem open to empathy and appear unnatural. (577–78)

Psychiatrists will be rewarded to read further as Jaspers goes on to provide classic detailed descriptions of the phenomenology of depression and mania (596–97) and to critique the main nosological schema of schizophrenia in the 1940s, that of Kurt Schneider (586–92).

12. Part 5, "The Abnormal Psyche in Society and History"

Part 5 assesses social and historical aspects of psychiatry; here Jaspers briefly makes some comments about religion, mass psychology, war, and culture (709–46). Of particular interest is his subtle discussion of the strengths and weaknesses of statistics in general and especially when applied to "socio-historical facts" (713–16).

13. Part 6, "The Human Being as a Whole"

Part 6 terminates the text of the book and is probably the most read segment, along with the introduction. Here Jaspers engages in his most clearly philosophical writing. He reviews the role of "psychopathology in retrospect" (747–55): "We do not accept any group of facts as genuine reality. We have opposed the tendency of all dogmatic theories of Being to build a structural whole and have pursued a systematic scrutiny of methods. The meaningful question for us is whether the differentiations are sufficiently clear and in what way they could be improved."

He discusses "the nature of man":

The retrospective survey of our psychopathology has been bringing us to the problem of human nature itself. . . . As with all sciences we have to find the limits of psychopathology as well, and see the concrete problem with which we are presented so that while we note the *wide expanse free for scientific enquiry* and its specific methods, we keep *within the limits of science* when we evaluate the findings and make use of them. It is just through science encountering its limits in this way that we can trace out [the ultimate nature of Man]. . . . What is of decisive importance for theory and practice in relation to Man is that there should be a basic philosophic attitude and no philosophical dogma. (756–57)

The human being is not merely a kind of animal nor is he any kind of purely spiritual creature of which we have no knowledge and which earlier times conceived to be angelic. Man is rather something *unique;* he partakes in the series of living things and in the series of angel, belonging to both and differing from both. . . . The human being is *open possibility,* incomplete and incompletable. Hence he is always *more and other than what he has brought to realisation in himself.* (765–66)

Jaspers goes on to make the most cogent argument for the relevance of philosophy for psychiatry:

> Where is the place for the many non-scientific discussions of traditional and contemporary psychopathology? Should we simply drop them as not belonging? Not so. They are the expressions of something inevitable, namely, that philosophy is operative in every living science and that without philosophy science is sterile and untrue and at best can only be partly correct.
>
> Many a psychiatrist has said that he did not want to burden himself with a philosophy and that this science has nothing to do with philosophy. Nothing can be said against that, inasmuch as the correctness of scientific insights in general and in psychiatry is not proved by philosophy. But the exclusion of philosophy would nevertheless be disastrous for psychiatry. . . . Since in psychopathology in particular scientific knowledge is not all of one kind, we have to distinguish the different modes of knowing and clarify our methods, the meaning and validity of our statements and the criteria of tests—and all this calls for philosophic logic. . . .
>
> The psychopathologist . . . must set his face against every attempt to create an absolute and to claim that particular methods of research are the only valid, single objectivities. . . . He must also take sides on behalf of meaningful understanding in the face of biologism, mechanism, and technics without denying them their validity within their own appropriate area. He has then to set his face against any attempt to turn scientific knowledge as a whole into an absolute so that consciousness may be kept free and with it the effectiveness of life at its source, which gives all practice its meaning. In this he stands on the side of differentiation as against a general confusion and of synthesis as against isolation. He is against the confusion of science with philosophy and of the physician's role with that of a saviour. But he is also against an isolation that plays off one thing against another instead of keeping them properly apart.
>
> To sum up: If anyone thinks he can exclude philosophy and leave it aside as useless he will eventually be defeated by it in some obscure form or other. (769–70)

Lastly, he discusses "the meaning of medical practice" (790–824), where he emphasizes the humanistic aspects of psychotherapy. First he criticizes "therapeutic nihilism" (an allusion to Kraepelin's school), which classifies and diagnoses carefully but provides little treatment, as well as "therapeutic overenthusiasm" (probably an allusion to psychoanalysis), which thinks it has the cure for every ailment. "In the long run effective practice can only be based on the certainties of knowledge" (791). He then describes the important factor of "existential communication" and the components of good psychotherapy, along with the characteristics of the "ideal" psychotherapist:

> The ultimate thing in the doctor-patient relationship is existential communication, which goes far beyond any therapy, that is, beyond anything that can be planned or methodically staged. The whole treatment is thus absorbed and defined within a community of two selves who live out the possibilities of Existence itself, as reasonable beings. . . . Doctor and patient are both human beings and as such are fellow-travelers in destiny. . . . There is no final solution. . . . (798–99)
>
> The final, decisive occurrence in any patient's therapy can be called "revelation." The patient becomes clear to himself, first by taking in the doctor's communicated knowledge and learning certain details about himself; secondly by seeing himself as it were in a mirror, and learning something of what he is like; thirdly, by bringing himself out further through an inner activity in which he gets to know himself more deeply, and fourthly by establishing and filling out the revelation of himself in the course of existential communication. . . . This process of clarification in the shape of the self-revelation of an individual extends far beyond what may be accessible to any psychotherapeutic plan. It carries one on into the philosophical realm of the individual growth of a self. . . . (799)
>
> Certainly a psychotherapist should have a training in somatic medicine and psychopathology . . . [but] science is only a part of his necessary equipment. Much more has to be added. Among the *personal prerequisites,* the width of his own horizon plays a part, so does the ability to be detached at times from any value-judgment, to be accepting and totally free of prejudice (an ability only found in those who generally possess very well defined values and a personality that is mature). Finally, there is the necessity for fundamental warmth and a natural kindness. It is therefore clear that a good psychotherapist can only be a rare phenomenon and even then he is usually only good *for a certain circle of people* for whom he is well suited. A psychotherapist for everyone is an impossibility. However, force of circumstance makes it the psychotherapist's duty to treat everyone who may ask his help. That fact should help him to keep his claims to modest proportions. (809)

14. The Appendix

Here the book ends, but as if he cannot leave the subject, Jaspers offers an appendix, with final thoughts on various topics, such as the method of interviewing psychiatric patients (*"A wealth of well-established viewpoints and an appropriate adaptation of them to the individual case* marks the ideal investigator" [825–30]), and further definition of psychotherapy and its types ("Psychotherapy is the name given to all those methods of treatment that affect both psyche and body by measures which proceed via the psyche. The cooperation of the patient is always required" [834–39]).

He then reviews "the history of psychopathology as a science" (844–59), again touching on by now familiar figures like Wernicke, Kraepelin, and Freud, and concluding with further expression of his conception of scientific method in psychiatry and the relevance of philosophy:

> Kraepelin was responsible for one of the most fruitful lines of research, the investigation of the whole life-history of the patient. He . . . laid the foundations for psycho-pharmacology. . . . But Kraepelin's basic conceptual world remained a somatic one which in the company of the majority of doctors he held as the only important one for medicine, not only as a matter of preference but in an absolute sense. The psychological discussions in his Textbook are brilliant in parts and he succeeded with them as it were unwittingly. He himself regarded them as temporary stopgaps until experiment, microscope and test-tube permitted objective investigation. . . . (853)
>
> The tenable observations [of Freud's psychoanalysis] . . . found a defender in [Eugen] Bleuler and a promoter. His critical penetration and its purging effect salvaged the tenable substance of Freud's teaching for the whole body of scientific psychiatry. . . . (855)
>
> The new element in the [contemporary] situation is the general uncommittedness and the breadth of approach possible today. We can ignore all theories, every established viewpoint and may investigate from any angle. . . . What our situation lacks is the absence of any over-all view, but this is only the negative side of something quite positive. The basic question is whether any fresh dogmatic idea will arise or what will take its place. Since 1913 my own effort has been to make a contribution here through an attempt to systematise methods. . . . (856)
>
> Everything creative usually tends to be converted into an absolute. The creator, however, experiences enthusiasm and a sense of fruitfulness—not the ruin. It is

his successor who pays for the enthusiasm, becomes one-sided and sterile and acquires a vested interest in the legacy, in being right because of it and in that power that lightly-won knowledge confers. . . . (857)

Scientific knowledge is precisely that which is independent of philosophy, opinion, and world-outlooks in general. It is valid for everyone, universal, and compelling. The vital thing therefore is whether our basic philosophical attitude contains the unconditioned will to get to know and therefore impels us to take the paths of science, or whether our philosophy makes conditions for our knowledge and unfailingly inhibits or destroys any scientific advance. (859)

Thus ends the *General Psychopathology.*

CHAPTER 6

What Is Scientific Method in Psychiatry?

> To observation, with reasoned thought, the Greeks added experiment . . .
> the instrument which has made science productive.
>
> —WILLIAM OSLER, 1889

I believe that Karl Jaspers has provided the most tightly reasoned analysis of scientific method for psychiatry. One might summarize his contribution in this regard in two main ideas: methodological pluralism and the understanding-explanation dichotomy.

1.

It is perhaps not an exaggeration to state that Jaspers was the first psychiatrist to clearly identify the need to be clear about one's methods. Jaspers took it as a given that each human being, including each patient, is unique. There is an aspect of each person that transcends any attempt to understand or capture that person by a certain way of knowing, whether it be science or anything else. This transcendence is the ultimate source of human freedom, Jaspers believed. Simply recognizing that we are each unique could also be understood biologically, I believe, as resulting from genetic differences, however small, between individuals. No matter how one views human freedom, Jaspers begins with this first intuition: that a human being can never be completely understood by a single method of knowledge. If one begins with this assumption, one is led inexorably to its corollary: every method of knowledge has its limitations. If no single method is sufficient, then multiple methods should be used. Complementary information should be obtained with multiple methods, leading to a better and better understanding of an individual's mental life or condition. Yet multiple methods never exhaust the uniqueness of individuals; hence clarity about one's methods is essential. Each method has an advantage and strength, capturing certain aspects more effectively and accurately than other methods; and each method has disadvantages and weaknesses, overlooking certain aspects. Each method begins with certain assumptions, thereby both honing its ability to capture certain aspects of reality and limiting its ability to capture other aspects of reality. *Methodological consciousness*, then, consists of recognizing the strengths and limits of each method and applying the ones that are best suited for specific circumstances (diseases, diagnoses, conditions). This was perhaps Jaspers's most important contribution to a theory of scientific method for psychiatry.

2.

This pluralism is closely tied to another idea that Jaspers introduced into psychiatry: *the understanding-explanation distinction*. This did not originate with Jaspers, but he was the first person to apply it systematically to psychiatry. By understanding *(Verstehen)*, Jaspers referred to "meaning," or the psychological intuition that an individual could have about the meaning of a psychological state or event for another individual. By explanation *(Erklaren)*, Jaspers referred to the more traditional concept of causal empirical experience, or the observable influence of one event or process on another that could be tested objectively. Thus, on the one hand, if one observes that throwing a rock breaks a window, and one conducts tests in which different individuals throw rocks at different windows, and each time the windows break, one is engaging in causal explanation and concludes that the throwing of rocks at windows causes the windows to break. On the other hand, if one observes that a certain person is throwing a rock at a particular window, and one wants to know why that person is throwing the rock, one might conjecture that that person is throwing the rock to get the attention of the person who lives inside that house. This line of thinking is an exercise in understanding, or trying to find meaning for an event. Wilhelm Dilthey argued that this explanation-understanding distinction applied to the natural versus the human sciences (Makkreel 1992). That is, in natural sciences (physics, chemistry, biology), causal explanation worked well and was sufficient to understand those fields of knowledge. However, in human sciences (Dilthey focused on history), understanding was required.

For instance, why did Napoleon invade Russia? A causal explanation approach would focus perhaps on economic factors that served as background for the events of the time, or even perhaps on Napoleon's physiological state (his bodily and brain function); yet this would seem insufficient. A historian following the understanding approach would try to place herself in Napoleon's place; faced with certain economic and political facts, and armed with her education, background, and beliefs, the historian could surmise that Napoleon might have had certain opinions about the advantages and disadvantages of invading Russia; ultimately, a certain line of thinking, which a historian engaged in understanding would provide, might explain Napoleon's invasion of Russia.

3.

The origin of this distinction in the work of the philosopher of history Wilhelm Dilthey is worth mentioning. History is the field where these ideas emerged, but even then Dilthey had their relevance to psychology very much in mind.

Dilthey began by emphasizing an essential difference between the object of natural science and the object of human sciences. In the natural sciences, objects in the external world could be broken down to their elements, such as atoms, and it was reasonable to view those underlying elements as the more fundamental features of natural existence. One could then work backward to develop general laws that could explain what is observed in natural existence after analysis of their underlying elements. Dilthey opposed this essentially analytic approach to the need to be holistic in the human sciences. Human individuals could not be broken down to constituent parts that explained the whole. In this belief, Dilthey held an opinion consistent with what we termed *emergence* in chapter 3 on current philosophy of mind. This nonreductive materialism, with which I agree, forces us to take seriously the human being as a whole, the person's psychology and social relations, separate from any underlying economic, biological, or other analyses that might claim to be more fundamental. Since Dilthey held hypotheses to be unique to natural sciences, he viewed them as unnecessary to the human sciences. His famous dictum was: "We explain *[erklaren]* nature, but we understand *[verstehen]* psychic life" (Makkreel 1992, 134). I will argue later in this chapter that hypotheses are needed for the understanding method, as modified by Max Weber to involve the concept of *ideal types*. Dilthey was somewhat more stark in the distinctions he drew. But the key to comprehending the roots of the method of understanding *(verstehen)* is to recognize its roots in a holistic view of human psychology: "In understanding we proceed from the context of the whole as given in its vitality, in order to make the part comprehensible on the basis of it. . . . All psychological thought contains the basic feature that the apprehension of the whole makes possible and determines the interpretation of the individual" (135).

4.

In some ways, this distinction between meaning and understanding appears to be common sense. But the vagueness and apparently limited objectivity of the understanding approach has troubled those who respect empirical science, such as Jaspers's mentor, the sociologist Max Weber (Gerth and Mills 1978). Could scientific approaches be brought to bear on the human sciences? And if so, would it be solely by causal explanation, or was there also a role for understanding?

The biological school of psychiatry, in Jaspers's era, sought to implement causal explanation to the exclusion of understanding, or psychological approaches, directed at the meaning of psychiatric states or conditions. Jaspers argued that this ideology was incomplete. Consistent with his methodological consciousness thesis, Jaspers favored a pluralistic approach in psychiatry that allowed for understanding as well as explanation.

These two major ideas, which Jaspers hammered home over and over again in the *GP*, were received with skepticism by psychiatry as a field initially, then ignored for decades, until they were again recently rediscovered by Havens and by McHugh and Slavney.

5.

Contemporary pluralistic models of psychiatry (those of Havens and of McHugh and Slavney) are consistent with, and indeed indebted to, Jaspers's earlier formulations. They provide a way above and beyond the historical seesaw between the dogmatisms of biological reductionism and psychoanalytic orthodoxy, without descent into the quagmire of biopsychosocial eclecticism. In this manner, Jaspers's ideas have been rediscovered and resonate again in psychiatry almost a century after he first propounded them.

Yet, while some academic thinkers in psychiatry may have come close to Jaspers's ideas, the psychiatric academicians and practitioners in the mainstream have not carefully followed these theoretical developments and have shown little interest in them. For this group, *eclecticism* is the catchword. They claim to be "ideologically neutral," by which in reality they mean that they simply ignore conceptual attempts to understand what they are doing when they study and practice psychiatry. They hide this lack of interest under the rubric of the biopsychosocial approach to medicine, initially introduced by George Engel as a means of attempting to include psychological and social factors in the largely medical disease model practiced in medicine. Today, the biopsychosocial approach, combined with eclecticism, has too frequently come to mean simply avoiding a discussion of methods and assumptions in one's psychiatric work.

Thus, a Jasperian pluralism conflicts with eclecticism, the mainstream philosophy of modern psychiatry. This is so because by eclecticism modern psychiatrists mean abjuring all talk of theories and methods, thus denying them all. Unable to place the rise and decline of biological psychiatry and of psychoanalysis in context, some have given up altogether on the attempt to comprehensively understand human nature. Since unified dogmas fail, no doctrines are allowed. This is an explanatory nihilism as sterile as the earlier therapeutic nihilism that Jaspers found irksome. Hidden under the rubric of a biopsychosocial approach to understanding human nature, this eclecticism takes no stands. It does not pay attention to the methods of biological, psychological, or social knowledge; it simply labels different theories under those concepts, appends them to each other, and does not attempt to weight their advantages or disadvantages critically. Therapeutically, it ends in the opposite of nihilism, a shooting from the hip with all types of treatments. Everyone gets medication and psychotherapy because everything is biological and psychosocial. But little work is done on specifying when and why medications work or do not work, when and why psychotherapy is effective or not, and when they might (or might not) work best together. Empirical research in psychiatry is beginning to ask these questions, but at the theoretical level, biopsychosocial eclecticism remains accepted doctrine, rather than the methodological pluralism proposed by Jaspers, Havens, or McHugh and Slavney.

The rediscovery of Karl Jaspers, however, may help modern psychiatry drop its presumed ideological neutrality, which actually hides a biopsychosocial eclecticism, and turn to principled methodological pluralism (see chapters 23 and 24).

6.

Jaspers's view of scientific method was largely derived from the sociologist Max Weber, who in turn had roots in the historian Wilhelm Dilthey's distinction between human sciences *(Geisteswissenschaften)* and natural sciences *(Naturwissenschaften)*. What is unique about Jaspers, however, is that he did not give up on a scientific worldview in making this distinction.

Unlike the version propounded by later hermeneutic heirs of this tradition, Jaspers's view of scientific method in psychiatry did not dissolve into a nonempirical relativism (Wiggins and Schwartz 1991).[1] I will argue that Jaspers's approach is consistent with modern philosophies of science in the tradition of Quine and Peirce but is inconsistent with Popper's view of science. I will show that the understanding-explanation distinction is critical to Jaspers's view of science but requires the abandonment of Popperian definitions of scientific method.

7.

As noted, Jaspers came to philosophy from psychiatry. Thus what he has to say regarding philosophy of science should have direct bearing on psychiatry.

The first fact to think about is that Jaspers believed that Max Weber was the greatest philosopher of his age. This is remarkable, given that it is sometimes held that Jaspers acceded that status to his sometimes friend Martin Heidegger. One cannot ascribe Jaspers's statement about Weber solely to personal friendship, either, given his equally important and indeed longer personal relationship with Heidegger. In fact there would appear to be more natural affinities between Jaspers and Heidegger in the subjects of phenomenology and existentialism, whereas Weber was an empiricist, analytically minded, and in many ways closer to the Anglo-American school of philosophy than the Continental school, with which Heidegger and Jaspers are often identified. (Clearly Jaspers cannot be easily categorized in either school of thought.) What in Weber's work was so impressive that it merited Jaspers's judgment of him as the greatest philosopher of the age? In his lectures on modern philosophy, Jaspers does not provide the reader with an easy clue. He makes his judgment in favor of Weber's intellect and philosophical status, but he mainly refers to Weber's work as being limited to the applied social sciences. The better source for the connection between Weber and Jaspers is the *General Psychopathology,* where, in parts 2 and 6, Jaspers makes the understanding-explanation distinction central to his understanding of psychiatry.

In beginning his discussion of meaning in psychiatry, Jaspers, in a footnote, makes the personal link we are looking for: "The work of Max Weber was mostly responsible for my deliberate use of understanding as a method which would be in keeping with our great cultural traditions. . . . This present book [was] greeted as something radically new, although all I had done was to link psychiatric reality with the traditional humanities. Looking back now, it seems astonishing that these had been so forgotten and had grown so alien to psychiatry" ([1913] 1997, 301–2).

Jaspers goes to some length to point out the limits of the understanding method in psychiatry; this is particularly important because, if left unchecked, the use of understanding in science would lead to a rather robust relativism. This drift has happened in fact with the hermeneutic tradition after Jaspers. It is thus important to show how Jaspers used hermeneutic ideas without succumbing to blatant relativism.

Jaspers always emphasized the importance and value of empirical science (explanation, *erklaren*). In the *GP*, his tone seems directed at his psychiatric colleagues, most of whom were empiricists; so he took the merits of empirical science for granted. He was trying to show them that another role still existed for understanding. Thus, he granted the importance of explanation in psychiatry. But he also assumed that we had to grant the importance of human freedom. Jaspers does not expound on this factor much in part 2 of the *GP*, but his later work clarifies what he means. If human beings are free, which most of us, including empirical scientists, would admit, then there are certain aspects of human beings that are beyond understanding *or* explanation. Jaspers calls this "the spontaneous freedom of Existence." So Jaspers places explanation at one pole and Existence at the other. Understanding, in his usage, mediates between the two.

Understanding is not on an equal footing with explanation, then; it cannot stand on its own as a method of science, producing facts and truths as the method of explanation can. Neither is understanding the repository of human freedom, the source of what makes each of us unique; each human Existence plays that role. Understanding lies midway between explanation and Existence; it does not exist separately as a body of knowledge (e.g., Freudian or Marxian doctrine). "Psychological understanding only serves psychopathology in so far as it makes something visible to our experience and fosters our observation" (Jaspers [1913] 1997, 312). Understanding throws light on specific facts or events; the knowledge gained may lead to new interpretations based on understanding or to new explanations of empirical facts that add to our objective explanatory knowledge.

Hence Jaspers does not view understanding as an equal, much less as a superior (as modern relativists would assert) method of knowledge comparable to explanation. He sees understanding as a necessary mediation in human beings between brute facts and human freedom, and the interpretations that arise as a result should provide meaning for what is observed and encourage further observations of fact and new interpretations.

8.

If psychiatry, as conceived by Jaspers, is a science, it is not one in Karl Popper's sense. As discussed in chapter 4, Popper sought to provide a deductive definition of science to replace the more traditional inductive definition. In the older view, science seemed to involve the accumulation of facts; the more facts, the more science. The problem with this inductive view traced back to David Hume, who showed that this approach could never, with complete certainty, prove anything. Induction relies instead on probability, and although something might be 99.99 percent likely based on induction, there is always at least the slightest chance that it may not be the case. Popper sought complete certainty for science, and he thought he had it with Einstein's discoveries. Einstein was able to make certain predictions based on his theories; if those predictions were wrong, then his theory was wrong. Only one mistake was required to disprove his entire theory. Thus, Popper argued that science could best be understood as an activity whose theories could be definitively disproved but never definitively proved. The best scientific theories, then, would be those that would make falsifiable propositions; if they were not subsequently falsified, those theories might be true. Popper accused Freud and Marx of having claimed to provide scientific theories when in fact their ideas were in no way falsifiable. This approach has caught on in modern science. It has the disadvantage, however, of making one part of science, physics, the ultimate paradigm of science, and this is something that Weber and his tradition had long warned everyone against. Freud and Marx are, in some sense, easy targets; Darwin's theory could just as well be rejected for being unfalsifiable.

Ultimately, Popper did not solve the Humean riddle. For Popper's view tells us not which theories are true, but which ones are not. And it does not even do that, unless one is willing to deny any evidence other than empirical data. If understanding is allowed, as Weber and Jaspers insist, then the interpretations based on understanding are not falsifiable; they cannot be definitively disproved, just as they cannot be definitively proved. And then we are left again with the problem of an impoverished psychology. Some, like Paul Churchland, would greet this turn of events gladly; "folk psychology" is essentially the use of understanding as a means of knowledge, and Churchland would deny its utility. But his brand of eliminative materialism is too narrow and dry for our purposes.

Jaspers draws this direct conclusion, years before Popper: "In the psychology of meaningful phenomena, the application of directly perceived, understandable connections to an individual case never leads to deductive proof but only to probabilities" ([1913] 1997, 313).

This leaves us with an inductive philosophy of science, like that of Peirce, but not exactly in the traditional sense again. To review, Peirce accepted induction as the method of science, acknowledged that it led to increasing probabilities of truth, and argued that these probabilities came so close to the limits of certainty that it was almost mathematically meaningless to deny certainty to them at some point of accumulated evidence. Peirce also added that this accumulation of near-certain inductive knowledge was a process that spanned generations of scientists and that the community of scientists that added to this fund of knowledge would eventually reach consensus on what was likely to be true based on those data. Jaspers's view of understanding differs from Peirce's in that Jaspers does not view the knowledge obtained from understanding as being similarly concrete. Interpretations based on understanding should not be passed along, whole and unchallenged, from one generation of scientists to another; they should not simply be built upon or added to; and they should not rely on a consensus of opinion as to their validity. All of these processes in fact happened with that one system of interpretations that Jaspers so vehemently criticized as ossified dogma: Freudianism. Jaspers viewed understanding as something more fluid and less empirical: "Psychological understanding cannot be used mechanically as a sort of generalised knowledge but a fresh, personal intuition is needed on every occasion" ([1913] 1997, 313). He approvingly quoted Eugen Bleuler (a respected mainstream academic psychiatrist, but also an open-minded man who befriended Freud but rejected his dogmatism): "Interpretation is a science only in principle, in its application it is always an art."

9.

Jaspers outlined his view of scientific method in the *GP* as follows:

> Science is knowledge that is generally valid and compelling. It is based on methods that are designed deliberately and which can be tested by anyone and it is always related to individual objects. . . . In the name of science we have been wrongly satisfied with mere *conceptualisation*, with mere logical method, mere clarity of thinking. . . . When simple thinking is confused with an objective knowledge science becomes lost in empty speculation and the resultant endless possibilities. Science is wrongly identified with *Natural Science*. . . . Natural science is indeed the groundwork of psychopathology and an essential element in it but the humanities are equally so and, with this, psychopathology does not become in any way less scientific but scientific in another way. . . . The scientific attitude is ready to adopt any methods and asks only for those universal scientific criteria; general validity, convincing insights (which can be proved), clarity of method and the possibility for a meaningful discussion. ([1913] 1997, 768)

It might appear that these latter criteria of science would exclude meaningful understanding, which might seem less than universally valid and not provable in the same sense as empirical methods. Although Jaspers did see understanding as being less reliable than causal explanation in the sense of the hallmarks of empirical science, he still saw understanding as being scientific in many ways. Leonard Ehrlich, who has translated and compiled many of Jaspers's works into English, has pointed out that when discussing science, Jaspers uses the German word *Wissenschaft,* which "refers to any disciplined, methodical inquiry. It does not only refer to the natural sciences." Ehrlich suggests a retranslation of the above section from page 768 as follows: "Science is cognition that is universally valid and cogent. It is founded on method deliberately engaged in, testable by anyone, and always referring to specific objects. . . . Whatever is cognized scientifically can be demonstrated or proven in such a manner that any intellect that is at all capable of grasping the matter at hand, cannot evade the cogency of its correctness." Ehrlich comments: "The heart of the matter is what Jaspers calls methodological consciousness. This means not only a methodical doing, a methodical procedure, but method accompanied by a consciousness of what the method presupposes, of the assumptions defining the method, what its possibilities and limits are, how it differs from other methods, why it is chosen, how it is relevant to the object of investigation, what its test of experience is, what its results are" (Ehrlich 1999).[2]

In further communication with me, Ehrlich has clarified what Jaspers meant by the term *universal validity,* in a manner that makes its applicability to the method of understanding more comprehensible:

> [Universal validity] does not refer to the idea that an item of scientific knowledge applies to all pertinent cases, which would be a very trivial principle. Instead, it means that what is known is valid for anyone, i.e., for any other person who is able to undertake the research or inquiry at the given scientific knowledge. It is the criterion of "objectivity" in the sense of "inter-subjectivity." . . . When it comes to diagnosis, prognosis, and to treatment, the physician knows what is scientifically involved in arriving at that knowledge. It is "universally valid" because it will be recognized as valid by any other person as qualified a scientist as he/she is. . . . Especially in medicine, "universal validity" is as a mark, as a criterion of science, an "aim" as Jaspers says, i.e., a measure, against which the scientist measures the degree of the validity of his findings and his knowledge. It is not a criterion to which knowledge must "conform." (personal communication, 2000)

In my opinion, this short section of the *GP* is among the most important, as it lays out most clearly Jaspers's important contribution to identifying scientific method for psychiatry, that is, the understanding-explanation methodological distinction, and the emphasis on methodological consciousness and pluralism.[3]

10.

Hence, Jaspers held a view of science as implying universal validity, though including within its purview the method of understanding as well as explanation. I will suggest here a few other sources of thinking about scientific method that merge with and complement Jaspers's views.

The first is Claude Bernard's work on the experimental method (Olmsted and Olmsted 1961). In the mid–nineteenth century, it was still an open question whether biology, the study of living beings, could be an empirical science, amenable to causal explanation alone, like physics or chemistry. Vitalists believed that this was not the case, and until a series of experimental advances in physiology led by Bernard, Magendie, and their colleagues showed otherwise, vitalism was the mainstream view among scientists. Bernard, who later published a book on the experimental method in medicine, can be credited with bringing biology, and with it medicine, into the camp of empirical science. Bernard's experiences shed light on the later debate about whether social sciences, and particularly psychology or psychiatry, could be empirical sciences.

First, Bernard established the skeptical attitude, in a way that Jaspers restated in detail, as the basis of the scientific attitude: "The theories which embody our scientific ideas . . . are by no means immutable truths, one must always be ready to abandon them, to alter them, or to replace them, as soon as they cease to represent the truth. In a word, we must alter theory to adapt it to nature, but not nature to adapt it to theory" (quoted in Olmsted and Olmsted 1961, 132). Thus, first and foremost, scientific method requires holding one's theories lightly (as Leston Havens says) and being willing to test them by experience and discard or change them based on the results. Thus, Bernard's view of science appears to approximate Peirce's later view, the gradual verification of theories that is never complete. Yet Bernard does believe in one absolute principle, scientific determinism, described by Olmsted and Olmsted as follows: "Under identical conditions, the resultant phenomena will be identical" (133). In response to Hume's challenge to causality, then, Bernard would reply that while we cannot be sure that the sun will rise tomorrow, we can know that it will rise tomorrow under the same conditions that it rose today. This allows Bernard to accept the inherent limits of verifying theories, without slipping into relativism.

Adapting Bernard's view, we might ask of the method of understanding the following questions: Does an interpretation based on understanding produce testable hypotheses? Can we test it by experience? We have abandoned Popper, so our interpretations do not need to be falsifiable. We are not looking for certainty. But if they are testable, if experience can seem consistent or inconsistent based on them, then they can add or subtract from the overall likelihood of the interpretations' truth. To say that something is testable is to view understanding as a mediator between Existence (in Jaspers's meaning of free unique human individuality) and empirical fact, rather than as a different world equal to and separate from explanation. Hence, insights based on understanding can be proved (in a non-Popperian sense, i.e., never with undoubted certainty) and have general validity (in a Peircian sense, i.e., being reproducible to some extent, or notable by a community of scientists). This latter aspect requires a community of open-minded investigators, who view validated interpretations as empirical scientists view facts—that is, as the data of experience with which they work, data that may be conceptualized in different ways and which need to be answerable to the evidence of further experience. This community of investigators should not be dogmatists (like orthodox Freudians), who would view interpretations in the way positivists view facts—as unchangeable absolute truths.

11.

It is also useful to return to Charles Peirce's definition of experiment, since the experimental attitude was so central to Peirce's thought. "What are the essential ingredients of an experiment? First of course, an experimenter of flesh and blood. Secondly, a verifiable hypothesis. This is a proposition relating to the universe environing the experimenter, or to some well-known part of it and affirming or denying of this only some experimental possibility or impossibility. The third indispensable ingredient is a sincere doubt in the experimenter's mind as to the truth of the hypothesis" (Peirce [1905] 1958, 198).

Hence the experimental attitude that is central to scientific method includes a verifiable hypothesis; this is perhaps the most important contribution of Peirce on this subject. There has to be some hypothesis that is being tested. To some extent, when dealing with human meanings, we might interpret Jaspers's view of the method of understanding as a means of generating hypotheses, which could then be tested to some degree, most adequately by the causal explanation method. He still allowed for the possibility that such interpretive hypotheses could not be tested with the method of explanation, however. This view of things seems to closely resemble Weber's view on the use of ideal types in social science research (see below). Again, the importance of doubt when engaging in scientific method, including the method of understanding, is restated by Peirce, and, as we see below, doubt may be even more important with the method of understanding than with the method of explanation.

12.

Another source that helps me understand what Jaspers means by understanding *(verstehen)* is a recent paper by a philosopher, Osborne Wiggins, and a psychiatrist, Michael Schwartz, in which they try to define the outlines of a science of meaning (1991). Wiggins and Schwartz first define science as "that kind of knowledge which is capable of the most rigorous justification or defense. If we wish to establish a science regarding some particular domain of reality, we must ask, How can we best justify and defend our claims to knowledge regarding that domain of reality?" (48). This general definition of science does not tie it to a specific kind of science, such as physics or biology; it is analogous to Jaspers's definition of science as "generally valid and compelling." Wiggins and Schwartz go on to explain scientific ideas along Peircean, rather than Popperian, terms: "Scientific belief . . . is a matter of degree. The extent of belief depends upon the extent of the supporting evidence. Scientific beliefs consist, accordingly, in degrees of likelihood of truth." They then define meanings as "mental processes and their intended objects" (49). They describe "understanding" as "the way in which one person experiences the 'meanings' of another person" (50). This depends on "expressions" by persons of their meaning, such as speaking about them or nonverbal facial gestures. Wiggins and Schwartz argue that expressions are objective forms of evidence that can serve as the scientific foundation of meanings.

Although meaning is by nature ambiguous, and thus one interpretation of a meaning can never be definitively established, this is not in principle different from any other branch of science. Even in the empirical sciences of causal explanation, as noted by Bernard, there is always space for doubt. Thus, the doubt inherent in understanding meanings does not disqualify understanding from being a science. There may be more room for doubt and less ability to get closer to certainty, but these are differences in amount, rather than type, of scientific evidence. Wiggins and Schwartz thus admit the ambiguity and multiplicity of interpretations that might be given to meanings, but they assert that there is a role, nonetheless, for the empirical evidence of expressions; certain interpretations will be more or less likely than others, and that, in itself, is the scientific method. Given that much about a person's mental processes is hidden from outer expression, and perhaps even to the person himself, the science of meaning will be limited. Many aspects of a person's mental life will not be able to be described or known with scientific or near-scientific certainty. Wiggins and Schwartz conclude along lines that could have been written by Bernard: "The only hope for diminishing this difficulty lies in a firmer dedication to the critical attitude in the human sciences. Suspiciousness and doubt, especially regarding one's own ideas, are doubly recommended" (53). Jaspers would undoubtedly agree with most of this exegesis of his thought. It would be interesting for a scholar also to think about the connection between Jaspers's view of understanding and Weber's ideal typess, however. Jaspers would likely agree that external expressions of meanings (statements, behaviors) are necessary to provide evidence for certain interpretations, but one wonders if Jaspers would also argue that we should use Weber's ideal types as a source of evidence for or against certain interpretations. Jaspers described ideal types as "cognitive instruments of approaching actuality" (Ehrlich, Ehrlich, and Pepper 1994, 482), something like certain interpretations against which further experience is tested. They are hypotheses that are conceptual constructs and are not viewed as valid but as ways to clarify the meanings of what is experienced. Without doubt, Jaspers considered Weber's concept of ideal types as central to the method of understanding, and he emphasized the value of this aspect of Weber's thought. In sum, there are sources of evidence for interpretations, and that in itself is an important lesson to draw in support of the scientific value of the method of understanding.

13.

Jaspers elegantly expressed the terms of the problem: if psychiatry is a science, it is a science that relies on understanding meanings, in addition to causal explanation. Understanding is just as much a scientific endeavor as causal explanation, however, and does not relegate psychiatry to relativism. This is because the method of understanding can be applied to psychiatry while one remains faithful to two basic aspects of scientific method: the use of whatever evidence is available to test one's theories both affirmatively and negatively, and the skeptical attitude of doubt. There is evidence for understanding that to some extent is reliable and generalizable, such as the speech and observable behavior of individuals, and this can serve to provide a scientific basis for the method of understanding. However, these sources of evidence are always limited, and thus, theories or interpretations based on them are never completely provable. However, interpretations are susceptible to more or less likelihood of explaining the available evidence. As a result, too strict definitions of science, like Popper's falsifiability criterion, must be abandoned. But lacking such a strict definition, an even more firm dedication to the skeptical attitude toward ideas is necessary to maintain scientific integrity.

14.

Jaspers's view of scientific method, derived from Max Weber, did not give up on a scientific worldview in making a distinction between understanding and causal explanation. Unlike the later hermeneutic thinkers, Jaspers's view of scientific method in psychiatry did not degenerate into "postmodern" relativism, although it requires the jettisoning of Popperian dogma.

Jaspers provides us with a means of reexamining what we mean by scientific method and how we can apply it to psychiatry. I conclude that we must get away from an oversimplified version of scientific method, the positivistic assumption that we can avoid any kind of belief and that we can know things with absolute certainty. This is not the case in life, and not even the case in specific sciences, since all sciences have certain conceptual assumptions. But for a field that deals with the mental life of living humans, like psychiatry, it is even less the case. Yet science does not require such strict disciplines. Psychiatry can live up to the standards of science and still use understanding to make interpretations about the meanings of individuals' mental processes.

15.

This discussion of scientific method will remain unconvincing, I fear, to two groups. There will be those, mostly psychotherapists, who will argue that the search for proof in psychiatry is misguided; psychiatry is an art, and pretenses to science are simply pretenses. The other group, hard-nosed neuroscientists perhaps, will be uneasy with talk of subjective meaning and will insist that psychiatry must adhere to the strict disciplines of quantifiability and objectivity. I hope I have sufficiently discussed the limitations of these extreme views to make the reader unsympathetic to them. In particular, I trust that most readers will feel little need to give up any inclination to scientific method in psychiatry altogether, thus rejecting the extreme antiscience viewpoint. However, I offer a further discussion of the limits of the strict empirical viewpoint in chapter 19, if for no other reason than the great apparent advances made in recent years in the empirical approach to psychiatry.

CHAPTER 7

Darwin's Dangerous Method

The Essentialist Fallacy

> As Darwinian thinking gets closer and closer to home—where we live—
> tempers run higher, and the rhetoric tends to swamp the analysis. But so-
> ciobiologists, beginning with Hobbes and continuing through Nietzsche
> to the present day, have seen that only an evolutionary analysis of the
> origins—and transformations—of ethical norms could ever properly make
> sense of them. Greedy reductionists have taken their usual first stumbling
> steps into this new territory, and been duly chastened by the defenders
> of complexity. We can learn from these errors without turning our backs
> on them. —DANIEL DENNETT, 1995

1.

My discussion of scientific method has touched little on the groundbreaking work of Charles Darwin. The philosopher Daniel Dennett has suggested
that philosophy, psychology, and other disciplines would also benefit from taking seriously the ideas of Darwin. Yet I have not discussed what arguably could
be the single most influential theory in modern biology: evolutionary theory.
Dennett (1995) argues that "Darwin's dangerous idea" can serve as a form of
"universal acid" that can clear away much murkiness in other fields, yet many
thinkers seem resistant to it.[1] So let us turn to Darwinian concepts and examine what relevance they may have for understanding psychiatry.

As a scientific model for psychiatry, Darwinian ideas have much more utility than other common scientific models, such as models derived from Einstein
and physics. Recall that Karl Popper was quite critical of Freud (and Marx) for
being "unscientific," since they produced rather broad theories that could not
be refuted. It is worth noting that Popper was also rather skeptical about Darwinism, since Darwin's methods seemed all too similar to Freud's and Marx's
in that they did not consist of simple refutable hypotheses. Yet Dennett makes

the point that Darwin was not completely unaware of the need for hypothesis-testing as part of the scientific process. Popper simply goes too far by making refutability the sole criterion of whether a method is scientific. Writes Dennett: "It is sometimes suggested that Darwin's theory is systematically irrefutable (and hence scientifically vacuous), but Darwin was forthright about what sort of finding it would take to refute the theory. 'Though nature grants vast periods of time for the work of natural selection, she does not grant an indefinite period,' so if the geological evidence mounted to show that not enough time had elapsed, his whole theory would be refuted" (1995, 46). Yet Dennett also makes the connection between Darwinian method and Peirce's philosophy of science: "It is reasonable to believe that an idea that was ultimately false would surely have succumbed by now to such an unremitting campaign of attacks. That is not a conclusive proof, of course, just a mighty persuasive consideration" (47).

The difference, to answer Popper, is that Darwin did produce many hypotheses that could be tested by empirical means, whereas Freud and Marx were either uninterested in empirical testing or saw their theoretical work as abstractly true rather than as concrete hypotheses vulnerable to empirical refutation. Darwin's defenders also sometimes argue that biology differs from physics in this sense: when the subject of interest is the origin of species, many of which are extinct, one has to make judgments based on events that occurred in the past (Irvine 1959). Scientific ideas are not limited to the here and now of the experimental setting (as they more often are in classical physics and quantum mechanics). Thus, since it deals with past events, evolutionary biology is in many ways more similar to the humanities discipline of history than to physics. As we discussed previously, psychiatry also may be considered a historical discipline. Thus, it might be asked what evolutionary theory has to teach psychiatry or, put another way, whether we might not better understand psychiatry with insights from evolutionary biology.

2.

There are a number of ways this process can occur. One approach is to take a general view of evolutionary theory in its content and then try to apply that theory directly to psychiatric phenomena. This method, used by some authors, does not seem particularly appealing to me. It consists of making many historical (and prehistorical) assumptions about the psychological state of humanity's ancestors and then extrapolating from those assumptions to current psychiatric conditions (Glantz and Pearce 1989; Stevens and Price 2000). This kind of theorizing is more like Marx and less like Darwin, more abstract speculation than empirically testable hypothesis generation. For instance, it might be argued that we function biologically at a basically hunter-gatherer level of existence, and yet civilized life puts many restrictions on those biological urges. Thus, the male dominance hierarchies that might have been evolutionarily useful in the prehistoric past are less acceptable in many Western industrial countries. As a result, it might be argued, various kinds of conflict occur, such as antisocial personality traits or interpersonal spousal conflict. The problem with this approach is that it assumes far too much: it assumes what prehistoric man was like, and it assumes that those features have not changed. Further, this approach to evolutionary biology is constantly guessing at what was useful from the perspective of natural selection, in a manner that is far less obvious than in many other animal species. Stephen Gould has rightly referred to this approach as "just-so" stories, warning against their overapplication: "The standard foundation of Darwinian just-so stories does not apply to humans. That foundation is the implication: if adaptive, then genetic" (1989, 259). In fact, Gould argues, many human adaptations are cultural and not explainable by evolutionary means.

Daniel Dennett agrees with Gould, and he specifically points this criticism at some proponents of "sociobiology," for example E. O. Wilson.

> Wilson declares that sociobiology has shown us that "Morality, or more strictly our belief in morality, is merely adaptation put in place to further our reproductive ends." Nonsense. Our reproductive ends may have been the ends that kept us in the running till we could develop culture, and they may still play a powerful—sometimes overpowering—role in our thinking, but that does not license any conclusion at all about our current values. It does not follow from the fact that our reproductive ends were the ultimate historical *source* of our present values, that they are the ultimate (and still principal) *beneficiary* of our ethical actions. [Those who] think otherwise . . . are committing the "genetic" fallacy Nietzsche (and Darwin) warned us about. (Dennett 1995, 470)

If one replaces the term *morality* in this quote with *human behavior*, we can see how Dennett's observations directly relate to the inappropriate use of evolutionary ideas in relation to psychiatry and psychology. Yet Dennett wrote an entire book about Darwinism in order to emphasize the importance of Darwinian ideas for philosophy and the humanities in general. He claims that evolutionary ideas can be useful in psychology (though he mainly emphasizes cognitive psychology rather than clinical psychology and psychiatry) if they point out specific hypotheses that can be tested: "There is plenty of good work in sociobiology and evolutionary psychology, and there is plenty of bad work, as in any field" (Dennett 1995, 491).

Taking a pluralistic approach, I am less interested in examining the utility of evolutionary biology from the perspective of the content of such theories, and I am more interested in thinking about the *methods* of Darwin himself, and how those methods might be helpful to psychiatrists.

3.

Darwin faced a dilemma that is not too different from some of the dilemmas facing contemporary psychiatry. Darwin's dilemma was the problem of whether animals and plants were always throughout time exactly as they are, or whether they evolved in some manner to become as they are. And if they evolved, how did they evolve, under the influence of what factors?

Darwin was interested in this matter from a strictly biological viewpoint. But his work was to butt into serious philosophical and religious beliefs.

The prevailing viewpoint was *essentialism*. Essentialism means that entities are what they are because of their essences, because there is something inherently unique about them without which they would not be what they are. This philosophical idea dates back to Aristotle, who divided all the characteristics of any thing in the world into essences (the unique necessary constituents) and accidents (features that exist but are not necessary to the existence of a thing). We might say that the essence of persons is that they are rational animals; whether they have red hair or black hair (or any hair at all) is an accidental characteristic. We cannot, however, conceive of anyone who does not possess the faculty of reason and the characteristic of being at some point a living being (an animal). Essentialism applied to species held that all species are essentially what they are because of their unique essences. There always would be something necessary and unique to each species which by definition could never change. The theological codicil to this essentialism was that God ordained the essence of each thing in the act of Creation.

Thus essentialism, and traditional theism, required that species never change. However, many observations made by Darwin (and others) convinced some biologists that species changed over time, and that they evolved in such a manner that they could markedly change, with no evidence of an unalterable necessary essence. The problem with this view of species, from the philosophical standpoint, was that it broke with millennia of accepted biological teaching dating to Aristotle, and it contradicted Christian theology.

It may be difficult, a century and a half later, to appreciate how much courage Darwin, Huxley, and their colleagues needed to possess to break with such powerful bonds of tradition. Yet they did (Irvine 1959).

It should be clear from this exposition that this break was not simply a matter of a new biological theory. It was a major epistemological and philosophical change in thinking about mankind and science. It is this aspect of Darwin's work that I think is most relevant to modern psychiatry. What did Darwin do in terms of his thinking that was so revolutionary?

4.

The big break, I believe, was with essentialism.[2] Once Darwin accepted evolution, he had to discard essentialism. One could no longer think about biology, and indeed science, in essentialist terms. Ernst Mayr describes this process well:

> Of the . . . ideologies challenged by Darwin's theories, none was more deeply entrenched than the philosophy of essentialism. Essentialism had dominated Western thinking for more than 2000 years, going back to the geometric thinking of the Pythagoreans. They pointed out that a triangle, regardless of the combination of angles, always has the form of a triangle. It is discontinuously different from a quadrangle or any other kind of polygon. The triangle is one of the limited number of possible forms of a polygon. In an analogous manner, all the variable phenomena of nature, according to this thinking, are a reflection of a limited number of constant and sharply delimited *eide* or essences. . . .
>
> Virtually all philosophers up to Darwin's time were essentialists. Whether they were realists or idealists, materialists or nominalists, they all saw species of organisms with the eyes of an essentialist. They considered species as "natural kinds," defined by constant characteristics and sharply separated from one another by bridgeless gaps. . . . Essentialism's influence was great in part because its principle is anchored in our language, in our use of a single noun in the singular to designate highly variable phenomena in our environment, such as mountain, home, water, horse, or honesty. . . .

In daily life we largely proceed essentialistically (typologically) and become aware of variation only when we compare individuals. He who speaks of "the Prussian," "the Jew," "the intellectual" reveals essentialistic thinking. Such language ignores the fact that every human is unique; no other individual is identical to him.

It was Darwin's genius to see that this uniqueness of each individual is not limited to the human species but is equally true for every sexually reproducing species of animal and plant. Indeed the discovery of the importance of the individual became the cornerstone of Darwin's theory of natural selection. It eventually resulted in the replacement of essentialism by population thinking, which emphasized the uniqueness of the individual and the critical role of individuality in evolution. Darwin no longer asked, as had Agassiz, Lyell, and the philosophers, "What is good for the species?" but "What is good for the individual?" And variation, which had become irrelevant and accidental for the essentialist, now became one of the crucial phenomena of living nature. (1991, 400–402)

Darwin killed essentialism not only in biology, and not only in religion, but also in philosophy. To the extent that philosophy seeks to explain anything about human beings, it can no longer be essentialist. In psychiatry, clinicians live and work as essentialists, as if nothing like this happened. We speak of schizophrenia or other diseases as if our descriptions of them pick out a natural kind, with certain essential characteristics. Some speak of a patient as "schizophrenic" as if the label describes his essence. Others deny any validity to such talk, believing that humans are essentially incapable of being mentally ill. So, many in psychiatry live with a dead philosophy, one that Darwin slew over a century ago. It is time we took notice.

Essentialism is dead in philosophy, and it should be dead in psychiatry. But what should replace it? Darwin did not have a philosophical plan to answer this question. But other philosophers and scientists, mostly across the Atlantic, took up this challenge.[3] Their answer was pragmatism, which we will discuss below. But, first, let us emphasize how a rejection of essentialism is relevant to contemporary psychiatry.

As pointed out by the psychologist Peter Zachar (2000, 2001), essentialism in medicine and psychiatry is revealed in the belief that our nosologies can "carve nature at its joints" (to use a phrase apparently original with Plato). This well-worn idea is based on the idea that illnesses are "natural kinds," entities that exist in nature as independent entities with unchanging characteristics.

Natural kinds have essences, and the task of science is to discover these essences. This is a view of scientific method common among many psychiatrists, as well as others. Zachar notes that we are intuitively predisposed to this view: "Children adopt 'the essentialist bias' with respect to the biological world by the time they are four years old. Four-year-olds are intuitive Aristotelians who assume that organisms have an internal essence. The essence makes organisms be what they are and behave as they do. . . . This bias is . . . intractable, meaning that it is adopted so early and generalizes so easily that evidence against it has limited impact on how people think" (2001, 191).

Daniel Dennett also emphasizes how difficult it can be to give up essentialist tendencies:

> Nothing complicated enough to be really interesting could have an essence. This anti-essentialist theme was recognized by Darwin as a truly revolutionary epistemological or metaphysical accompaniment to his science; we should not be surprised by how hard it is for people to swallow. Ever since Socrates taught Plato (and all the rest of us) how to play the game of asking for necessary and sufficient conditions, we have seen the task of "defining your terms" as a proper preamble to all serious investigations, and this has sent us off on interminable bouts of essence-mongering. We *want* to draw lines; we often *need* to draw lines—just so we can terminate or forestall sterile explorations in a timely fashion. . . . Darwin shows us that evolution does not need what we need; the real world can get along just fine with the *de facto* divergences that emerge over time, leaving lots of emptiness between clusters of actuality. (Dennett 1995, 201–2)

I think this characterization of species can be just as well applied to psychiatric diagnoses.

What did Darwin do? Darwin contradicted essentialism, and he asserted that the nature of species depends on many different characteristics, which change over time. The influence of the environment in selecting out individuals with particularly useful characteristics is what produces the constellation of characteristics we see in a species. But this constellation is ever changing.

Later biologists, such as Ernst Mayr (1991), introduced population thinking into the concept of species, as mentioned above. A species is a population of ever-changing individuals. Although very dissimilar species will have major differences between them, it may prove very difficult to distinguish one species from another that is very similar to it, especially since minor differences between them may be undergoing change on a gradual basis.

Zachar suggests that psychiatric diagnoses are also such entities; they are collections of characteristics that overlap with similar collections but are dissimilar from some other very different collections. Thus, they have value in terms of differentiating unlike conditions, but they are not clean-cut and easily separable from all other conditions. Sometimes observers assume that the lack of clean separability among psychiatric diagnoses reflects the underlying inaccuracy of the current psychiatric diagnostic system (the DSM system). However, it may be that the diagnostic system simply reflects the reality of psychiatric illnesses, just as evolutionary theory reflects the reality of biological species.

Sometimes those with essentialist leanings hold onto them tightly because of a misconception: they fear that if they give up the concept of natural kinds, they will be forced to accept "artificial kinds," and then they will have to accept that psychiatric diagnoses (or other conditions) are not real. In other words, are the only two choices essentialism or joining the camp of postmodernism and antipsychiatry (like Foucault, Szasz, and others who claim that mental illnesses are myths [Foucault 1994; Szasz 1974])?[4] Indeed, many of the postmodernist criticisms of psychiatry consist of a legitimate critique of essentialism. But Darwin long before them made the same critique in relation to biology, without in the least giving up the concept that animal species are real entities. We can hold that psychiatric illnesses are real entities, while at the same time holding that their characteristics are not understandable in terms of essences but rather in terms of populations of changing features. To some extent, by rejecting essentialism we are saying that as human beings we can only know things from a partial perspective, with a collection of facts that change over time. This is the pluralist point. But in terms of what really exists (ontology), we are not thereby committed to saying that since we cannot know the essences of things, those things do not exist. Even if the whole concept of essences and accidents is misguided, the world and its contents will continue to go on existing.

5.

Thus, Darwin's major contribution to psychiatry, and to philosophy of science in general, is, in my opinion, having fostered a rejection of essentialism. I mentioned that this rejection led to a philosophical movement toward a theory to replace essentialism, a theory mostly born and bred in the United

States and called pragmatism. I have already discussed some of the ideas of Charles Sanders Peirce and William James, the first founders of pragmatism. I will just point out here that taking a pragmatic view of truth and science provides one a perspective that can be helpful in the post-essentialist assessment of psychiatry. I have contrasted Peirce and Popper and their definitions of science; many contemporary dogmatisms stem from essentialism and an unthinking acceptance of Popper's views. In the course of this book, I will often turn to Peirce, and I partly do so because I will be presuming a rejection of essentialism and thus a need for alternative perspectives.

One need not be a pragmatist to reject essentialism; Darwin certainly had no such overt philosophies. Yet, some of the concepts of pragmatism seem useful to me as I try to conceptualize what we do in psychiatry. In chapters 10–13, I discuss psychiatric nosology, and the role of ideal types I expound there has some similarities to pragmatic notions of truth.

Thus, much of what follows can be seen to be influenced by pragmatism, which is partly justified, in my opinion, by taking Darwin's contribution to science seriously and thus rejecting essentialism. But in referring to pragmatism in this book, I am not referring simply to the pragmatic theory of truth, that what is true is what is useful. This is one definition, advanced by James and easily criticized by many. Pragmatic approaches to philosophy also entail the concept that it is very difficult to know the truth, and thus our knowledge of the truth is always an approximation, based on inductive empirical experience and a consensus among inquirers, as advanced by Peirce. Further, pragmatism entails pluralism; since we cannot know the truth easily from one avenue of knowledge, we must be open to others. The whole pluralistic perspective on psychiatry is very consistent with a general pragmatic philosophy, since no simple revelation of truth from only one perspective is allowed by pragmatism. Pragmatism can also be used to support eclectic models of psychiatry, as Adolf Meyer did, but in that case the eclectics are breaking James's fundamental rule of philosophy: they have given up on trying to engage in an "unusually stubborn effort to think clearly" about their methods. This is the eclectic error, which keeps rearing its head wherever we go. One can accept multiple methods and perspectives without giving them all equal validity. Eclectics who seek to claim pragmatism have not understood Peirce's essay "The Fixation of Belief." They are not scientific but rather vacillate between their own solipsistic wishes, the authority of others, and various systems of reason that happen to appeal to them. Scientific method, understood in the philosophy of pragmatism, is much more rigorous than eclectics allow, and in fact, I argue, it entails an explicit rejection of eclecticism. If we are to take James and Peirce seriously in psychiatry, we have to reject the biopsychosocial model. I suggest that pluralism would be the most supportable other approach to psychiatry (though integrationism also remains an option; see chapters 23 and 24). Indeed, William James is probably the one person who most expounded both pragmatism and pluralism in equal degrees as a way of thinking about ourselves and the world around us. It is in these senses, not simply on the criterion of utility, that I support pragmatism.

6.

Besides examining what psychiatric reality is (philosophy of mind, ontology) and how we know about it (epistemology), we are left with the question of how we are to value it (ethics). What does it mean to us, as human beings? This brings us to the ethical aspects of psychiatry.

CHAPTER 8

What We Value

The Ethics of Psychiatry

> With all my devotion to the Union and the feeling of loyalty and duty of
> an American citizen, I have not been able to make up my mind to raise
> my hand against my relatives, my children, my home. . . . I know you
> will blame me; but you must think as kindly of me as you can, and be-
> lieve that I have endeavored to do what I thought right.
>
> —ROBERT E. LEE, TO HIS SISTER

1.

In the psychoanalytic heyday, ethical discussions about psychiatry were
rare. Freud insisted that he was simply engaging in medical science and that
medicine was value-free. The only value, if any, for physicians was the general
goal of preserving life and ridding people of disease.

Patients in psychoanalytic psychotherapy generally were not at risk of losing their lives, however, as long as they were not suicidal. Psychoanalysts
sought instead to improve the way patients lived their lives, psychologically
rather than in the physical sense that applied to other medical disciplines. Yet,
as they went through years of psychoanalysis, did analysts and their patients
have a sense of why certain ways of living life were better than others? Most of
these patients were not diagnosable with diseases; indeed psychoanalysts generally eschewed the whole concept of making psychiatric diagnoses. They saw
the human lot as neurosis, and they saw themselves as seeking to ameliorate the
general neurosis of mankind. But how? And why in the specific way they did?

What did Freud say about the purpose of psychoanalysis? He did not say
much, in fact, presumably because he assumed it was clear that neurotic patients suffered and he was easing their suffering. But he did make a famous
brief statement that lived on to become a mantra that I would suggest makes
up the core of the ethics of psychoanalysis: He said that the goal of psycho-

analysis was to allow a person to engage in the chief tasks of life: to work and to love *(arbeiten und lieben)*.[1] What does this mean?

If working is seen as a task of life, one must assume that Freud had in mind freely chosen self-fulfilling labor, not just any kind of work. Surely he did not mean that the back-breaking labor of a factory worker with low wages and no benefits should qualify as a goal of psychotherapy. One must assume he meant work that one enjoys doing. Love also clearly is based on pleasure, with an erotic component presumably and, in our culture, certain accoutrements like family and children.

A Marxist might object, of course, that work is alienated in capitalist society and can never be completely pleasurable. But we might allow Freud a margin of error on that idea if we assume that some form of reasonably pleasurable, unalienated work is possible for many people in capitalist society. The conception of love also seems fraught with bourgeois overtones: marriage, family, monogamy—these all seem assumed in the orthodox Freudian notion of love. Although Freud himself may be exonerated from expecting too much interpretation of what was after all just one pithy statement, his orthodox followers seem to have encumbered it with middle-class overtones of the most restrictive kind. Over the middle decades of the last century, it was almost assumed that the effective outcome of an orthodox psychoanalysis would involve conventional success in one's employment and steps toward a typical monogamous love relationship, preferably in the institution of marriage. Some psychoanalysts no doubt were more liberal, as Freud himself was, but I am referring to the general trend of the profession as a whole. As a result, there existed a subtle but powerful directionality to the work of the psychoanalyst: the patient was sent in a certain direction, toward conventional notions of work and love, that betrayed an ethical value judgment on the part of the analyst.

I do not intend to argue that work and love are unworthy values, although I do believe that in their most conventional forms they contain many cultural and political assumptions. I wish to point out that psychoanalysis, as it has been practiced in the United States at least for most of the past century, was suffused with ethical assumptions, while it pretended not to be. Psychoanalysts, following Freud, assumed that the work of analysis was objective and would lead simply to freer expression of the patient's repressed psyche.

If orthodox psychoanalysis has a hidden ethical agenda, does psychiatry as a whole have one also? What of biological psychiatry, the mainstream medical model? Does it have an implicit set of values that it imposes on patients?

2.

Most psychiatrists, and most physicians, would argue that conventional medicine has minimal or no ethical assumptions, maybe simply the value of health and the disvalue of suffering. These basic values might be reflected in a "reverence for life" (as Albert Schweitzer [1969] put it) and certain rules, such as "first, do no harm" and in some cases injunctions against abortion. Scholars engaged in philosophy of medicine might argue for much more than this. Medicine, like any human activity, implies constant value judgments, frequently falling along the traditional ethical fault lines described by philosophers for centuries. For our purposes, it is enough to emphasize that even biological psychiatry shares these constant ethical judgments.

William Fulford is a psychiatrist and philosopher who has carefully addressed this subject as it relates to psychiatry (1989). I will limit my comments to his work, since it is perhaps the most systematic effort on this topic in current psychiatry, though there is a much larger literature on the topic in medicine in general, and others have written about it in psychiatry (Sadler 2002; Sadler, Wiggins, and Schwartz 1994). I will also limit this discussion somewhat because I return to it in the chapter on the nature of mental illness (chapter 10).

What matters here is the question of whether there is an ethical or evaluative component to the standard medical approach in psychiatry, just as there is in psychotherapeutic methods like psychoanalysis. Fulford argues that this is the case.

Fulford starts with the criticisms of Thomas Szasz that mental illnesses are not diseases because mental illnesses contain an ethical or evaluative component that is missing from "physical" illnesses in other branches of medicine (Szasz 1974). For example, having a broken leg seems like a brute fact, which has no ethical aspects and is amenable to the strictly scientific (non–value based) approaches of standard medicine (diagnosis, treatment). However, if someone is judged to be experiencing a delusion, and that person is then labeled with the diagnosis of schizophrenia and treated with antipsychotic medication by a biologically oriented psychiatrist, some value judgments have been made. It has been judged that the delusion is wrong somehow and that the person is unable to function psychologically in certain ways. Those ways in which the person is deemed to be psychologically impaired or to have false beliefs involve some value judgments, according to this view. In assessing the many value judgments inherent in such psychiatric diagnosis and treatment, and in contrasting them with physical illness, Szasz argues that mental illnesses are not diseases and should not be treated as medical conditions. Rather, they are a matter of ethical value judgments, much like crime, and belong to the sphere of legal, social, and political decisions. Opponents of Szasz, such as the psychiatrist R. E. Kendell (1989), emphasize the similarities of major mental illnesses to other physical illnesses, which they argue will become more obvious with more knowledge about the brain basis of mental illness. Kendell and others argue that mental illnesses are simple facts, like other physical illnesses, rather than a matter of value judgments.

Fulford grants Szasz's argument but extends it to physical illnesses also. Fulford is influenced by contemporary discussions in philosophy regarding two major problems that touch on this controversy: the *fact-value* distinction, and the *is-ought* dilemma.

The fact-value distinction refers to the assumption that facts and values are separable. In common language, we often assume that there are such things as facts, which have no relation to how we value them, and there are values, which are not necessarily related to any facts in the external world. Historically, moral philosophy has accepted this fact-value distinction. For instance, Kant and Mill in different ways both sought to develop rational theories of ethics that did not rely on actual facts of human history, psychology, or biology. (There is a notable exception: Aristotle's virtue theory, described later in this chapter.) These classical moral philosophers sought to develop a "normative" ethics, one that was based on reason, did not require empirical proof, and was not liable to empirical refutation. Facts are different from values. Szasz could then argue that physical illnesses are based on facts and mental conditions on values. One belonged to medicine and biology, the other to the law and society. But many modern philosophers argue that the fact-value distinction is not valid. Their main argument is that all facts have some evaluative component, however small. This is to some extent an epistemological point, which we discussed earlier in reference to Peirce and Jaspers. Any fact is observed through some method; some theory or hypothesis is required to observe any fact. Since any theory, method, or hypothesis is chosen for a specific reason by a living human being, some level of evaluative judgment is involved. If one is extremist about this point, as are postmodernists, one could claim to refute all reliable scientific knowledge. Peirce showed that one did not need to go to this extreme.

The second controversy is the is-ought dilemma. This discussion goes back to David Hume, who argued that *ought* does not follow from *is*. In other words, one could not base a normative ethical statement on a fact. For example, one could not argue that the Soviet Union was an excellent political system in 1975 based on the simple brute fact that it existed. Hume asserted that, although facts could be involved, any ethical statement at some level did not rest on facts but only rested on ethical grounds held for some other reasons.

Hence, contemporary philosophers have weakened the notion that facts exist independent of values, and, influenced by Hume, many current philosophers emphasize that ethical viewpoints are independent and can never be reduced to nonevaluative facts.

Fulford accepts that facts are also evaluative, thus undercutting Szasz's critique of mental illness as being particularly inferior to physical illnesses. But physical illnesses would then seem to be compromised. Fulford argues that any physical illness, like a mental illness, involves an initial value judgment, the recognition by a person that some ability to do something is impaired. This is not simply a functional impairment, viewed externally; Fulford calls it an "action failure," viewed internally from the person's subjective perspective. Even if a person does not experience any symptoms initially, and the physician merely recognizes some abnormal laboratory value that portends later illness, the judgment of the physician is based on the likely action failures that the patient will experience in the future.

Fulford does not feel that allowing evaluative elements a place in mental and physical illness invalidates disease concepts. I agree and will expand on this issue in chapter 10. For our purposes here, the main point is that not only biologically oriented psychiatry but all of medicine has an ethical component that is central to its practice. Biological psychiatry cannot dispense with a discussion of ethics.

3.

What are the main kinds of ethical standpoints that bear on psychiatry? Philosophers have identified two basic approaches: utilitarianism and deontology.[2] Utilitarianism, often identified with the British philosopher John Stuart Mill, is the ethical philosophy of choice of many of us in modern society; it is a familiar approach that has developed along with the growth of democratic institutions. According to this theory, an act is right or wrong based on its consequences. If its overall consequences are good, then the act is good, and vice versa. The utility of the act determines its ethical value.

Mill's version of utilitarianism focused on those acts which produced the greatest happiness of the greatest number of persons. In this sense, Mill's theory is hedonistic; it is also quantitative and more focused on the overall outcome of acts than on the consequences to the individual who acts. Most of us who act in a utilitarian manner tend to take an instinctively individualistic approach, however. Each time you are faced with a decision and you ask yourself what act would result in the most happiness for me, you are making a utilitarian ethical judgment.

The utilitarian approach has been criticized on many grounds. The purely individualistic approach seems too egoistic. Often, acts that make me happy make others miserable. This is a cold-hearted philosophy (which Mill realized, and as a result he turned to focus on the happiness of the greatest number). There are those who claim that if everyone pursues his own happiness, the aggregate end result will be the greatest happiness for the greatest number. This is, in a way, an ethical counterpart of Adam Smith's "invisible hand" theory in economics. Just as with Smith, however, this approach assumes quite an optimistic attitude toward the results of the ethical free-for-all implied. Mill's focus on the overall greatest good has also been subject to criticism, for it seems to allow all sorts of individual acts of pain and apparent injustice, in the name of a greater good. We rightly condemn those politicians and generals who sacrificed soldiers and civilians in pursuit of an "ends justifies the means" approach to life. At its extremes, this was the defense of such men as Lenin, Trotsky, Stalin, and Hitler.

Another major problem with strict utilitarianism is that it requires a level of certainty about the consequences of one's actions that is frequently impractical. Most often, the possible consequences of an action are numerous, and one cannot easily foretell what might happen. This is a common cause of indecision among modern individuals. We are all so used to thinking in terms of consequences—utilitarianism has seeped into our bones—that we wonder and wonder about whether to do something (Should I marry? Should I take this job? Should I move?), conjuring up unpredictable and vague probable outcomes. Utilitarianism suffers from the fact that we cannot know the future, at least not well enough to base all of our major ethical life decisions on this approach.

A final criticism that can be made of utilitarianism is that it ignores motivations and focuses on actions. This may seem laudable in some senses; although we cannot often know a person's motivations, her actions are empirically observable. But it has the unfortunate consequence that we need to accept as ethical actions that produce good results, even if they grow out of unethical intentions. For instance, Mussolini made the trains run on time; suppose he did this so that he could strengthen his grip on public opinion in Italy in order to entrench fascism further. One would have to grant that Mussolini was an ethical man, in the absence of other data, if all we knew were those facts. Conversely, someone may have good intentions and mistakenly produce unpleasant consequences, and we would have to morally condemn this person. Suppose a doctor diagnoses a potentially fatal appendicitis and operates. During the operation, the patient has an allergic reaction to the anesthetic, which no one could have predicted, and does not survive. We would have to morally condemn the doctor. This certainly runs counter to most of our ethical intuitions.

4.

For these reasons, utilitarianism is not as straightforward and helpful as it might seem at first glance. Again, living in a modern democratic society, we are predisposed to it, but as a general ethical theory, it has many limitations.

Its main opponent in ethical theory is called deontology. Deontology, which is less familiar these days than it may have been to our forefathers, is associated in philosophy with Kant. Deontology refers to a system of ethics based on duties. An act is good or bad if it is consistent or inconsistent with a sense of duty that one possesses.

The system of duties has an outside source: this has traditionally been religious, but it could also be based on another ideology (nationalism), or on other traditions (aristocracy). Traditional duties that often are referred to include fidelity (keeping promises), justice (treating others as one would treat oneself), beneficence (helping others), and non-maleficence (not hurting others). The latter two duties are enshrined in the medical maxims of Hippocrates. When faced with a sick patient, a doctor is not supposed to calculate whether his actions will result in the greatest happiness of the greatest number of people, or even in the happiness of the patient himself. The doctor is simply supposed to follow the duties of helping the patient and not harming him. A great example of a list of duties would be Jesus' Sermon on the Mount. A sense of duty might be felt by force of tradition or family instruction as well.

Often, a deontological approach seems unreasonable on utilitarian grounds. When General Robert E. Lee was offered command of the Union armies in

1861 at the outbreak of the American Civil War, a sober estimation of the likelihood of the outcome of that conflict might have led him to make a utilitarian judgment that he should accept the post. However, he refused and took a position in the Confederate government, which his native state of Virginia had joined, because he had a sense of duty to his state. He was not happy about it, and he never gave any explanation other than his sense of duty.

This has indeed caused some confusion for historians. Lee apparently opposed slavery, yet he fought for a government that upheld it. A utilitarian judgment might have been that since slavery is wrong and produces unhappiness, Lee should join the side that fights against it. Again, in that era, it seemed natural for Lee, raised with an aristocratic sense of duties, to simply choose the most important duty that he sensed and follow it above all others. Duties might conflict, the duty to his state and his duty to help slaves, for instance, but a hierarchy of duties requires that priority be given to those that are felt to be the most important. Who establishes this hierarchy is problematic at times, however. Should his duty to free slaves have been higher than his duty to his state? Today it would be, but in 1861 it was not. Thus, duties can be culturally bound, and deontology has been criticized for failing to provide universal ethical principles.

Kant felt he had described a few duties that had universal relevance, because they could be derived from reason alone, rather than religion or tradition. This was his categorical imperative: "Act only on that maxim whereby you can at the same time will that it should become a universal law," which translates into always treating others as ends in themselves rather than as means. Kant emphasized that this duty-based approach should hold, irrespective of one's inclinations. One might be unhappy about it, but one had to follow one's duties. Ultimately, all duties derived from the categorical imperative, which was the one ethical law that applied to everyone.

Although it is logically coherent, Kant's approach has seemed quite austere to many. Human happiness is relatively unaccounted for in it. Yet it is worthwhile to note that in general the deontological approach has many merits, a fact that is often lost in modern democratic society. Utilitarianism has meshed well with democratic intuitions, although, like fascism, it contains the seed of a tyrannical mind-set within it. By contrast, deontological ethics are taught to us in houses of worship and religious education programs and in the course of learning to act on certain virtues of character; yet deontological ethics too carry the seed of ideological bias, based on which duties are prioritized over others.

5.

In philosophy, therefore, the contrast between utilitarian and deontological ethics has been an unending one. There is a third approach, older than either of these two, which has recently experienced a renaissance: virtue theory. Virtue theory is usually traced to Aristotle, who provided its outlines centuries before Christ. Basically, it involves the recognition of a series of virtues, which are acquisitions of one's character in the course of one's upbringing and life experiences. The virtues are such things as courage, truthfulness, frugality, generosity, industry. They are unrelated to a reckoning of the consequences of an act, unlike utilitarianism.

Thus, a soldier in battle does not make a calculation of the risks and benefits of engaging in battle before deciding to fight or run: He shows courage in all situations; in some he will be put in danger and in others he will not. In the long run, the consequences would be best if he always demonstrated courage, rather than if he calculated those consequences in each case before acting. Virtue theory also differs from deontology in that it is not based on a simple reliance on duty. It is not related to a series of admonitions, whether religious or otherwise. Rather, it is a learned way of living; it is part of one's personality, learned but intuitive. It is something that is automatic, after it is practiced, not a matter of referring to rules or external duties. A simple analogy would be riding a bicycle, which is like a learned virtue, rather than reference to a book of rules, which is like the admonitions of deontology. One learns how to ride a bicycle initially by learning certain rules, then by practice one no longer needs to recall as many rules explicitly, and eventually riding a bicycle becomes a habit. Aristotle saw virtues as habits of this kind.

Aristotle further defined how one recognizes a virtue. Take the courageous soldier again: he should not engage in reckless folly, nor should he show cowardice. The virtue of courage is the mean between these two extremes. Aristotle's famed Golden Mean was actually a definition of virtue.

Some have mistaken the Golden Mean to encourage moderation in all things. It is not, in fact, so simple. Aristotle repeatedly emphasized that the virtues were exercises in "practical reason," by which he meant that they are learned in practice, by example, not by verbal discussion. Thus, one cannot define any specific virtue in clear terms verbally in such a way that the definition applies for everyone. Each individual needs to learn how to recognize a virtue in real, practical situations. And the Golden Mean refers to recognizing when to apply which virtues, in what circumstances, in what manner.

In the *Nicomachean Ethics,* Aristotle held that the virtues could be inculcated in children and young adults and practiced throughout adulthood and ultimately would lead to an ethical life. He emphasized that the virtues were learned and had to be practiced; they were not innate or discovered by contemplation. One learned the virtues in practice, by example, not in theory or by words. This Aristotelian theory of ethics was superseded in the West by the more deontological aspects of Christian ethics, although the virtues were incorporated into Catholic thinking to some extent in the Middle Ages (e.g., charity, chastity). Liberal Protestant theology also gave some rebirth to virtue theory in the Enlightenment era; such was the predisposition of the American deists, like Benjamin Franklin and Thomas Jefferson. In fact, Franklin's *Autobiography* (1996) is almost a classic text of virtue theory–oriented reasoning.[3]

In the nineteenth century, Kantian deontology, followed by Mill's utilitarianism, largely submerged the virtue theory tradition again. After the world wars of the twentieth century, however, utilitarianism fell into disrepute in some circles, since fascism and communism both had been defended by many on utilitarian grounds: war and dictatorship were the means to a better future society. Deontology also seemed limited by its religious ties, as well as its potential association with similar totalitarian ideologies. For instance, members of the German SS sought to defend themselves on grounds that they were driven by a sense of duty to their organization. Virtue theory reemerged as an attractive alternative. It shared with deontology an opposition to the utilitarian focus on consequences. It shared with utilitarianism a rational basis free from religious principles. Probably the philosopher most associated with modern virtue theory is Alasdair MacIntyre (1984), who explicitly connects ideas from Aristotle and from Marx in his ethics.[4]

6.

I think virtue theory has many attractions as an ethical underpinning for psychiatry. It is based on virtues understood as part of human personality and learned in the course of human development, under the influence of parents and the larger culture. This is exactly the setting that psychiatrists and psychologists have long examined. Freud, for instance, defined the superego, or the ego-ideal, as just this kind of ethical mechanism derived from one's family and society. Thus, virtue theory meshes with the thinking and research of developmental psychology in general and psychoanalysis in particular.

I believe that psychotherapists should help their patients understand what ethical system they follow: whether utilitarianism, deontology, or virtue theory. Based on their personal and religious backgrounds, patients might prefer a particular approach. I think that careful, consistent, and conscious application of one of the ethical theories, within the limits of reason and with a spirit of tolerance, makes for a happier life. I believe that the greatest portion of unhappiness and indecision among patients in psychotherapy comes from the confused, erratic use of different ethical methods. In general, virtue theory, in my opinion, has fewer limitations than the other approaches and provides a particularly helpful way of conceptualizing how we should live our lives.

7.

Ultimately, I believe the goal of psychotherapy in particular, and all psychiatric treatment in general, should be the *liberation* of the individual. But here we run into the paradox of making someone free. You cannot *force* someone to be free. Thus, the clinician must always defer to the patient's agency, and conversely, no patient can be liberated without having the ability to be liberated herself, that is, without wanting freedom. And there are some people who do not want to be free. For psychiatry, those individuals are major problems. For instance, many persons with serious psychosis or mania refuse to recognize their illness, have poor insight, and never are able to free themselves from the imperatives of their illnesses. It is almost impossible to help them. Nonetheless, the psychiatrist must try, if possible, with the help of the law and society in general, if necessary, against the patient's expressed wish.

But this should be the exception rather than the rule, especially with less severe psychiatric conditions. Most patients want to be free of their psychological problems. Freeing them is the ultimate goal of treatment. Leston Havens has captured this aspect of psychotherapy, as has Karl Jaspers.[5]

Recognition by patients of the ethical methods that most liberate them to act with their free will is the ethical goal of psychiatric treatment. By free will I mean that they choose consciously the actions that are most in accord with their wishes, values, and purposes in life, and that they are free to choose otherwise if they wish. All of this, of course, as with anything in human life, must be within the limits of the law and general norms of morality (e.g., the patient may not choose to commit murder). This latter constraint should not seem excessive: all freedom comes with some measure of responsibility.

8.

While Aristotelian virtue theory seems to have many advantages as an ethic for psychiatry, later Hellenistic philosophies (Stoicism, Epicureanism) and alternative Eastern traditions (Hinduism, Sufism) can lay claim to providing other, and possibly better, approaches. I now turn to them.

CHAPTER 9

Desire and Self

Hellenistic and Eastern Approaches

> Empty is that philosopher's argument by which no human suffering is
> therapeutically treated. For just as there is no use in a medical art that
> does not cast out the sickness of bodies, so too there is no use in philoso-
> phy, unless it casts out the suffering of the soul. —EPICURUS

> Lamps are many; light is one. —RUMI

1.

In psychiatric training, as one learns to do psychotherapy, one soon realizes
that there is an ethical component to psychotherapy. The therapist is inti-
mately involved with trying to understand what the patient values, what the
patient does in life, and why he does it; and what might be different. Freud denied that psychoanalysis was value-laden or that the work of his brand of psychotherapy involved ethics or value judgments. Yet, the new psychotherapist
is faced with the clear impression that such is not the case. The question is,
then, What is the ethical basis of psychotherapy?

Besides traditional Hippocratic ethics on the one hand and standard moral
philosophy (utilitarianism versus deontology) on the other, there is a system
of ethics that has even more direct implications for the ethics of psychotherapy: Hellenistic ethics.

2.

The schools of Hellenistic philosophy are quite unusual from the modern
perspective. Today, philosophy often involves logic, attempts to prove arguments, and abstract systems of thought. Philosophy rarely has a therapeutic

orientation. It is a fascinating historical fact that there was a time (the Hellenistic period) when philosophy was largely identified with ethics and seen to have an important role in the lives of human beings, a role that was analogous to medicine's role. The Hellenistic schools saw philosophy as a field similar to medicine, where philosophers healed the soul as physicians healed the body. The explicit goal of philosophy for these schools was to promote human flourishing, *eudaemonia*.

The first matter that one comes up against in considering the relevance of Hellenistic philosophy to psychotherapy is the issue of whether rational argument is useful in psychotherapy. The Freudian school would likely argue not; it might say that the patient ends up in therapy because rational argument has been ineffective in influencing her feelings or behavior. Otherwise, the advice of friends and family would have been sufficient. Besides, psychoanalytic theory would argue that the basis for much psychopathology is unconscious, instinctive, and emotional and thus not influenced by rational discussion. Even if one accepts this psychoanalytic notion, allowing for the important influence of emotional factors in psychotherapy, one is still faced with the problem that Freud identified as *resistance*, the difficulty of effecting real emotional change in a person's life.

The Hellenistic philosophers addressed this issue head-on. In fact, Aristotle had previously laid out the same objection: to read discussions of ethics did not make one a more ethical person. The Hellenistic philosophers argued that reason influenced one's emotions and that emotions were affected by true or false cognitive judgments. These days, this discussion would be supported by cognitive-behavioral theory and the empirically demonstrable effectiveness of cognitive-behavioral psychotherapy in many psychiatric conditions. Furthermore, research in neuroscience tends to blur the traditional distinction between reason and emotion. For instance, the frontal lobes are a part of the neocortex (which is generally associated with rational cognitive faculties) but have many connections to the limbic cortex (which is generally associated with emotional function). Thus, from the empirical standpoint, whether of clinical psychiatry or of neuroscience, a sharp distinction between reason and emotion does not exist. Among some philosophers as well, the view that reason and emotion are entirely separate realms has lost credence.

3.

As a result, the assumption, held by many psychiatrists, that reason has little influence on emotional conditions is less obvious than it may at first seem. If reason has a connection to emotion, then philosophy may have a role in psychotherapy. This is exactly what the Hellenistic philosophers supposed.

The two main schools of Hellenistic philosophy were the Epicureans and the Stoics.[1] I will focus on the school of Epicurus, since its potential links to current psychiatric theories are numerous.

Epicurus, who was apparently a charismatic man, led a community of students in his "Garden" school of philosophy. He held a number of views with direct relevance to psychiatry. For instance, Epicurus believed that his approach to life, based on his maxims, could not exert a sufficient influence upon the soul without memorization. Because he felt that merely hearing his views, the simple influence of reason, was insufficient, he admonished his students to memorize his maxims so that they became part of their mind-sets. The philosopher Martha Nussbaum (1994) has suggested that Epicurus hit on the required influence of unconscious ideas on one's way of living, beyond simple conscious rational explanation.

Epicurus also emphasized that his students should follow his example as their leader and encouraged strong emotional attachments to himself, in a manner quite different from that of previous philosophers. Epicurus encouraged such emotional connection again as a means of influencing his students beyond pure abstract reasoning. Nussbaum suggests that this method has similarities to what Freud later called transference, that is, the emotional attachment between therapist and patient that is necessary for deep effects of therapeutic interpretations on the patient's psyche.

Epicurus encouraged his students to approach philosophy by providing narratives of their lives. He did not see philosophy as a subject matter laid out in books, but as a way of looking at how one lives, and thus best elucidated by examining a narrative of one's own life. This has similarities to McHugh and Slavney's life story perspective, which they saw as the essential feature of psychotherapies.

4.

Thus, one can see aspects of psychotherapy in Epicurus's ideas. But he went further. Like the Stoics, he provided a different perspective on life that can have utility for psychotherapy. In general, Epicurus held that the secret to eudaemonia was fewer emotional attachments. He taught that we would be happier if we had fewer desires, and if we held those we had less strongly. He especially applied this idea to three major matters: sex, death, and anger.

Unlike orthodox Freudianism, Epicurus opposed marriage in general. He felt that sexual need could be satisfied simply and healthily outside of marriage and that marriage produced numerous attachments and responsibilities inimical to eudaemonia.

A central tenet for him was the absence of fear of death. "Death has no meaning for us" was his central maxim, emphasizing that since we cease to exist when we are dead, there is nothing to fear there. By not fearing death, we cease yearning for immortality and continued attachments to transitory things of the world. Paradoxically, we can then enjoy the things we have, rather than fret about losing them in the future. In this view, Epicurus goes directly against the existentialist approach, which is to see death as the ultimate fact of life, one of which we must be conscious, and the basis of authentic decision-making about what truly matters in life.

Anger, aggression, and war all stem from too many attachments, the Epicureans held. If we had fewer desires, we would show less anger and fight less frequently. We would then solve our problems "with words, not arms" *(Dictus, non armis),* as the Epicurean Lucretius famously wrote. Here too one might contrast the Epicureans with Freud, who saw aggression as innate and unavoidable in humanity. In answer to letters from Albert Einstein regarding the possibilities for pacifism, Freud was extremely pessimistic and held that humans were doomed to war (Einstein and Freud [1933] 1978).

5.

The school of Epicurus contained ideas later commonplace in psychiatry and also took a general approach to life at odds in many ways with the views of schools of psychiatry such as psychoanalysis and existentialism. Psychiatrists today could profitably study some of these Epicurean notions as contrasting tonics to the accepted axioms of current psychotherapy schools.

In general, the notion of fewer emotional attachments, upheld by both the Epicureans and the Stoics, as a source of mental health is a viewpoint not often discussed in contemporary psychotherapy. And perhaps with reason, given that social isolation is associated with many forms of psychopathology! Perhaps there are different senses of attachment upon which one might place value: one sense in which too many attachments would be problematic and another sense in which too few would produce difficulties. I also think that Eastern and Western approaches sometimes differ in the kinds of attachments with which they concern themselves.

6.

Do Eastern ways of thinking also provide an alternative perspective on psychiatry?

This subject is in itself large and, though I must discuss it, I cannot pretend to do full justice to it here. If I could simply allude to aspects of Eastern ways of thinking that have been identified as potentially relevant to psychiatry, I could provide a list like the following: suspicion of reason and science; respect for religion; a sense of spirituality; the absence of a robust concept of the individual self; a focus on the needs of larger society; strong attachment to the extended family, patriarchy, and authority; belief in intuition as a source of knowledge; interest in other worlds before or after life on earth; disinterest in desires such as sexuality and material prosperity; meditation; and yoga.

From this list, the reader will have a sense of the variety of perspectives often identified with Eastern cultures. I will emphasize certain aspects of Islamic philosophy as an example of the kinds of ideas from Eastern cultures that might be relevant for psychiatry.

7.

I will focus on Sufism and Shiite illuminationism as two aspects of Eastern philosophy that may be relevant to better understanding the mind, mental illness, and psychiatry. I am not discussing many other aspects of Islamic philosophy: various Sunni schools, specific theologies, or fundamentalist belief systems. I make these choices deliberately. On the one hand, they are derived from my experience and exposure through my family and cultural background. On the other hand, I am trying to highlight perspectives that are useful in helping us examine and critique the current approaches in psychiatry outlined in the first chapter (dogmatism, eclecticism, pluralism, and integrationism). And also, these perspectives go against the assumptions often made in the West, more so recently, that Islam is by nature fundamentalist and dogmatic. As I will discuss here, Islamic views can also be pluralist, rationalist, and existentialist in ways not unlike many Western perspectives. In fact, some of these Islamic perspectives can be seen as complementary to many Western views and not at all in conflict with them.

Let us begin with Sufism, which will perhaps be the Eastern viewpoint most familiar to Western readers, since it is quite similar to some Buddhist and Hindu views that have entered Western culture in recent years. In fact, Sufism itself is an amalgam of Indian (Buddhist, Hindu), Greek (Neoplatonic), and Islamic influences. It is important to note that one need not be a Muslim to be a Sufi. One can belong to any formal religion; Sufism is considered the underlying meaning of all religions, according to its adherents. Yet it is true that Sufi sects have developed in the Islamic world. And most Sufi circles trace their historical origins to the thought and practice of the great founder of Shiite Islam, Imam Ali. Ali was the son-in-law and first cousin of the prophet Muhammad. He was famous for many skills: as a warrior, a scholar of the Quran, and a political leader (he was the fourth Caliph). But Sufis view him as a spiritual leader, the first person to present Islamic ideas in a mystical manner. He was a uniquely uncategorizable man, a military and political leader who in the middle of battles would give sermons about human desires. (Perhaps the Western figure with the most similar character traits was the Stoic Roman emperor Marcus Aurelius.)

Imam Ali was a spellbinding and poetic Arabic speaker whose sermons and sayings have been collected in a classic text of Shiite Islam called the *Peak of Eloquence* (Nahj-ul-Balagha) (Ali 1984). In that text, one finds many sayings that presage later Sufi perspectives. In a testament to his oldest son, Hasan, after Ali lost one of his final battles, Ali wrote:

> Know with certainty that you cannot achieve your desire and cannot exceed your destined life. You are on the track of those before you. Therefore be humble in seeking and moderate in earning because seeking often leads to deprivation. Every seeker of livelihood does not get it, nor is everyone who is moderate in seeking deprived. Keep yourself away from every low thing even though they may take you to your desired aims, because you will not get any return for your own

respect which you spend. Do not be the slave of others for Allah has made you free. There is no good in good which is achieved through evil and no good in comfort that is achieved through hardship. . . . Know, O my child, that livelihood is of two kinds—a livelihood that you seek and a livelihood that seeks you, which is such that if you do not reach for it, it will come to you. How bad it is to bend down at the time of need and to be harsh in riches. You should have from this world only that with which you can adorn your permanent abode. If you cry over what has gone out of your hands then also cry for what has not at all come to you. (502–4)

This disinterest in desires and attachments is a central feature of Sufism. We also saw that it was a central feature of Epicurean philosophy, and it is well known that Stoic philosophers took a similar view. We will return to the topic of attachments and desires. First, though, I would like to turn to another central feature of Sufi thought, its pluralism. This aspect, which is entirely in keeping with the discussion of pluralism in psychiatry throughout this book, is best exemplified by another parable, the story of the elephant. First propounded by the Persian Sufi poet Jalaluddin Rumi (Jalaluddin Mohammad Balkhi, also known as Mowlavi), the story of the elephant has become a somewhat commonplace story even in the West.

8.

The parable of the elephant in the dark:

Some Hindus have an elephant to show.
No one here has ever seen an elephant.
They bring it at night to a dark room

One by one, we go in the dark and come out
Saying how we experience the animal.

One of us happens to touch the trunk.
"A water-pipe kind of creature."

Another, the ear. "A very strong, always moving
Back and forth, fan-animal."

Another, the leg. "I find it still,
Like a column on a temple."

Another touches the curved back.
"A leather throne."

Another, the cleverest, feels the tusk.
"A rounded sword made of porcelain."
He's proud of his description.

Each of us touches one place
And understands the whole in that way.

The palm and the fingers feeling in the dark are
How the senses explore the reality of the elephant.

If each of us held a candle there,
And if we went in together,
We would see it. (Rumi 1995, 252)[2]

9.

I think it is accurate to state that Karl Jaspers was making the same argument for psychiatry that Rumi was making for Sufism. And indeed Kety's parable, with which I began this book, can be seen as a modern adaptation of Rumi's Sufi fable. The similarities between Rumi's parable and many of the discussions in previous chapters are in fact quite striking. The story is straightforwardly pluralistic. There are multiple methods, each with their own limits and weaknesses. Further, the philosophers are not humble; they become dogmatic with each of their methods. If they all went together with the *best* method (a candle), they could see the elephant. This is reminiscent of Peirce's approximation to reality. Absolute knowledge is beyond the natural realm and belongs to the divine, if anywhere.

In another poem on desire, Rumi highlights how hard this process is:

Show me your face
The garden of roses is what I desire
Open your lips
Sweet sugar is what I desire
O sun of beauty, Come forth from the clouds
Your radiant face is what I desire
"Leave me, go!" you say in anger
Just that "Leave me, go!" is what I desire

This circle of bread and water is a disloyal torrent

I am a fish, a whale, the sea is what I desire

Like Jacob, I wail and flail about

The vision of young Joseph is what I desire

Without you, the city is my prison

The exile of mountain and desert is what I desire

Yesterday, the Shaikh took a lantern around the city

Saying, "Beast and devil tire me, Humanity is what I desire"

"He is not to be found," they said. "We have searched."

"That which is not to be found," he answered,

"That is what I desire." (sec. 31, Divani Shams)[3]

10.

The relevance of Sufism to psychiatry has been extensively discussed by the psychiatrist Mohammad Shafii (1998). Shafii emphasizes the release of desires and the dropping of attachments as the core of the Sufi approach. Rumi and other poets, such as Hafiz and Saadi, provide numerous parables to exemplify this approach, in addition to the one I quoted above. Shafii provides some detail on what Sufis call the Path, the process by which one moves toward the final stage of Fana, or ultimate loss of attachments, which Shafii calls "freedom from the self." The six stages before Fana consist of Repentance, Abstinence, Renunciation, Poverty, Patience, and Reliance on God. Contentment is the final stage, that of Fana, or freedom from the self. It can be seen that the Sufis' method does not consist of simply a philosophy of exhortation toward contentment, but rather a practice of habits and character that leads in experience through spiritual stages to the final goal of Contentment. In this sense, the Sufi Path is similar to the approach of Aristotle's virtue theory and also has similarities to the Epicurean approach to philosophy.

In his book, Shafii emphasizes similarities and differences between psychoanalytic theory and Sufism, but he downplays the similarities between Sufism and existentialism. I believe that the links between Western existentialism and Sufism (as well as illuminationism, discussed below) are the strongest and most interesting. It is important to note that there are different varieties in both approaches. Shafii tends to view Sufism from the theistic angle (like Ghazali), and he views existentialism from its more atheist sources (like Sartre). Yet there are also Sufi-oriented thinkers who are not particularly theistic (like Omar Khayyam), and of course existentialists who are theistic (like Jaspers). What the two approaches (Sufism and existentialism) share in common is a recognition of the need to view human life from the perspective of an individual's existence, a distrust of excessive reliance on reason, a disinterest in rational or theological theories, a sharp recognition of the limits of human existence and the reality of death, and a focus on the present rather than the future or the past. Theistic Sufis tend to also emphasize the ultimate divine reality, whereas nontheistic Sufis emphasize the cyclic nature of existence and the ultimate reality of Nature. Sufi sects differ from existentialism in recommending participation in a circle of fellow Sufis and engaging in a defined Path toward enlightenment, whereas existentialists tend to view the path to authenticity as one that needs to be taken individually by each person. Many Sufis also tend to emphasize the ultimate goal of contentment through loss of attachments, while many existentialists emphasize the need to become focused on and content with present attachments. Many Sufis also see the self as something to be transcended, while many existentialists view the self as something to be actualized authentically.

There are enough similarities and differences here to suggest a creative dialogue between these different approaches to philosophy, as well as these different approaches to understanding human behavior, which is relevant to psychiatry. Much depends on whether the Sufi or the existentialist is approaching his respective philosophy from a theistic or from a nontheistic perspective. It seems to me that the decision whether to believe in divinity comes from outside of these philosophies; as William James argued, such religious belief comes from one's own makeup. But the kind of Sufism or existentialism that one encounters is highly influenced by whether one approaches those viewpoints from theistic assumptions or not. For psychiatry, as a practical discipline, it would seem to me that a nontheistic approach to Sufism could have some utility and could link up with a nontheistic approach to existential methods. Taking such an approach, one would not focus on Sufi views regarding divine Reality, or the stages of the Path, or the specific sects and their methods. Rather, one would focus on Sufi views regarding the ill effects of many desires and attachments on human existence, the limits of life, the importance of pluralism, and the need for being present-centered.

11.

In addition to Sufism, two other trends in Islamic philosophy may have relevance for Western culture, and specifically for psychiatry. The first trend is not distinctively Eastern, but it is worth mentioning since some Westerners assume its absence in the East, and that is the rational-empiricist approach to knowledge. The second trend, which is more Eastern, and which I shall discuss more fully here, is the intuitionist (or illuminationist) approach to knowledge. The history of Islamic philosophy is mainly a back-and-forth struggle between these two approaches, with the ultimate defeat of the rational-empiricist approach—not in the battlefield of ideas but rather owing to political repression.

Islamic philosophy was born in Arabic-speaking lands soon after the expansion of Islam as a religion and a political force into areas that had been influenced by Hellenic culture. The Muslims discovered the philosophical works of the Greeks, especially Aristotle, when those works had lain fallow for centuries after the declining days of Roman rule. Aristotle became the most famous teacher of philosophy of the age, and great Islamic thinkers sprouted up by meditating upon his words. Most of the early Islamic philosophers, taken together, began to create what came to be known as the school of Knowledge (Hikmat).[4] They included Farabi, Avicenna, Kindi, and others; in general, they expounded a largely rationalist perspective of philosophy that had much in common with later Western rationalists, such as Descartes, Kant, and Leibniz. They also possessed an empiricist streak, however, which was taken up in the ninth century A.D. by their more overtly empiricist students, called the Mutazilah, whose ideas would not have been foreign to later empiricists such as Locke and Hume. But they drew the ire of some of the religious authorities, who became uncomfortable with the theological implications of empiricism and condemned the rationalists and empiricists altogether. As a result, the initial period of excitement in Islamic philosophy ended after two centuries. Although the nascent empiricist movement was dealt a severe blow, Islamic philosophy did not disappear entirely. These early giants of Islamic philosophy—for example, Avicenna in his Quranic commentaries—also advanced some Neoplatonic ideas that would later inspire others to derive illuminationist theories from them. After a century or two of quiet, philosophical thinking gradually reemerged on the fringes of Islamic civilization. Much of the Aristotelian rationalist heritage migrated West to the new frontier of Islamic civilization in Spain, with thinkers such as the eleventh-century Averroes. To the

East, in Iran, it evolved into the more Platonist illuminationist tradition, led by Suhrawardi and Ibn al-Arabi in the twelfth century and Sadr al-Din Shirazi (also known as Mulla Sadra) in the sixteenth century. This last group built upon the Platonic tradition of knowledge by "intellectual vision" of divine forms and held that all reality was analogous to a divine light and knowledge consisted of being illuminated by the ontological reality of light. In Spain, as is well known, Islamic philosophy passed Greek rationalism along to European thinkers like Aquinas and Bacon in the fourteenth century. In Iran, the illuminationist tradition continues to the present day, alongside Shiite theology.

12.

One of the few expositions of illuminationist philosophy in English is Mehdi Hairi Yazdi's *Principles of Epistemology in Islamic Philosophy* (1992).[5] According to the illuminationist school, knowledge is of two types: knowledge by presence *(shuhud),* which is immediate, nonrepresentational, and has no reference to external objects; and knowledge by correspondence, which involves the traditional notion of true justified belief concerning the correct apprehension by a subject of an external object. Seven centuries ago, the founder of illuminationism, Suhrawardi, used the phenomenon of pain to exemplify the characteristics of knowledge by presence. He emphasized (as the American analytic philosopher Saul Kripke did in the twentieth century [1972])[6] that the knowledge of pain does not appear to be separate from the experience of pain. One cannot be had without the other. Hairi notes that Wittgenstein made observations similar to Suhrawardi's on this subject. Hairi also comments that Bertrand Russell once advocated a similar idea (in an empiricist vein) with his doctrine of knowledge by acquaintance. But for the illuminationist, unlike the empiricist, knowledge by presence is the epistemological expression of true ontological reality, where, as shown with the example of the phenomenon of pain, there is no difference between knowing something and experiencing something. Ontology and epistemology converge on a single point.

Knowledge by presence is an epistemological fact. But, Hairi concludes, if it is something we do, if it is an epistemological reality, then it also must be an ontological reality, for ontology and epistemology are identical in the case of knowledge by presence, as established by the example of the phenomenon of pain. But what is the ontological reality that is revealed by knowledge by presence? Here the illuminationist school of philosophy transforms itself into what Hairi calls an existentialist school of thought. What we know and what we are is the same when we know by presence. Mystical experience represents the most fundamental type of knowledge by presence.

13.

Hairi offers two lines of evidence for the existence of this kind of knowledge.

The first type of evidence he offers is empirical evidence, which centers on sensory phenomena. Interestingly, the example that Hairi uses, dating back to a direct reference to this example by Suhrawardi, is pain, an illustrious phenomenon that has been the focus of much philosophical controversy in this day as well. Hairi extends Suhrawardi's position, emphasizing that in sensory phenomena such as pain, the objective knowledge of possessing pain does not seem to differ from the subjective experience of the pain itself. Such phenomena, Hairi implies, reduce the objective-subjective distinction to nothing, and one is left with empirical evidence of a different way of knowing, a way in which subjective experience and objective analysis are not separate. This is what he calls knowledge by presence; what we know simply is present before us in our experience; it is not separate from us, nor are we from it. He identifies this type of knowledge with the intuitive mystical knowledge *(shuhud)* which always was the core feature of illuminationism. The central conclusion that Hairi draws from this description of the phenomenon of pain is that knowledge by presence is a legitimate type of knowledge.

Yet this phenomenon has been analyzed in other ways that might be just as plausible as concluding that it provides evidence for knowledge by presence. Since the philosopher J. J. C. Smart's paper "Sensations and Brain Processes" ([1959] 1991), pain has been a favorite subject of controversy in the mind-body problem. Smart advanced the idea that the subjective, or mental, phenomenon of pain *is the same as* the objective brain-based phenomenon of the "firing of C-fibers," which has been associated with the occurrence of pain. This idea of "psychophysical identity" came under attack from numerous directions. One critic was Saul Kripke (1972), who held that pain cannot be identical to C-fiber firings or any brain event because the *experience* of pain cannot be translated into an objective phenomenon (C-fiber firing) without losing the quality of pain itself ("it hurts"). This line of criticism has hurt the psychophysical identity theory and has much in common with Hairi's critique. But other conclusions have been made by philosophers, as discussed earlier in chapter 2. Some philosophers have taken a "property dualism" argument to be the best alternative. In this approach, the subjective quality of pain and the objective brain events are taken to be two *different properties,* which might belong to the same event. One cannot be *reduced* to the other. They are simply different *properties* that the painlike event produces. Another approach to the dilemma of pain has been a materialist-functionalist approach, which, in a manner similar to that of property dualism, denies that the psychological phenomenon of pain can be reduced to brain events but asserts a dependence of the psychological phenomena on the existence of central primary brain events. In other words, given certain input (a noxious stimulus), certain mental events (the memory of past pain), and certain output (removing a limb from a hot pot), the functionalist description of pain would claim to account for all the mental phenomena without any direct (token-token) correlation to the underlying brain events, while claiming, *at the same time,* that without the brain events, the subjective experience of pain could not occur. Hence although Hairi uses the controversies surrounding subjective phenomena such as pain to suggest the possibility of knowledge by presence, he does not establish it with his argument, nor does he address alternative explanations.

14.

Hairi offers a second line of evidence in support of the validity of knowledge by presence: mystical experience. A number of apparently reliable individuals have reported repeatedly that they have certain experiences of a feeling of unity with an all-pervading existence, often described in terms of an all-encompassing sense of light. These mystical experiences can provide evidence for the validity of knowledge by presence, Hairi writes. Hairi admits that mystical experience could be criticized, however, in terms of representing abnormal physical phenomena, such as illusions or hallucinations. He dismisses this possibility by citing other investigations, such as the remarkable work of William James ([1901] 1958). But all James showed was that such experiences are common and have characteristics that are similar to normal psychological phenomena. It remains an open question whether mystical experiences represent abnormal physical phenomena. On the one hand, given that mystical experiences are known to occur with the auras of temporal-lobe epilepsy, and that religious preoccupation can be a core personality trait related to an epileptic focus in the same part of the brain, it is not impossible for mystical experience to be due to biological abnormalities. On the other hand, just because some religious experiences may represent pathological aspects of brain function, one cannot conclude that *all* religious experiences are therefore aspects of psychopathology. Indeed, it would seem to be an overexaggeration of the effect of the brain on human beings to make such an assertion; the role of culture seems to be larger in uncovering the source of the birth and growth of religions. What remains unclear is whether we can account for *all* mystical experiences in biological, psychological, and cultural terms, or whether *any* mystical experience is true; if *any* mystical experience is true, it might provide evidence for knowledge by presence. But again, this claim, though possibly true, needs to be proved. It has been asserted often that one must *experience* such phenomena to be convinced of them, but that begs the question. Hairi, to his credit, goes beyond that typical response and tries to show that mystical experience can be described logically through a "metamystical" language (Irfan), which can explain the claim of such experience to *existential* validity. This effort needs to be successful for mystical experience to serve as a source of evidence. Perhaps because of space limitations or perhaps owing to the complexity of the problem, this task was not completed in Hairi's book.

15.

The implications for modern philosophy and psychiatry of the possible validity of the illuminationist argument are numerous.

Historically, illuminationism developed in a philosophical vacuum left by the rejection of rationalist and empiricist philosophy. Knowledge by presence was assumed to be a fact in illuminationist thought. But the illuminationist critique of rationalism and empiricism may not prove convincing to adherents of modern doctrines. Like Sufism, illuminationism might find some allies in this regard among phenomenological and religiously oriented existentialist philosophies, which also have been dissatisfied with the course of traditional rationalist-empiricist philosophy.[7] Hairi makes a connection with this group when he describes the evolution of illuminationist thought as culminating in Mulla Sadra's "Islamic philosophy of existence," or "Islamic existentialism."

A central feature of both Western existentialism and Mulla Sadra's version is that the most primary concept of philosophical explanation is the category of existence. This perspective has led, through many variations, to a central insight of Western existentialism (summarized along these lines by Thomas

Nagel [1986]): that there is a gulf between the seriousness with which each individual pursues his or her own life subjectively, from the first-person perspective, and the lack of importance of each individual's life and actions when viewed objectively, from the third-person perspective.

For Mulla Sadra, the primacy of the category of existence leads to an attempt to resolve the apparent gulf between the existence of God (eternal, all-powerful, and pure) and humans and other beings (transitory, weak, and corrupted) (Nasr 1976). He asserted that there is no qualitative difference between the existence of God and human existence, and hence in principle the apparent gulf between God and humanity is a continuum that can be *traveled* (his main philosophical work is called *Kitab al-Asfar*, or *The Book of Travels*); once it is breached, humanity and God can be united in one all-encompassing existence. Epistemologically, explains Hairi, this notion was instrumental in developing the field of Irfan ("the linguistic methodology of introspective knowledge") to reconcile the different forms of knowledge Hairi discusses: knowledge by presence (which is the source of mysticism) and knowledge by representation (which is the source of rationalism and empiricism). In this regard, Mulla Sadra contributed the concept of "transexistentiation" (al-harakat al-jawhariyah), which refers to the ability to *translate* mystical experience (obtained through knowledge by presence) into the *language* of reason or empirical evidence. This transexistentiation allows *communication* to occur between our different ways of knowing, Hairi writes, and thus allows us to bridge the epistemological as well as the existential divides. In this effort, Hairi argues with originality that illuminationist thought, derived from Mulla Sadra, really is proposing a new existentialist philosophy.

It is this concept of epistemological and ontological divides that makes the contributions of illuminationism in the East and phenomenology in the West of interest. But it also poses a large challenge to these schools of philosophy. Given the definitive progress of science, there is certainly much evidence to commend rationalist-empiricist philosophy, perhaps with some criticisms of its excesses (such as psychophysical identity) along the lines suggested by its opponents. Although illuminationism and phenomenology may bring useful perspectives to the topic, the burden of proof seems to lie with them to show where rationalist-empiricist philosophy fails and to prove how and why their own alternatives are superior.

16.

There are many aspects of overlap among Epicurean, Stoic, and Sufi approaches to philosophy and ethics. I think the overlap suggests that these views share roots in a basic approach to philosophy and ethics that differs from that of the Western traditions discussed in chapter 8. In Sufism, there is a relationship to Epicurean ideas: the effort to decrease worldly attachments, an emphasis on avoiding anger, and the use of dance and song to elicit states of spiritual rapture. Like the Stoics, Sufis try to limit their appetites, whether for food or sex. And like Hinduism, Sufism emphasizes harsh living *(riazat)* and meditation, as well as respect for religion and tolerance of religious denominations.[8]

I believe Hellenistic schools and Islamic philosophy can be relevant to current views on the ethics of psychiatry. The Hellenistic and Islamic schools have in common an emphasis on reduction of attachments. This approach is quite different from the essentially bourgeois ethos of orthodox psychoanalysis, and also outside of the mainstream of Western culture in general. It has many similarities to Western existentialist approaches, however, and I suggest that a dialogue between Western existentialism and these Hellenistic and Eastern approaches can be creative and useful. Besides reducing attachments, relevant concepts for psychiatry include focusing on the present, recognizing the limits of reason, examining the role of intuitive knowledge, and realizing the benefits of a pluralistic attitude.

Part II / Practice
What Clinicians Do and Why

In the first half of this book, I have tried to explain how psychiatry has to answer certain problems in ontology, epistemology, and ethics: what exists in psychiatric practice, how do we know about it, and how do we value it? Yet, to answer these questions, it is important to have a clear understanding of the actual phenomena of psychopathology. In the next part, I turn to a conceptual analysis of psychiatric nosology, psychotherapy, and psychopathology, that is, the actual phenomena of psychiatric practice. I apply a pluralistic approach to psychiatry, in the spirit of Karl Jaspers, and I attempt to show how conceptual clarity about what we do in practice can shed light on the real-world questions with which clinicians and patients struggle daily.

CHAPTER 10

On the Nature of Mental Illness

Disease or Myth?

1.

What is mental illness? Is it a disease entity, as in the standard medical model, or a myth, as in postmodern critiques, or something in between?

A discussion of mental illness needs to begin with a discussion of illness in general, followed by specific matters related to psychiatric conditions. In this chapter I review this general issue conceptually, and in the following chapters I discuss specific types of classification systems (nosologies) in psychiatry.

Illness can be defined as something distinct from health. A common view, perhaps the most parsimonious, in medicine is that illness is the absence of health. Hence illness is defined negatively: the opposite of health. A potential problem with this view is that it shifts the burden to defining what health is, and there are as many different views about the nature of health as there are about the nature of illness.

An alternative is to define illness based on a specific set of requirements, leaving aside any definition of health. On this perspective, health is the absence of illness. Illness is defined positively, and health negatively. The psychiatrist Aubrey Lewis (1967) took this approach and contrasted it to the other one.[1] He begins by quoting the World Health Organization's broad definition of health as "a state of complete, physical, mental, and social well-being and not merely the absence of disease or infirmity" (180). Lewis opposes this view:

> A proposition could hardly be more comprehensive than that, or more meaningless. But to condemn it because it is meaningless is to ignore the history and complexity of the idea behind it . . . an ancient formula of unattainable wholeness of body, mind and soul, realized in the Golden Age but long since forfeited. . . . Now if the various organs work well enough not to draw attention to themselves, and their owner is free from pain or discomfort, he usually supposes that he is in good health. The criterion is then a subjective one. But if he avails himself of the mass

X-ray service and in consequence learns that his lung shows strong evidence of tuberculous disease, he ceases to consider that he is in good health: the criterion he now adopts is an extraneous one, viz. the assertion of a physician who relies on objective or pathological data. It is evident that the physician's criteria of physical health are not the same as the patient's, and that, in practice, it is the presence of disease that can be recognized, not the presence of health. There are no positive indications of health which can be relied upon, and we consider everyone healthy who is free from any evidence of disease or infirmity. (180–81)

Lewis goes on to provide criteria for illness based on the process of medical practice: "The criteria of physical illness and health depend upon: first, the patient's account of how and what he feels, i.e., upon subjective statements; secondly, manifest signs of satisfactory or impaired function or structure; and thirdly, occult signs of such adequacy or impairment, detected by special instruments or procedures." Up to this point, Lewis has not discussed psychological or social aspects of physical illness. He does not feel that such aspects are necessary parts of the definition of physical illness, but they are nonetheless important:

I have spoken of organs and systems; but these are, of course, strictly, artificial abstractions from the total living organism. . . . The physician must rely on estimation of the total performance of the patient, as well as on the performance of separate parts of him, isolated for convenience as organs or systems: all should be working in responsive harmony. A great many pathologists and physicians have sought to make this the touchstone of health, which they define, or rather sum up, as "a state of physiological and psychological equilibrium," whereas they view disease as the organism's reaction to a disturbance of its inner equilibrium. . . . At this point we are again adrift, away from objective, well-studied norms. The adequate performance of the body working as a whole is highly individual; the range of variability in the human species is wide. . . .

So even in regard to physical illness, we cannot disregard total behavior, which is a psychological concept, and the environment, which, so far as it consists of human beings and their institutions, includes a social concept. (182–83)

In this discussion, Lewis approaches Engel's biopsychosocial model of medicine, as opposed to what Engel called the "biomedical reductionist" model, which would allow only biological definitions of disease. Yet Lewis does not completely go along with Engel, for Lewis feels that biological aspects of disease are necessary, though not sufficient, for understanding illness, whereas the psychosocial aspects of illness are contingent. In other words, Lewis allows for a biopsychosocial model, but with the biological component being essential and more central.

Lewis then goes on to define mental illness:

> In general discussion it is customary to assume a monistic standpoint, and infer a physical aspect to all mental health and illness, just as we infer a psychological aspect to all physical illness; but in practice the limits set to our observations and knowledge compel us to talk a dualist language. . . . (183)
>
> Mental health, ideally, might be a state of perfect equipoise in an unstable system. It has been described by some as a state in which one's potential capacities are fully realized. But unless some capacities are characterized as morbid and excluded from the generalization, this is absurd. We all have deplorable potentialities as well as desirable ones. It is hardly necessary to dwell on the emptiness of an ideal notion of mental health, perfect and unattainable. The serviceable criterion commonly employed to define mental health is absence of mental illness. This shifts the difficulty, and slightly lessens it. (183)
>
> What then is mental illness? Can it be recognized, as physical disease often is, by the qualitatively altered function of some part of the total, by disturbance of thinking, for example, or disturbance of perception? This is possible: we very frequently recognize a man to be mentally ill because he has delusions or hallucinations. But not always, for if the disturbance of part-functions is without influence on his conduct, or falls within certain categories which we regard as "normal," we do not infer "mental illness" from their presence. . . . if a man expresses an irrational belief, e.g., that he has been bewitched, we do not call it a delusion, a sign of disease, unless we are satisfied that the manner in which he came by it is morbid . . . [that is] through highly individual, devious, suspicion-laden mental processes. . . . (184)
>
> Two criteria have apparently been applied, then, to changes in function: a psychopathological one paying attention to the process, and a statistical one paying regard to the frequency of its occurrence. (184)

I will expand on these notions regarding delusion and psychosis in chapter 14. But for my purposes here it is sufficient to follow Lewis's line of argument that mental illness involves, like physical illness, assessment of some disturbance of a function, in this case the function of normal thought processes. In addition, however, one has what Lewis calls a "statistical" criterion, that is, that something is uncommon and unusual. Although this latter aspect would seem to imply an inherent social component of mental illness, Lewis asserts that the disturbance of psychological function is the essential feature:

> The concept of disease, then—and of health—has physiological and psychological components, but no essential social ones. In examining it, we cannot ignore social considerations, because they may be needed for the assessment of physiological and psychological adequacy, but we are not bound to consider whether behavior is socially deviant: though illness may lead to such behavior, there are many forms of social deviation which are not illness, many forms of illness which are not social deviation. . . . To deny a social content in the idea of health in no sense implies denying a social context. (189–92)

Lewis summarizes his view:

> If I now try to pull together my argument, it is this. Health is a single concept: it is not possible to set up essentially different criteria for physical health and mental health. We commonly assume a break between health and ill-health, for which there is no counterpart in the phenomena but which we cannot yet replace by a continuum because we lack means of measuring some of the necessary dimensions. Besides subjective feelings and degree of total efficiency, the criterion of health is adequate performance of functions, physiological and psychological. We can therefore usually tell whether an individual is physically healthy, but we cannot tell with the same confidence and consensus of many observers, whether he is mentally healthy. (194)

2.

Leston Havens takes the opposing view. He feels that illness in general, and mental illness in particular, needs to be defined in terms of absence of health. In other words, controversies in psychiatric nosology—disagreements about the nature of psychiatric illnesses, how to classify them, whether they are diseases or not—have their root in confusion or ignorance about the nature of mental health. If we cannot delimit what is health relatively clearly, then we will disagree about what is illness.

Here is Havens's own argument:

> Contemporary psychiatry seeks symptoms and signs and the collection of these into syndromes or disease states. Health is considered to be an absence of these

disease states, a preponderance of what are called negative findings. The foundation of the psychiatric disease concepts is therefore a largely negative description of health.

It might appear that this is also true of the physical disease concept, but it is not, because physical disease is always defined against a literally palpable awareness of health. . . . Physical diseases are defined against standards of normal functioning, by departures from normal levels of blood pressure, pulse, visual acuity, and so on. It is the detailed knowledge of at least acceptable standards of physiological functioning that allows for consensual validation of concepts of disease. In essence the doctor of physical disease not only excludes disease but tests for health. . . .

It is true that the mental status or psychological examination, the chief diagnostic tool of the disease school, includes some tests of mental health . . . [like] memory, grasp, orientation, and calculation. It is no accident that these are the parts of the psychological examination closest to neurology, which is so replete with other tests of neural health. However, the psychological examination is weakest where it is most needed by the psychiatrist: in tests of normal affect, sociability, self-image, capacity for self-protection, and coping, among others. (1984, 1208)

Havens has been impressed with the evolution of neurology, where the introduction of techniques like the pinprick, the reflex hammer, and the tuning fork in the late nineteenth century led to major clinical progress. Neurologists could then define health more clearly and thus, by extension, circumscribe disease more decisively. Havens emphasizes that disease is a circumscribed entity in medicine, whereas it is fluid and overwhelming in psychiatry. When a patient goes to an internist or a neurologist, the physician, in the course of the physical examination, reassures the patient about all those aspects of the examination that are normal. Abnormalities are identified in the context of the normal, and the patient and the doctor are able to objectify those abnormalities. The disease becomes an "it" (Pellegrino and Thomasma 1981), and the patient is seen as *having* the disease. In the case of psychiatry, the clinician all too often searches the patient's mind for evidence of infirmity, rather than seeking evidence of health. More often than not, patients emerge from psychiatric examinations with speculations about abnormality but very little reassurance of areas that are functioning well. Consequently, the proposed illness seems large and menacing, and the patient is often identified with the illness. The patient *is* the illness, in this scenario, rather than *having* it. Hence it is no accident that we speak of the schizophrenic or the manic patient so loosely, instead of the patient who has these conditions.

If we compare Havens's description of the process of medical practice with that of Lewis, we notice a major difference. For Lewis, even in physical medicine, little can be said of health, and disease can be well enough understood as abnormalities of physiological functions of organs and systems by those who are trained to have enough specialized knowledge of the process. In psychiatry, Lewis simply adds the factor of psychological dysfunction, as in the illogical thought processes leading to a delusion. For Havens, in physical medicine, much is said of health, and illness is the circumscribed entity left over when the mainly healthy aspects of a person are reconfirmed. In contrast, in psychiatry, health is ignored and illness looms excessively large, leading to disagreements about definitions of illness, as well as an increased component of stigma.

This disagreement between Lewis and Havens reflects a key point for the understanding of mental illness. Are we to approach mental illness primarily by seeking for the presence of disease, with health being left aside (as Lewis advocates), or by identifying health primarily, with disease being the circumscribed remainder (as Havens suggests)?

3.

It is interesting to note that Lewis and Havens both approach their conceptions of what is illness and what is health primarily by meditating on what it is that doctors do in medical practice. They focus on the process of diagnosis to determine what we mean by disease. This is a useful practical approach, but different conclusions may arise in other hands or with other approaches. Both Lewis and Havens are psychiatrists. Let us examine what comes to the attention of Edmund Pellegrino and David Thomasma (1981), nonpsychiatrist physicians and philosophers, William Fulford (1989), a psychiatrist and also a trained philosopher, and Norman Daniels (1985), a philosopher who specializes in health care ethics.

In their classic text *A Philosophical Basis of Medical Practice* (1981), Pellegrino and Thomasma decide to apply the phenomenological idea of the "lived body" to their understanding of disease. In other words, not only do they focus on the body as an object, or on its parts or organs; they also view the body as seen through the subjective experience of the owner of it. They thus see disease as "a relational structure between sickness, the sick person, the physician, and society. The ill person enters three relations—one to the self, another to the physician, and still another to society and environment—all of which are governed by the need to help. The physician also enters three relations—one of responsibility to the sick person, another to the disease (what is the case? what to do?), and another to society" (74). They continue:

> Disease [is] the presence of a subjective, clinical, or social need for help in persons whose physical, psychic, or psychophysical balance of boundaries in the organism is disrupted. Health, or well-being, on the other hand, is characterized by the presence of order and balance in the organism and no perceived or actual need for help. . . . In the realm of the lived body, dis-ease is an interpretation of the disruption, an interruption in the ability to cope. Dis-ease is not a symptom but a sign of dysfunction. As such, it is heavily value-laden. . . . Concepts of disease are also therefore intrinsically and extrinsically evaluative. That is, they depend on organic dysfunction, a perceived need for help, and physician intervention. . . . The goal of medicine is primarily the relief of perceived lived body disruption, not scientific explanation. Cure of the organic dysfunction is a necessary but not a sufficient step toward this goal. (76)

One might think that this approach to disease, which adds a strong subjective component not present in Lewis's definition, might be quite amenable to defining mental illness. Yet the authors single out psychiatry (along with religion!) as not falling within this definition of the practice of medicine.

> Although psychiatry is usually considered a branch of medicine, it shares with religion a primary focus on the lived self, the symbolic integration as a person. . . . [But] medicine focuses primarily on perceived needs of the lived body, rather than on the lived self. Thus psychiatry shares with religion the methodology of verbal therapy. Psychiatry is primarily a persuasive art whose therapy consists of understanding, interpretation, and coping. . . . Insofar as psychiatry discovers organic causes of dis-ease, it is medicine. . . . Mental illness is primarily a symbolic disorder, not an organic one. (Pellegrino and Thomasma 1981, 78)

It is striking that, despite their differences, Lewis and Havens appear to agree on trying to find common ground between medicine and psychiatry, between conceptions of physical and mental illness. Pellegrino and Thomasma, in contrast, define the medical aspects of psychiatry away. Readers at this point should have no difficulty recognizing the error of Pellegrino and Thomasma. In pluralist terms, they completely identify psychiatry with McHugh and Slavney's life story perspective, and they completely ignore the other perspectives of psychiatry. Alternatively, they argue that any other approach in psychiatry is not, therefore, psychiatry and is part of medicine. This is quite circular logic indeed.

Yet Pellegrino and Thomasma offer us the concept of the lived body, and they point out the need to recognize illness and disease as things that occur in individual lives and bodies. They argue that we cannot abstract the organic dysfunction outside of this context and thus that there is always an evaluative component to notions of disease.

4.

The psychiatrist and philosopher William Fulford agrees. In his book *Moral Theory and Medical Practice* (1989), Fulford engages in a tightly reasoned exposition of the nature of psychiatric diagnosis. He begins with the simple but powerful critique by Thomas Szasz (1974), who argued that physical disease concepts are facts, whereas mental illness concepts are value-laden. Since medical disease requires the absence of value judgments, mental illness is not a medical disease, according to Szasz. Pellegrino and Thomasma showed, however, that, from one perspective, medical disease concepts are also value-laden. In that respect, one cannot differentiate concepts of physical and mental illness. Fulford focused on the concept of "action failure" as being the common thread. In both mental and physical illness, the patient experiences an inability to function in daily living owing to physical or psychological difficulties.[2] Fulford alters the conventional view that disease stems from a dysfunction of some thing (organ or system); he says instead that disease arises indirectly from action failure. He makes this argument based on a logical discussion of the meaning and relations of the terms *dysfunction, illness,* and *disease.*

The problem for understanding mental illness is obvious on this view. The notion of disease is tightly bound to the notion of dysfunction. Concepts of physical illness flow from the disease = dysfunction relationship. Yet, mental illness is one step further removed, and if distinctions between mental and physical illness are highlighted, the relation of mental illness to disease seems even more distant.

Fulford's alternative is to view action failure as logically primary, with concepts of illness, whether mental or physical, derived from action failure; disease concepts are then derived from concepts of illness.

Fulford's argument needs to be read in its entirety to appreciate the full force of his approach. Yet, although it satisfies the rigors of analytic philosophical reasoning, I suspect that many clinicians will want to supplement Fulford's approach with more clinical reasoning along the lines of Pellegrino and Thomasma. In either case, these writers emphasize the ethical or evaluative aspects of all illness concepts, whether physical or mental. In that sense, the common accusation against concepts of mental illness as being value-laden is rendered less weighty. Rather, the ethical components of all medical practice are highlighted. The dogmatism (limiting psychiatry to the life story perspective) of Pellegrino and Thomasma notwithstanding, psychiatry does not seem too different from medicine from these perspectives.

5.

The philosopher Norman Daniels takes a more straightforward approach derived from biological considerations, as well as ethical perspectives derived from the philosopher John Rawls. Daniels begins by assessing what kinds of needs are relevant to notions of health and illness (1985). He follows David Braybrooke in dividing needs into "course-of-life" and "adventitious." Course-of-life needs are those that people "have all through their lives or at certain stages of life through which they must pass," and adventitious needs are based on contingent projects. Thus, examples of course-of-life needs would be food, shelter, clothing, and so on. "A deficiency with respect to them 'endangers the normal functioning of the subject of need *considered as a member of a natural species*,'" writes Daniels, quoting Braybrooke. Daniels uses the biological concept of "species-typical normal functioning" as central to notions of health. He then goes on to lay out its implications: "I shall begin with a narrow, if not uncontroversial, 'biomedical' model: the basic idea is that health is the absence of disease, and diseases . . . are *deviations from the natural functional organization of a typical member of a species*. The task of characterizing this natural functional organization falls to the biomedical sciences. . . . The concept of disease that results is not merely a statistical notion—deviation from the statistical norm. Rather, it draws on a theoretical account of the design of the organism" (28).

This approach, like that of Lewis, focuses on functional abnormalities, but it extends the concept from that of the usual state of an organ or an individual to the natural state of a typical member of the species. Recalling our discussion of essentialism in chapter 7, this approach has an advantage. Lewis engaged in an essentialist argument. He stated that organ dysfunction was essential to notions of disease. Daniels is avoiding such essentialist terms by returning to the population-based approach to typologies. He takes a species and then abstracts a *typical* member from it, an approach that is similar to Max Weber's ideal-type approach. This becomes his model of the normal, which is what Havens insisted on. He then defines disease as against this model of the normal. In so doing, Daniels is avoiding many of the weaknesses of the other approaches discussed so far.

He goes on to extend his discussion to mental illness: "Adding mental disease and health into the picture, which we must do, complicates the issue further. We have a less well-developed theory of species-typical mental functions and functional organization. The biomedical model clearly presupposes we can eventually develop this missing account and that a reasonable part of what we now take to be psychopathology will show up as diseases within the model" (Daniels 1985, 29).

Hence Daniels identifies mental and physical illness, though admitting the need to base such identification on evidence for a biological basis for mental illness. He concludes by agreeing with Lewis's critique of the broad WHO definition of health. "The biomedical model has controversial features. First, some insist it too narrowly defines health as the absence of disease. . . . In contrast, some . . . [like WHO] view health as an idealized level of well-being. But health is not happiness, and confusing the two over-medicalizes social philosophy. Nor does a 'narrow' biomedical view of disease mean that we should ignore its social etiology" (1985, 29).

Up to now, it would appear that Daniels's view takes steps to resolve the Lewis-Havens conflict, looking at mental illness from a primarily medical viewpoint, yet he has not addressed the ethical claims of Pellegrino and Thomasma and of Fulford. Daniels is not unaware of those claims:

> Some pure forms of the biomedical model also involve a deeper claim, namely that species-normal functional organization can itself be characterized without invoking normative or value judgments. Here the debate turns on hard issues of philosophy of biology. . . . My discussion does not turn on this deeper, strong claim about non-normativeness advanced by some advocates of the biomedical model. It is enough for my purposes that the line between disease and absence of

disease is, for the general run of cases, uncontroversial and ascertainable through publicly acceptable methods, such as those of the biomedical sciences. It will not matter if what counts as a disease category is relative to some features of social roles in a given society, and thus to some normative judgments, provided the core of the notion of species-normal functioning is left intact. (1985, 30)

Daniels's main project, to which this discussion led, was an examination of public policy regarding fair provision of health care. For my purpose, though, his discussion is also useful in tying together the loose threads of some of the previous discussion of health and illness and of the nature of mental illness.

6.

Daniels's discussion points a way forward, I think. Daniels oscillates between the Lewis and Havens alternatives. Like Lewis, Daniels argues against a broad definition of health. Yet, like Havens, he bases the definition of disease on an understanding of health. If we broaden our view of disease to involve normal species-functioning, then we will focus on defining what is normal, while avoiding the broad, vague entities that Lewis feared. Something along these lines would seem to be of central importance for psychiatry, as Havens argued, so as to reduce stigma. It is perhaps no accident that diagnosis and classification in psychiatry is often interpreted as "labeling" and dehumanizing. Perhaps psychiatric diagnosis tends in this direction because the field of psychiatry fails to recognize the importance of defining disease in terms of health, as Havens suggests.

We can also admit an ethical and evaluative component to concepts of mental illness and to psychiatry in general, while not thereby reducing the status of concepts of mental illness or psychiatry compared to concepts of physical illness or medicine. The process of medical practice is shot through with evaluative judgments, as Pellegrino and Thomasma demonstrate, and the same is true of psychiatry. Yet, admitting such normative components does not mean that we have to retreat from a definition of health and disease along the lines suggested by Daniels. For practical purposes, for the physician treating a patient, and for researchers defining diagnoses, what matters is consensual agreement. All physicians engage in evaluative judgments in the course of diagnosis. As long as we all agree on how we make those judgments, why, and in what circumstances, there will be a level of consensual agreement that will be sufficient for medical practice. Similarly, all diagnoses made for research purposes also include evaluative judgments; again, as long as the judgments are based on similar considerations, there is no inherent loss of reliability. Acknowledging that there are evaluative judgments does not invalidate the whole process, nor does it remove any connection between the concepts of disease and the underlying realities in the biological processes in which they are based. Medical or psychiatric diagnoses do not carve nature at the joints (see chapter 7), yet they can be quite adequate for approximating the natural world.

7.

I have used the words *illness* and *disease* almost interchangeably throughout this chapter. But it is relevant to note that the two words are not identical in meaning. Among the writers reviewed so far, Fulford makes the clearest distinction, seeing illness as primary to disease, with illness being derived from the experience of an action failure, a failure in ordinary doing in daily life. The illness is then understood in terms of disease concepts applied to the features of the action failures that occur. The anthropologist and psychiatrist Arthur Kleinman (1988) suggests a related definition of these terms: "*Illness* refers to the patient's perception, experience, expression, and pattern of coping with symptoms, while *disease* refers to the way practitioners recast illness in terms of their theoretical models of pathology. Thus, a psychiatric diagnosis is an *interpretation* of a person's experience" (7).

Kleinman's distinctions appear to tie into the concepts of lived experience at the basis of views of health and illness, as also advocated by Pellegrino and Thomasma. Like Fulford, Kleinman emphasizes that disease concepts are theoretical models, somewhat distant from their roots in the actual lived experiences of the person (Fulford's action failures). It is likely that all the writers referred to in this section would agree that the concept of disease involves moving a certain level of abstraction away from the originating processes of either organ dysfunction or failed functioning. Kleinman seeks to emphasize the more subjective experiences, and the more experientially primary experiences, of the person through definition of the word *illness* as equivalent to such subjective experiences. This approach has achieved some popularity and seems not without some utility. It also has the advantage of reminding the doctor that the illness is not the same thing as the disease and that the patient's experience of disease is an important matter.

8.

I believe I can summarize a few important points from this chapter. This analysis of discussions of health and illness, and especially mental illness, highlights the point that I am not assuming that mental illness is simply a biomedical phenomenon with nothing more to be said on the matter. Rather, there are clearly evaluative components to concepts of mental illness. But this fact does not distinguish, in principle, mental illness from physical illness, which is also a value-laden concept.

There are clear divergences of opinion on how to define health and illness in relation to each other. I lean toward the view that it is important to define illness in terms of health, rather than the common assumption to the contrary. Like Daniels, I think this can be done with a rather circumscribed perspective on health, such as that of normal species-functioning. Like Havens, I think this approach is very important in helping us get beyond differences about which conditions represent mental illnesses and which do not, and in reducing potentially stigmatizing and dehumanizing applications of psychiatric diagnoses.

If I have convinced the reader that the concept of mental illness is not entirely without justification, and that a biological perspective on it is also acceptable, allowing for an evaluative aspect, I can now turn from the question of whether there is such a thing as mental illness to the question of how we can classify mental illness. What psychiatric diagnoses exist, how do we classify them, and why?

CHAPTER 11

Order out of Chaos?

The Evolution of Psychiatric Nosology

> Studies of invalid constructs will probably generate invalid results, however sophisticated the methodology used might have been.
> —HERMANN VAN PRAAG, 1999

1.

In the eighteenth century, there was only one mental illness: insanity. The diagnosis of insanity meant roughly what clinicians currently mean by the word *psychosis* or what is referred to colloquially by "crazy." *Insanity* denoted that patients had somehow lost touch with reality, often with delusions or hallucinations or with severe melancholia or states of elation. Although these symptomatic states were described, and had been for ages dating back to the Greeks, physicians who treated these patients did not consider them to represent different diseases or diagnoses. The general condition of insanity was applied to all.

Physicians who specialized in these patients were largely identified by their work in the mental asylum, usually in rural areas. Another group, as the nineteenth century progressed, was physicians who worked in cities and towns, treating patients in their homes, in the physician's office, or in a hospital clinic. As a classic example of the mental asylum physicians, sometimes called "alienists," one could cite Philippe Pinel, the Frenchman who is known for taking shackles off asylum patients after the French Revolution in the 1790s. Pinel introduced "moral therapy," the concept that insanity was a disease and that patients needed to be assisted in their recovery, not through shackles or medicines, but through calm, pleasant surroundings and understanding care. Pinel belonged to the Hippocratic school of treatment, which viewed medical therapy as the handmaiden to nature. Nature caused illnesses, and nature cured illnesses; the physician's job was to not hinder, and perhaps help, nature in the process. This was a very different view from the interventionist school in medicine, which focused on treatments (medicines, bleeding, tinctures of this and that) for symptoms. An American revolutionary, Dr. Benjamin Rush, one of the signers of the Declaration of Independence, is often seen as a proponent of the anti-Hippocratic view in psychiatry (Ghaemi 2002). (Ironically, Rush is viewed as the founder of American psychiatry, and his figure is on the seal of the American Psychiatric Association.) Although figures such as Rush and Pinel, both of whom wrote texts on insanity, could disagree on how to treat mental illness, they agreed on the diagnostic schema: one diagnosis—insanity.

This simple nosology, one illness of insanity, held sway in the United States and most of Europe throughout most of the nineteenth century. The exception was mainly in France, where Pinel's successors engaged in a fervent effort to split the concept of insanity into its different components, viewed as bona fide medical diagnoses. As the disease model in medicine spread quickly in the late nineteenth century (influenced by the discovery of the bacterium and the rise of Darwinian materialism), the German schools of psychiatry unified the French "splitting" approach and the one-illness "lumping" approach. Emil Kraepelin was the key unifier, with his schema of two major mental illnesses, dementia praecox (soon relabeled schizophrenia by Eugen Bleuler) and manic-depressive illness (also labeled affective illness by Bleuler). Some opposed Kraepelin's splitting of insanity in two, and these critics upheld a "one psychosis" *(Einheit psychosen)* model, also called the continuum model (current proponents include Timothy Crow).

Aubrey Lewis describes this period:

> [The German psychiatrist] Hoche pointed out that Kraepelin had relegated melancholia from . . . a disease to a clinical picture and that it no longer mattered whether there was mania or melancholia, occurrence once in life, or many times, at irregular or at regular intervals, whether late or early, with predominance of these symptoms or those—it was still manic-depressive insanity. This standpoint Hoche attacked on theoretical and practical grounds, and proceeded to his general thesis—that clinically distinguishable diseases do not exist. . . . The influence of these views . . . was great, and Kraepelin himself in 1920 made considerable concessions. (1967, 92)

As early as 1906, when Kraepelin was gaining steam internationally, Adolf Meyer (1948) was opposed to Kraepelin's approach:

The superstition about the value of a diagnosis of a disease prompts many to believe that a diagnosis once made puts them into a position to solve the queries about the case not with the facts presented by it and naturally considered in the light of principles based on experiment and on clinical experiences with a concrete series of cases, but by a system of rules and deductions from the meaning of the newly defined disease entities. . . .

What we act on should be facts. If the facts do not constitute a diagnosis we nevertheless must act on the facts. To jump from the facts at an arbitrary diagnosis and then to act on that abstract diagnosis is a procedure . . . bound to lead to self-deceit and confusion. (154, 168)

Whereas Kraepelin deemphasized melancholia and focused on the overall manic-depressive syndrome, Meyer moved in the direction of emphasizing *depression,* a term he emphasized, and Meyer's emphasis remains more influential on mood diagnoses in the United States even today.

If instead of melancholia, we applied the term depression to the whole class, it would designate in an unassuming way exactly what is meant by the . . . term melancholia. In the large group of depressions we would naturally distinguish our cases according to aetiology, the symptom-complex, the course of the disease and the results. . . . Besides the manic-depressive depressions, the anxiety psychosis, the depressive deliria . . . and hallucinations, the depressive episodes of dementia praecox, the symptomatic depressions, non-differentiated depressions will occur. (1948, 147)

Kraepelin's nosology spread quickly and took over the psychiatric world from roughly the 1880s to the 1930s. With the rise of psychoanalysis as a new and exciting theory as well as treatment, the Kraepelinian nosology was dealt a severe blow, however, and it was all but left for dead. Meyer's views gained greater support, and Karl Menninger expressed the general view that Kraepelinian psychiatry was both therapeutically nihilistic, since it offered no hope for treatment, and dehumanizing: "Kraepelin's application of the principle of prognosis as a nosological criterion provided a most practical tool for the clinical worker . . . but the intimate association of prognosis with diagnosis tended to encourage a fatalistic and dogmatic attitude not conducive to wholehearted therapeutic efforts" (1967, 463).[1]

Kraepelin's therapeutic nihilism especially contrasted with both Meyer's pragmatic American optimism and the psychoanalytic school's therapeutic claims. As Karl Jaspers put it in describing the state of German psychiatry in the Kraepelinian era, "We were therapeutically hopeless but kind" ([1957] 1986, 5).

From the 1940s until the 1970s, especially in the United States (less so in England and some other parts of Europe), there was a reversion to essentially the insanity model, except that it was relabeled as the neurosis-psychosis continuum. Everyone, patient or not, sick or healthy, fell on that continuum somewhere. The disease tradition in medicine was not considered central in psychiatry.

A major change began to occur in the 1950s. Chlorpromazine was developed and tested in schizophrenia, imipramine and reserpine in depression, and lithium in mania. These medications were increasingly used and validated in clinical trials in the 1960s, and by the 1970s, a very practical problem led to a reassessment of the Freudian consensus on the neurosis-psychosis model. The birth of psychopharmacology suggested that, at least for medication treatment, Kraepelin's schema seemed quite serviceable.

And then the "neo-Kraepelinians," those mostly American researchers who were impressed by this process, began to test Kraepelin's nosology with new psychometric methods, and they began to demonstrate its reliability and utility. In the famous U.S.-U.K. study of 1970, researchers showed that American psychiatrists diagnosed almost every condition they saw in New York as schizophrenia, whereas British psychiatrists in London diagnosed fewer conditions as schizophrenia and diagnosed others as mood or anxiety conditions (Kendell et al. 1971). The American approach seemed extremely broad, and the new medications suggested that making finer distinctions was practically important.

Thus occurred the revolution of DSM-III in 1980. DSM-III was, to some extent, a conscious attempt to answer the criticisms of Kraepelin's nosology. Gerald Klerman (1986), a key figure in the development of modern psychiatry, who had trained in the psychoanalytic era but helped lead the movement toward psychopharmacology, summarized four critiques made of Kraepelin's views.[2]

First, some of Kraepelin's opponents felt that psychiatry was not a legitimate part of medicine. A recent proponent of this view is Thomas Szasz, who held that there are no mental illnesses. Obviously, if there is no such thing as "real" mental illness, then a nosology would be superfluous. I discussed the limitations of this view in the previous chapter. Second, some criticized the Kraepelinian nosology as being unreliable; psychiatrists simply could not agree on diagnoses, and if they did agree, they could not pick out the same patients. Klerman argues, justly, that DSM-III essentially fixed this problem. Third, some, like Meyer and Menninger, worried about the social and psychological consequences of the process of diagnosing, specifically being critical of the dehumanizing manner in which diagnoses are employed. Yet, as I will emphasize also later, the proponents of DSM-III can justifiably argue that they were not proposing a diagnostic process but rather a means of organizing our definitions at the conclusion of the diagnostic process. Diagnoses need not be labels; they are only labels if misused reductionistically. Hence, this is a criticism about an extreme approach to nosology, rather than a criticism of the utility of nosology per se. The fourth critique comes from those, often experimental psychologists, who view the entire categorical approach that underlies Kraepelin's nosology as wrongheaded. These individuals accept the reality of mental illness, as well as the need to diagnose, but they argue that such diagnosis should use dimensions rather than categories. Klerman appears to view this as an empirical debate within nosology, and I would tend to agree. One view would be that a single psychosis continuum model fits the facts more accurately than Kraepelin's schemas, but this is a matter for empirical research. Another view, proposed by recent researchers discussed later in this chapter, is more nuanced and, in my opinion, very important.

DSM-III was a restoration more than a revolution, returning to psychiatry's Kraepelinian heritage. This change, along with the rise of psychopharmacology, is often viewed by critics as the major mistake of modern psychiatry. There are, in my view, both positive and negative aspects to the DSM-III restoration/revolution, but to understand those aspects, we need to have a sense of how this restoration happened.

2.

In 1982, two years after the adoption of DSM-III, the American Psychiatric Association held a debate in Toronto about the validity of it. Klerman was in favor. Also in favor was Robert Spitzer, the chairman of the DSM-III committee, who had organized the revision and who was perhaps the key specialist in nosology who led the movement to DSM-III and later revisions. Against were Robert Michels, a well-known academic and psychoanalyst, and George Vaillant, a prominent psychoanalytically trained researcher who specialized in research on psychoanalytic concepts like defense mechanisms.

Klerman spoke first:

In my opinion, the development of DSM-III represents a fateful point in the history of the American psychiatric profession. . . . In 1950–1954, psychiatry made an important decision with regard to its destiny when chlorpromazine and the other psychopharmacologic agents became available. In previous eras, when an effective treatment for a mental disorder became available, psychiatrists gave up interest in that disorder, and responsibility was transferred to other professions. . . . When chlorpromazine became available, American psychiatry reversed its pattern and accepted psychopharmacology as its domain, albeit with internal controversy and acrimony. (Klerman et al. 1984, 539)[3]

So Klerman makes the point that a major impetus for the shift in diagnostic schema in psychiatry in 1980 was the development of psychopharmacology. We will see that many issues in nosology take us back to the battle of dogmatisms we described in chapter 1, psychopharmacology versus psychotherapy, or biology versus psychosocial models.

Klerman then outlines the benefits of DSM-III:

First, it embodies the concept of multiple disorders, reaffirming psychiatry's acceptance of the modern medical model of disease.

Second, and for the first time, an official nomenclature has incorporated operational criteria with exclusion and inclusion criteria . . . based on manifest descriptive psychopathology rather than on presumed etiology—psychodynamic, social, or biological. This reliance on descriptive rather than etiological criteria does not represent an abandonment of the ideal of modern scientific medicine that classification and diagnosis should be by causation. Rather, it represents a strategic mode of dealing with the frustrating reality that, for most of the disorders we currently treat, there is only limited evidence for their etiologies. . . .

Third, DSM-III underwent field testing for reliability. Never before have practitioners of a medical specialty participated in a test of the reliability of their nomenclature. . . .

Fourth, a multiaxial system was introduced to accommodate the diverse aspects of our patients' existence.

Fifth, there is implicit in the creation of DSM-III . . . the necessity for change— the push for DSM-IV is already apparent. The changes that appear in DSM-IV should be determined by the state of evidence rather than the assertions of competing ideological camps. (540)

Klerman's list is not unimpressive. To summarize it, one might say that DSM-III, once and for all, made the commitment that psychiatry was a medical specialty. Since we do not know the etiologies of mental illnesses, nor with certainty how to define them, we should take one approach, define them in a way that is consensually reliable, and then embark on research to confirm, validate, or change those diagnostic definitions, while at the same time seeking for etiologies that might be incorporated into the diagnostic system later if empirically proven. This description of the course of thinking that led to DSM-III is, I think, accurate and scientifically defensible and still remains acceptable.

DSM-III and IV have many critics. In some ways, I think this just reflects human nature. We have plenty of rebels against the status quo, and thank goodness. But the critics should not lose sight of these basic facts about the evolution of DSM-III. For all its weaknesses, and I will enumerate those, the move to DSM-III had some major advantages.

Klerman continues: "The problem of reliability having been solved, one must acknowledge that there are two unresolved problems: validity and the uniqueness of individual patients. Reliability does not guarantee validity. However, reliability is a necessary precursor to establishing the validity of diagnostic classes" (541).

Reliability reflects whether different persons can agree on how to define and recognize a syndrome. Validity reflects the idea of whether that definition of the syndrome accurately represents the reality of that disease or condition. This is perhaps the most common, and most justified, criticism of the DSM-III system. But its developers simply claim that they could not establish validity based on the state of knowledge at the time, and so they took a humble, agnostic approach, admitted their lack of knowledge regarding etiology, and proceeded to establish reliability at the very least. They would argue that the issue is not reliability *versus* validity, but reliability *before* validity. Klerman basically states that we need to wait for further research on etiologies to become definitive.

Readers may recognize that I have already laid the groundwork of how to deal with this problem in previous chapters. The concept of reliability is straightforward, but the concept of validity is a bit murky. It is an epistemological assumption. Does a nosology "correspond" to a real disease in some one-to-one manner if it is valid? This is not something one can assume. Rather it is a thorny problem of epistemology with which philosophers continue to struggle. Unexamined, the concept of validity would seem to accept the notion that our nosologies "carve nature at its joints," an assumption that I tried to show is itself invalid in chapter 7. At best, our nosologies are something on the order of species, classifications of groups with similarities on many matters but with individual variations as well. The Darwinian notion of species best applies, as does the Weberian concept of an ideal type (see chapter 12). The diagnostic schema is an ideal paradigm of the underlying species. It is not true or false, in a Popperian sense, but more or less true or false, in a Peircean sense (see chapters 4 and 6). Controversies on this subject often come down to unexamined assumptions or commitments in epistemology or philosophy of science.

Klerman addresses the issue of the uniqueness of individual patients well:

> Most American psychiatrists, trained in the Meyerian tradition, have been reluctant to rely on diagnostic distinctions because of the acknowledged diversity of human attributes. Furthermore, in making clinical decisions about patients, diagnosis—reliable or not, valid or not—is only one criterion in decision-making. . . . A diagnosis alone is not sufficient to account for all decision-making; other attributes of the individual are crucial in the clinical context. No diagnostic system can encompass all these multiple attributes. The development of the multiaxial system represents a novel attempt to acknowledge this clinical experience. . . . For scientific investigation in medicine and psychiatry, the unit of investigation is the disorder, while for clinical practice the unit is the individual. (541)

Meyer had made exactly the same criticism of Kraepelin's nosology that many were making of DSM-III. One continues to hear this criticism today. Klerman's comment makes it clear that the developers of DSM-III were not unaware of this potential problem. He distinguishes between diagnosis and decision-making. A diagnosis is necessary, but not sufficient, for decision-making, he says. What old-fashioned Marxists would have called a "vulgar" version of DSM-III-ism would be to consider the nosology necessary and sufficient for clinical decision-making. Now most clinicians would not make such an assertion, but the question is whether clinicians *act* that way. In other words, does practice, in many settings, consist of listing symptoms, making a diagnosis, and then prescribing a treatment, without any further considerations? This frequently seems to happen, perhaps more in the era of managed care, when time limits (imposed by others or by oneself for financial gain) lead to less emphasis on individual differences among persons. Insurance agents are vulgar DSM-III-ists; they love lists and they love to apply them without ever knowing the person behind the list. But one cannot blame the developers of DSM-III for this problem. Managed care happened later. Nevertheless, DSM-IV, in the current economic climate in the United States, certainly can be misused.

One might distinguish between the makers of DSM-III, erudite people like

Klerman who clearly had thought through many of these issues, and the un-informed persons who apply DSM-IV crudely. This would be much like exon-erating Marx for the errors of Stalin or Hitler, or declaring Freud innocent of the excesses of his American heirs. "Moi, je ne suis pas Marxiste" (I am not a Marxist), Marx reportedly declared in trying to make the same distinction. Yet careful readers might note that I did not let the founders of biopsychosocial eclecticism, like Engel, off the hook on similar grounds. The excesses of the fol-lowers reflect on the master.

And, for all the awareness of the problem on the part of its makers, the DSM-III nosology lent, and lends, itself to serving as a dehumanizing system of la-bels, as Meyer warned, rather than a thoughtful nomenclature, as Klerman urged. I sympathize with Klerman and Spitzer and their colleagues, though. All in all, DSM-III and IV have done much more good than harm. The same can-not be said of Marxism, psychoanalytic orthodoxy, or, I fear, of the eclectic error.

Klerman's last sentence above also makes an important point, to which I will return below. He suggests that research and clinical practice may require two different nosologies. I think one of the reasons there is so much conflict around the current nosology is that Klerman and Spitzer and colleagues tried to meet these two purposes in one nosology. But experience now suggests that perhaps we need two or more nosologies (see below).

Klerman concludes on a pluralist note, derived almost word for word from the work of Leston Havens, whom he knew well:

> Part of the strength of American psychiatry has been the existence of many com-peting schools: psychoanalytic, interpersonal, behavioral, biological, existential. These schools have not only been our strength but at times have contributed to our weakness. We seem to spend more time fighting ideological battles than gen-erating data. . . . This debate is already an anachronism. . . . I invite our colleagues to acknowledge the achievements of DSM-III and to join with us in gathering data based on science to revise it—on to DSM-IV! (542)

The reference to pluralistic schools of thought is encouraging, and it sug-gests that Klerman perhaps approached his support for the DSM-III nosology from a pluralistic conceptual base. I think this may well be true. Yet later in the debate, his opponents, particularly Michels, claimed to defend the pluralism of American psychiatry and argued that DSM-III was a one-sided view that did violence to the plural views in the field. Michels's critique consists of the com-mon, and dangerous, confusion of pluralism with eclecticism, as we will see.

3.

The psychoanalyst Robert Michels made a powerful rebuttal:

I hope that whatever happens in this debate, we do not lose all that is of value in American psychiatry that does not fit in 300 pages of operational criteria. . . . In constructing a nosology, we must first decide whether we want to define the domain of the discussion as that which we can describe precisely or that which we believe to be relevant. DSM-III opts for the former. If this criterion for DSM-III had been employed in 1850, we would not have developed the concept of dementia praecox or schizophrenia by 1950; the initial formulation was too unreliable. The heterogeneity of our field is a potent argument for including, not excluding, a variety of concepts and ideas when developing nosology. (548)

I consider this to be Michels's most valid point, and this point is a general one about empiricism. It is the question of precision versus relevance. As I mentioned in chapter 4 on scientific method, one definition of scientific method insists that it include empirically testable hypotheses. However, some hypotheses are certainly very difficult, if not impossible, to test empirically. Those related to subjective states, as in psychiatry, are especially difficult to test objectively in the external world. What should we do with these subjective states and the hypotheses that involve them? Should we simply exclude them from the field of psychiatry, or perhaps include them but deny them any scientific validity (instead asserting that they are value judgments)? If we exclude them, we are in danger of creating what Michels calls "mindless psychiatry." If we say nothing or little about subjective states, psychiatry as a field would lose a great deal of relevance to what patients experience and for which they want assistance: their subjective states.

This process indeed seems to have taken place with the evolution of DSM-IV in the United States. In 1992, ten years after the Toronto debate, the psychiatrist Herman van Praag argued that Michels's concern had come true.

According to van Praag, DSM-III led to objectification: "coarsening of diagnosis; preoccupation with the obvious . . . oversimplification." He continued:

The DSM-III system and the psychometric instruments in use provide no more than rough-draft diagnoses, lacking not only detail and finesse but also disregarding elements essential for proper diagnosis, namely those that are subjective. A painting by Vermeer in which the blues have been left out may be Vermeer-like,

but it is not a Vermeer. Similarly, a rough-draft diagnosis, omitting important subjective components, provides not much more than a global diagnostic outline.
The preoccupation with the objective did not subside over the years; on the contrary, it seems to have intensified. It is no longer seen as a transitory phase on the
way to greater diagnostic refinement, but as an end-point. The so-called subjective is not seen as territory still to be conquered, using empirical methods, and has
become synonymous with non-operational, non-measurable, non-quantifiable—
a symbol of soft science at best. (1992, 266)

Back to Michels in 1982, as he tries to explain the origins of this problem in
DSM-III:

> The designers of DSM-III confused two fundamentally different tasks. One is de-
> ciding what the nomenclature is about, defining its goals, and developing the hi-
> erarchy of principles and values that will generate it. The other is implementing
> those goals in a specific nomenclature. They did a superb job of implementing a
> set of goals. The problem stems from the way in which they selected the goals.
> They never established what goals the profession wanted. They acted as if these
> goals were clear, and they proceeded to substitute the goals of the small and non-
> representative group who had a special interest in methodology and nosology for
> the goals and values of the entire profession. A recent paper has referred to this
> group as an invisible college. . . . True, it is a brilliant and productive one. . . . It
> has made important contributions to our thinking, but it represents only one way
> of thinking. The purpose of a nomenclature is to allow the profession as a whole
> to think, study, treat, and work together. (Klerman et al. 1984, 548–49)

Michels is making an eclectic, and potentially a pluralist, critique of the
DSM-III method. I of course agree with the general idea, but the designers of
DSM-III would likely respond again that they view their approach as simply
one attempt at a nomenclature, and not the only one. Yet, from a political perspective, there is no doubt that the imprimatur of the American Psychiatric Association and the economic use of the nomenclature for insurance purposes,
among others, have lent a special strength to DSM-III compared to other potential nosologies.

Michels goes on to make his eclectic leanings clear: "[DSM-III] moved back
to a narrow hyper-Kraepelinism, not really a neo-Kraepelinism but rather a version of Kraepelin that would have made Kraepelin himself quite uncomfortable. It is less interested than Kraepelin in patients as people, less interested

than Kraepelin in their lives and their experiences. . . . Modern psychiatry uses a biopsychosocial framework. Although it has been asserted that DSM-III reflects that biopsychosocial frame . . . there is virtually no room for psyche except in the form of disease" (549).

It is not clear to me that Michels is right here; he seems to have an idealized version of Kraepelin in mind. But the term *hyper-Kraepelinism* strikes a chord that does not seem too out of tune with some aspects of the evolution of DSM-III and beyond. In fact, as discussed above, Kraepelin was certainly no biopsychosocialist, and he was very committed to a biological framework to understand at least major psychoses. Yet it is true that the mature Kraepelin was more of a lumper than the designers of DSM-III were. It seems likely, however, as Robert Spitzer asserts in his rebuttal, that this was not simply a matter of choice on the part of the DSM-III committee:

> The essential fact is that we did not insist that there be evidence that a diagnostic category was reliable before it could be included in the classification. In fact, our basic concern was clinical relevance. The principle that we finally evolved was that if a group of clinicians believed that a clinical syndrome was important to their work—regardless of their theoretical view as to how the condition developed—we said, "Fine, we will work with you to make that category as descriptively accurate as possible, with the hope that it will be reliable, and we will include that category in the classification." . . . What was the reaction of this so-called neo-Kraepelinian group to including these categories in DSM-III? Many of them thought it was a big mistake. . . . However, eventually this neo-Kraepelinian group and the other task force members were convinced that the pluralistic nature of American psychiatry requires that these categories be in the classification. And they are. (552)

Spitzer is trying to explain the political aspects of the development of DSM-III. David Healy (1998, 235–37) has examined the political factors related to including the diagnosis of dysthymia, which van Praag (1993b), for example, often criticized as an unreliable entity that overlapped excessively with other conditions. Healy makes the point that the more Kraepelinian members of the committee wanted to include only "major depression" as a depressive diagnosis. Yet apparently, as the draft of DSM-III progressed, psychoanalytic interest groups became concerned that their bread-and-butter diagnosis, neurotic depression, was not captured by the criteria for major depression. Dysthymia was the political compromise that ensued. These political aspects of DSM-III should not be discounted. Whatever the wishes of the committee, their draft was not the DSM-III that was eventually published. Their draft had to go through other committees of the American Psychiatric Association, and then it had to be voted upon by its assembly, and it was altered along the way. Hence, DSM-III is partially the document created by the task force and partially the product of institutional compromises among interest groups in psychiatry. This process explains some of the differing and overlapping categories one finds in it.

Michels finishes by expressing a concern about the impact of DSM-III on psychiatric teaching:

> In teaching psychiatry one teaches concepts, not criteria. We want to give our students some sense of a big picture. What is the big picture provided by DSM-III, the tune you whistle after the show is over? I still remember the distinctions between psychosis, neurosis, and personality disorder that I learned in medical school. . . . The goal should not have been to make DSM-III as good as possible, but rather to make DSM-III as facilitating of the growth of psychiatry as possible. (550)

Spitzer's response:

> Dr. Michels has asked, What is the tune? What is the theme that a student might get from DSM-III? Students can misuse anything, and we certainly acknowledge that there is a danger that a student reading DSM-III might think that that is all there is to psychiatry. But it seems to me that there are some themes to DSM-III that make for memorable tunes. One theme is that we do not know everything about these disorders, and we know less than we wish we knew. Another theme is that when we talk to each other, we ought to use the same language in a way that really communicates. DSM-I and DSM-II did not do that very well. So I think there is a tune that the student learns from DSM-III, and it is a happy tune as well. (553)

I am sympathetic to Spitzer's response, but unfortunately many persons view DSM-IV as the "bible" of psychiatry, with a reverence similar to that usually reserved for revelation, rather than as a set of hypotheses that emphasize how much we do not know, as Spitzer wished.

I will let Michels finish his critique, where he ends with a flourish that has become oft-quoted:

> There was an error made several decades ago by another invisible college, the invisible college of psychoanalytic psychiatrists. Their error was not that they were interested in the mind and its workings—that was a brilliant contribution to

American and world psychiatry. Their error was that they failed to be interested in the social and biological as well as the psychological determinants of mental illness. DSM-III does not correct that error; it repeats it. Dr. Spitzer and his group have led us from the brainless psychiatry of the 1950s to the threat of a mindless psychiatry of the 1980s. We await the integration. (550–51)

Michels is dancing around some of the terms that I have brought together in the first chapter of this book as the methods of psychiatry. The force of Michels's critique is that DSM-III is reductionist, that it is not eclectic enough, and further, that psychiatry needed an integration of the psychoanalytic and biological/Kraepelinian approaches. The basic thrust of Spitzer's response was that DSM-III was indeed eclectic enough and that it represented a practical integration of different approaches in psychiatry. Although both used the word *pluralist,* neither meant by pluralism the definition I have given it in this book (or that derived from Jaspers, Havens, or McHugh and Slavney).

In reality, DSM-III was eclectic in its intentions and its content, and it has furthered the biopsychosocial eclecticism that has become part of the mainstream in psychiatry. The critiques of Michels and Vaillant (who mainly argued that DSM-III was "parochial," "reductionistic," and "adynamic" [542–44]) really represented a wish that DSM-III were even less amenable to biological approaches in psychiatry. This, it seems to me, was basically a reflexive reaction of psychoanalytic powers in the profession. Yet some of their critical predictions appear to have come true, and, to the extent that DSM-III evolved, it did so reductionistically in some ways that are harmful. Consequently, there are at least these three features of the evolution of our current nosology: first, it was powerful and helpful as an empirical approach to psychiatry, using that method well in a pluralistic sense, as in the refinement of the concept of schizophrenia compared to DSM-II; second, much of it (probably the parts that were most reflective of political compromise) is too eclectic and has led to confusion and lack of purpose in the profession; third, other parts of it have been interpreted reductionistically by many who forget that the nosology is meant to be heuristic rather than to reflect reality, a process rather than a conclusion.

This evolution of psychiatric nosology is an important aspect of the current state of psychiatry, and I will now turn to current representative perspectives on this topic from important thinkers in the field.

4.

Kenneth Kendler is one of the most thoughtful and prolific researchers in psychiatry today. His papers are among the most cited in the profession, and arguably they have had the most influence on discussions of nosology (Kendler and Walsh 1998; Kendler 1990; Kendler, Glazer, and Morgenstern 1983). Kendler is a psychiatrist who, along with his geneticist colleague Lyndon Eaves and others, has been a trailblazer in the field of psychiatric genetics (Eaves, Eysenck, and Martin 1989).[4] Because of his important contributions, Kendler is widely respected in the field and can be seen as something of a mainstream thinker in psychiatry today. This appellation again has to do with the respect he commands as a result of his work, not any political position he holds. Thus it was not inconsequential when he published a thoughtful paper in 1990 in the *Archives of General Psychiatry*, entitled "Toward a Scientific Psychiatric Nosology."

Kendler distinguishes two basic approaches to nosology in psychiatry in the past: "the great professor principle" and "the consensus of experts" (1990, 969). He contrasts these with what he hopes will be "scientific nosology" in the future. The great professor principle held sway before DSM-III in 1980. At first, Kraepelin's views were dominant because of his enormous influence; then Kraepelin was replaced by Freud and Meyer. With DSM-III, a group consensus of "experts," researchers and epidemiologists and political leaders, replaced reliance on the ideology of a great professor. The consensus of experts had advantages compared to the great professor principle, but it, too, was not scientific. By *scientific*, Kendler means a nosology that is based on "empirically testable hypotheses" (970) (see chapter 4).

Kendler's essay, without citing Jaspers or espousing pluralism per se, is an excellent example of the pluralistic approach to psychiatry in action. He goes on to discuss the strengths *and the limits* of a scientific nosology, just as Jaspers would have done. The strengths come first:

> The concept of a scientific nosology . . . offers the prospect of a single clear criterion by which proposed nosologic changes can be evaluated. . . . Second, a nosology based on empirical data would be buttressed against fluctuating changes in nosologic "fashion." . . . A third virtue of a scientific nosology is that it would keep us honest; that is, the application of scientific principles to psychiatric nosology should both clarify what we do know and outline what we do not know. By so

doing, the method should give us increased confidence in those nosologic areas where our knowledge is substantial and prevent premature reification of ideas in areas where that knowledge is meager. (1990, 970)

Then the limitations:

> These include (1) the potential exclusion from the nosologic process of historical tradition, clinical experience, and the realms of psychiatric practice that are less amenable to scientific study (intrapsychic factors); (2) the undesirability of complex criteria, even if they have the greatest reliability or validity, because of difficulties in learning and retaining them; (3) the need for complete diagnostic coverage and hence for individual categories for which no validating evidence exists; and (4) the need for a nosologic system that serves administrative purposes unrelated to scientific issues. (970)

Although these are important limitations, they are essentially practical ones, and Kendler focuses on others which are "inherent" to an empirical approach to psychiatric nosology. The first is the problem of construct validity. Kendler argues that if there is disagreement about the construct or "key defining features" of a diagnosis, then empirical testing cannot occur. For instance, since Kraepelin viewed dementia praecox as an illness *essentially* characterized by a chronic declining course, the course of illness would be a key validator of the diagnosis. Yet this logic is circular. If someone else had a different view of the illness, in which declining course was not an essential feature, then the course of illness would not be a key validator. So Kendler argues that there is no way to empirically test this question: "Therefore, one important limitation of a scientific nosology is that it cannot address the validity of a psychiatric disorder where there is disagreement about its proper construct. That is, data can only provide an answer if there is agreement about what the question is. . . . Empirical data *cannot* determine which . . . [of two constructs] is better, for this decision is essentially a value judgment as to which construct of the disorder is more conceptually appealing" (970–71).

Kendler's essay is carefully reasoned up to this point, but unfortunately I fear that Kendler has committed the essentialist error here (see chapter 7). He views diagnoses as containing essential properties, and if we disagree about those essential properties, he sees no way around those disagreements. Things then come down to aesthetic ("appealing") and personal ("value judgment") beliefs (1990, 972). Now, value judgments are involved in nosology, no doubt, as we discussed in chapter 10, since ethics are intertwined with medical practice in general. However, Kendler's use of this ethical and aesthetic terminology has an idiosyncratic flavor that would appear to make a truly scientific nosology quite unlikely. Of course, much hinges on the meaning of the term *scientific*, which I have discussed in detail in chapters 4 and 6. But what I want to focus on here is the essentialist problem, which rears its head again now.

There is no need to assert that any criteria or defining features are essential to the definition of any diagnosis. All criteria for all diagnoses are, in principle, changeable and liable to empirical support or refutation. As discussed in regard to species, diagnoses do not carve nature at the joints but rather represent constellations of individuals with differing features. Diagnoses are populations of such individuals and do not possess any essential or unchanging characteristics. Diagnoses possess characteristics that are more or less common, but none that are essential. To the extent that diagnoses represent classic presentations, they are merely abstractions from the real, ideal types in Jaspers's terminology (see chapter 12), and thus not real entities.

So Kendler's dilemma of disagreements about essential characteristics is based on an epistemological mistake, the essentialist error of thinking that there are such things as essential characteristics. That is not the case in biology, and it is not the case in medicine.

Rather, I think Kendler's argument might be made in a modified form in relation to the validators of diagnoses. In general medicine, it is now accepted that the ultimate validator is tissue pathology, or some similar laboratory specimen (a bacterial growth, for instance). One might argue that this belief, that tissue pathology is a diagnostic validator, must be agreed upon before any empirical assessments of medical diagnoses can be made. If physicians disagreed about this fact, we would seem to have a potentially nonempirical problem at the very root of medical nosology, along the lines Kendler suggests. As I discuss in chapter 13, Robins and Guze have proposed four basic validators for psychiatric diagnoses in the absence of tissue pathology: symptoms, course, genetics, and treatment response (or other laboratory or biological markers). Here again, one could make Kendler's argument: if psychiatrists cannot agree, for instance, on whether genetics or course are viable diagnostic validators, then we would not use empirical data gathered in those fields to assess the validity of a diagnosis.

Yet I do not find serious arguments, either logical or conceptual or empirical, that these four validators of diagnosis are not useful. The weakest seems to be treatment response, and, in fact, one could avoid or limit the use of that validator without losing much in the way of empirical data based on the other validators for a scientific psychiatric nosology. But in general, these validators are commonly accepted and are in line with medical and scientific tradition.

The key question, then, it seems to me, is not which validators are appropriate, since these validators seem reasonable, but rather, Do the validators all point in the same direction? Just as, in a general pluralistic model of psychiatry, one needs to use different methods because of their inherent limitations, so, too, one needs to use different validators because of their inherent limitations. None is perfect. The key is that the validators should all point in the same direction. They should agree with each other so as to suggest a real diagnostic entity that they outline.

Therefore, in the case of schizophrenia, it is indeed circular logic to define the illness as one with a declining course and then to use course data to validate it. But if one also has viable genetic and symptom and treatment data suggesting that the same group of patients is picked out by those criteria as by the course criterion, then the overall definition would seem more likely to be valid.

This brings us to the next limitation of a scientific nosology that Kendler describes: "What if the different validators do not agree?" Kendler's example involves different definitions of subtypes of schizophrenia, some of which better predict outcome and others of which better agree with genetic studies. So which criteria are superior, those that better match outcome or those that better match genetics? Although this problem can be difficult, if it occurs, I would suggest that it likely represents diagnostic definitions that are not sufficiently valid. The more valid the diagnosis, the less likely that different validators will disagree.

Kendler ends with a brief comment on the reliability-versus-validity conundrum, which was brought up repeatedly in the 1982 Toronto symposium. The reader will recall that the critics of DSM-III (Michels and Vaillant) argued that it sacrificed validity for reliability, and the proponents of DSM-III (Klerman and Spitzer) argued that reliability was a necessary precursor to validity. Kendler comments that the emphasis on reliability, which privileges more objective factors in diagnosis, is also a value judgment. Yet it seems to me that Klerman and Spitzer had a point. How could one know whether something is valid, in an empirical sense, if one could not use empirical scientific methods? Reliability simply means that different observers agree on the same terms; this would seem to be a necessity before any scientific research could be conducted.

Kendler's comment might be more relevant if we think about Jaspers's distinction between causal explanation and meaningful understanding. When we are engaged in causal explanatory approaches, that is, empirical psychiatry, reliability is needed; no validity can be shown without prior reliability. However, if we are engaged in attempting to meaningfully understand the thoughts or feelings of a single patient, then reliability is less relevant and in some cases may be unnecessary. As I discussed in chapter 6, though, meaningful understanding does not mean that empirical methods are completely put aside. Instead, standard empirical methods are simply more difficult to apply, and more limited in use, when we are engaged in meaningful understanding. In general, then, reliability is important and usually necessary in psychiatric methods. Hence, I think the importance of reliability is not simply a value judgment in any arbitrary sense.

Kendler concludes with reasonable comments along the lines of Jaspers's views:

> We need to guard against exaggerating the potential impact of science on our nosology. Many important nosologic questions in psychiatry are *fundamentally* nonempirical. As psychiatry takes up the "banner" of a scientific nosology, we must take care not to promise more than we can deliver. . . . We should not in our enthusiasm overlook the inherent limitations of the empirical method. There is a danger that this process will degenerate into pseudoscience, in which we pretend to be "objective" and "empirical" when, in reality, we are making informed value judgments. The fundamental problem is that the scientific method can only answer "little" questions. . . . By contrast, in nosology, we need answers to "big questions." . . . In many cases, obtaining answers to the little questions will not provide unambiguous answers to the big questions. Before the answers to the little questions can be applied to the big questions, there is an important intervening step. This step often requires answers to other sorts of questions that are usually nonempirical. (1990, 972)

Kendler's methodological caution is laudable and is in keeping with much of my discussion in previous chapters. Nonetheless, as I explain above, the specific issues he raises do not seem to me to be *fundamentally* nonempirical. Kendler's emphasis on applying the scientific method to the "little questions" would seem to reflect a Popperian influence, skepticism toward large theories. However, again, Darwinian theory in biology, as well as other large theories in physics and other fields, may belie excessive caution on this topic. A

Peircean approach would emphasize how consensus gradually can be obtained empirically, not, to be sure, in an absolute manner, but nonetheless sufficiently.

5.

Another important thinker regarding psychiatric nosology is the psychiatrist Hermann van Praag. Van Praag was one of the early biologically oriented psychiatrists in the 1960s, but as he saw the field move in the biological direction in the 1970s and 1980s, he strongly warned against certain excesses and misconceptions (most prominently in his 1993 book *"Make-Believes" in Psychiatry* [1993b]).

Van Praag's concerns stem from a few observations. First, he notes that biological research in psychiatry has not progressed far. He attributes this lack of progress to the lack of diagnostic specificity. In other words, we have not been able to identify clear biological bases for specific psychiatric disorders because our definitions of those disorders are not valid (1993a). To use the phrase I emphasized in chapter 7, van Praag is saying that since our biological research is not finding etiologies for our proposed diagnoses, those diagnoses are not carving nature at its joints. Van Praag is very concerned about this problem, and he proposes an alternative approach to nosology in psychiatry, which I will discuss soon. However, readers will note that our discussion in chapter 7 allows us to conclude that this problem of not carving nature at its joints is not unique to psychiatry and that in fact it is not a serious problem for psychiatric nosology. That is just the way things are; species definitions do not carve nature at its joints either. Yet definitions of species, or diagnoses, can still be accurate representations of the realities of nature, with their commonalities and their variabilities. Although van Praag may be right in asserting that our nosology *may be* invalid owing to the lack of clear biological confirmations of it, he is not right, I suggest, in implying that the current nosology *must be* invalid owing to this problem.

A corollary is that van Praag is rather unhappy with what he calls the "choice" method of diagnosis used in DSM-III and beyond (van Praag 1997). In this approach, a patient needs to have *x* of *y* criteria for an illness, and thus two patients may meet criteria for the same diagnosis while meeting somewhat different criteria. Van Praag is again concerned that this approach introduces too much heterogeneity into psychiatric diagnosis, making biological research that much more difficult (1996). He may have a point, but it seems to me unrealistic to think that we can make diagnoses in groups of patients *without any overlap*. In this assumption, I think van Praag is committing the essentialist error, looking for necessary and pathognomonic criteria only, whereas the biological reality is otherwise (see chapter 7). Similar critiques of heterogeneity are made by psychiatric geneticists, on the same grounds as those proposed by van Praag, but again I think such views should be carefully examined so as to avoid overly essentialist assumptions (see below).

I have previously discussed van Praag's critique of an overly objective approach to psychiatry, with which I largely agree (van Praag 1992). There is more to van Praag's extensive views on this subject, including his discussion of how the occurrence of comorbidities may simply reflect a poor nosology that fails to distinguish conditions well. Van Praag also coined the term *nosologomania* (1992) to emphasize the excessively "splitting" approach taken in successive revisions of DSM, with more and more diagnoses added to an already long list. He points out (1997) that DSM-I (1954) contained 106 diagnoses, DSM-II (1968) contained 182, DSM-III-R (1987), 292, and DSM-IV (1994), 297. His question is, Do we really need 297 diagnoses in psychiatry. Can we even fully validate one or two, much less almost 300?

Van Praag's critique of nosologomania should be placed in the context of the Toronto symposium. Readers will note that DSM-III and later editions, though they markedly increased the number of diagnoses, were not nosologies that came from strictly one perspective (such as an empirical neo-Kraepelinian orientation). Rather, all these nosologies are compromises that are affected by political and administrative considerations, or, as Kendler emphasizes, "value-judgments." One cannot with historical justification blame this nosologomania on the Kraepelinian approach to psychiatric diagnosis. In fact, as I discussed above, the neo-Kraepelinians involved with DSM-IV wanted to have few diagnoses. Indeed, the classic neo-Kraepelinian text written by leaders of the neo-Kraepelinian movement from Washington University at St. Louis, *Psychiatric Diagnosis* (Goodwin and Guze [1974] 1989), sought to describe only those diagnoses that had significant empirical support and was limited to chapters on the following topics in its last edition: affective disorders, schizophrenic disorders, panic disorder, hysteria, obsessive-compulsive disorder, phobic disorders, alcoholism, drug dependence, sociopathy, brain syndrome, and anorexia nervosa. These are eleven diagnostic categories. The authors, Donald Goodwin and Samuel Guze, make the point that they are not interested in more diagnoses, while at the same time revealing their Kraepelinian assumptions: "[This book] takes the position that only about a dozen diagnostic entities in adult psychiatry have been sufficiently studied to be useful. . . . In choosing these categories, the guiding rule was: diagnosis is prognosis. There are many diagnostic categories in psychiatry, but few are based on a clinical literature where the conditions are defined by explicit criteria and follow-up studies provide a guide to prognosis. . . . Not every patient can be diagnosed using the categories in this book. For the word 'undiagnosed' is, we feel, more appropriate than a label incorrectly implying more knowledge than exists" (viii–xi).

The nosologomania of DSM-III and beyond does not have to do with Kraepelinian ideology (in fact the mature Kraepelin was a great "lumper" rather than a "splitter"), but with the fact that the DSM schemas are trying to serve too many masters. They are being used for research, biological studies, genetics, administrative record-keeping, and insurance payments in private practice as well as government-funded settings. These are too many and too different purposes.

To accommodate these different purposes, it may be best to have multiple psychiatric nosologies, and this is what van Praag suggests when he recommends a "two-tier" system of psychiatric nosology (1990). The first tier is the standard DSM system, an inadequately valid system of many diagnoses, which is not very useful for biological research or treatment but which is useful for administrative and insurance (economic) needs of practicing clinicians. The second tier would consist of what van Praag calls "functional psychopathology." Here van Praag is referring to the lack of association between DSM diagnoses and biological findings. Van Praag reviews some evidence that links biological findings to psychopathological states, which then underlie different diagnoses. For instance, the psychopathological state of disturbed regulation of anxiety and aggression underlies many depressive syndromes, as well as other conditions. And the psychopathological state of disturbed regulation of mood but not anxiety and aggression produces a depressive diagnosis with a different biological basis than other depressive diagnoses.

The views of van Praag have not been commonly accepted in psychiatry, yet it seems to me that they are creative and have great potential. In bipolar disorder research, for instance, biological studies tend to find a great deal of relevance of mechanisms of recurrence (the tendency for episodes to repeat themselves) and the psychopathological state of impulsivity (Swann et al. 2002). These two features are likely to be important findings in biological research in bipolar disorder. However, the current DSM-IV nosology is entirely focused on polarity (is mania ever present or not?). If we take into account the psycho-pathological states that underlie our diagnoses, we may alter our diagnostic definitions so as to be more in line with the biology of these illnesses, but even if we do not wish to alter our nosology, it may still be useful to have a way of talking about psychiatric conditions that takes into account the underlying biology. Another example is psychosis. It is now a well-established fact that the biology of a psychotic episode is little different in many ways whether the episode is occurring as part of schizophrenia, bipolar disorder, unipolar major depression, or indeed perhaps other conditions (e.g., drug-induced psychosis). In all these cases, the biological findings include elevated cortisol levels in the blood and urine, for instance. Does this finding mean that all psychotic illnesses should become one large diagnosis (Crow 1990)? Or, if we grant other reasons to distinguish between schizophrenia and bipolar disorder, would it not make sense to also allow for similarities biologically related to the underlying psychopathology of psychosis?

In other words, the points that van Praag makes, with which I agree, are (1) that we need to pay attention to the underlying psychopathology (and its biological correlates) of psychiatric diagnoses and (2) that there is no special reason to try to stay with only one approach to psychiatric nosology. In fact, multiple approaches for multiple purposes would make sense, as long as we are always clear about what our purpose is when we are using a specific diagnosis. This approach is consistent with, and implied by, the general pluralist model of psychiatry that I am advocating in this book.

6.

Other recent discussions of psychiatric nosology are consistent with some of the themes I have just mentioned. There is growing interest in the psychiatric genetics community in the formulation of a "psychiatric genetic nosology" (Tsuang, Faraone, and Lyons 1993). This would be based on genetic findings and would be designed to maximally promote genetic studies. Thus, it is generally thought that such a psychiatric genetic nosology would tend to be quite homogeneous, trying to find the most classic phenotypes of our diagnostic categories so as to maximize the ability of geneticists to identify and replicate the identification of specific genes for those conditions.

The psychiatrist Assen Jablensky has recently offered a careful analysis of these issues, which I think highlights the relevance of a pluralist nosology

(1999). Jablensky begins by emphasizing the different purposes of psychiatric nosology. On one hand, we seek to classify diseases; on the other hand, we seek to treat people. We cannot avoid the fact, however, that psychiatric symptoms, used to classify disease, are based on the behaviors of individual persons. Hence, following previous suggestions by Essen-Moller, Jablensky argues for "a system of double diagnosis, one of etiology and one of syndrome" (140). This is similar to van Praag's call (1990) for two tiers of diagnosing, one clinical and one biological, as well as the recent proposals for a psychiatric genetic nosology (Tsuang, Faraone, and Lyons 1993). Jablensky then makes a wonderful analogy: "Perhaps the closest analogue to current psychiatric classifications can be found in the so-called indigenous or 'folk' classifications of living things (e.g., animals in traditional rural cultures) or other material objects. 'Folk' classifications do not consist of mutually exclusive categories and have no single rule of hierarchy. . . . Such naturalistic systems seem to retain their usefulness alongside the more rigorous scientific classifications because they are pragmatic and well adapted to the needs of everyday life" (1999, 143).

Readers of chapter 2 will note the analogy to discussions of folk psychology among philosophers of mind. One can think of DSM-III and beyond as a kind of folk psychiatry, without being in any sense pejorative. Again, keeping in mind the basic pluralistic maxim that all methods have both limits and strengths, the DSM-III nosology had the advantage of being a highly useful and pragmatically helpful folk nosology. It has not proved as useful for biological or genetic research. Thus, alternative adaptations of DSM-IV for those purposes would make sense, without seeking to replace the current DSM-IV nosology, which has its own clinical and administrative uses.[5]

7.

Why is there dissatisfaction with DSM-IV? It was there with the introduction of DSM-III, too. Although many agree that much progress has been made, there is a distinct sense of unease among many clinicians regarding the DSM system.

Jablensky suggests one problem, which I think underlies the concerns of many persons: the problem of "reification." The problem of reification is best illustrated by a recent conversation I had with psychiatrists in the Canadian province of Quebec. These clinicians, one or two generations older than I, were French-speaking and heavily influenced by French traditions in psychiatry.

Some of them had, in fact, studied in France in the 1950s and 1960s during the heyday of famous teachers such as Henri Ey, Jean DeLay, and Jacques Lacan. These French Canadian clinicians emphasized the extreme attention to detail in psychiatric symptoms that they were taught by these teachers. The textbook of Henri Ey, for instance, which I do not believe is yet translated into English, consists of very detailed descriptions of psychiatric syndromes, covering 1,015 pages. Yet, since the introduction of DSM-III in 1980, according to the French Canadians, few new psychiatrists study Ey's text; instead, they rely *almost entirely* on the categories and descriptions of DSM-IV for their knowledge of psychiatric nosology. Leaving aside the specific merits or demerits of Ey's text, this observation runs counter to the professed intentions of the formulators and proponents of DSM-III, as reviewed above. But if the proponents of DSM-III did not want this reification to happen, and the opponents of DSM-III did not want it to happen, why did it happen?

Let's define reification first. The idea goes back to Karl Marx and refers to treating an entity as a thing when it is not in fact a thing. For instance, the private marketplace for books treats me as a thing (a writer or a reader), though I am not simply a writer or a reader. In the case of psychiatric nosology, reification means that we treat our diagnoses as things, as objective realities, as entities that are proved and fixed. DSM-III was not meant to be seen this way. It was supposed to represent hypotheses, somewhat proved and somewhat unproved, that were reliably defined so as to be further studied and later further refined, proved, or disproved. Instead, as Jablensky wrote, there is "a dulling of the natural interest in exploring variations in the clinical phenomena, studying atypical forms of illness, or describing new syndromes" (1999, 142). He continues later: "It is almost certain that DSM-IV and ICD-10 do not represent classifications in the usual sense in which the term is applied in biology. Essentially, they are augmented nomenclatures (i.e., lists of names for conditions or behaviors, supplied with explicit rules as to how these names should be assigned). As such, they are useful tools of communication and can play an important role in psychiatric research, clinical management, and teaching. However, it is essential that neither DSM-IV nor ICD-10 be perceived as a complete, closed system of validated diagnostic entities in psychiatry" (143). Yet this is happening. Reification is a reality in psychiatric practice and research. Given that almost no one claims to support it, why is this the case?

One reason has to do with the problem of the multiple purposes of our nosology. As a researcher, I might be quite willing to view DSM-IV diagnoses as hypotheses, which might be better proved or disproved in the future. However, as a clinician, I might be concerned if the diagnostic label that allows me to be paid by an insurance company is no longer valid next year. This might mean that a large proportion of my patients would no longer be able to pay me for my clinical work. In reality, I would likely search for another diagnostic label, which would make payment of my fees possible. If I were an administrator in an insurance company, I might be upset by hearing that the entities for which I was paying money were only hypotheses and that they might not be real at all. As a hospital administrator, if I have to explain to my supervisors how many patients with various diagnoses are admitted and discharged each year, frequent changes in the diagnostic labels would make my job more difficult and my data harder to interpret. Therefore, when diagnoses are made for insurance payment or administrative labeling, reification is encouraged.

Another, perhaps more basic, reason why reification has happened may have to do with one of the basic themes of this book: the ideology of psychoanalysis was displaced by DSM-III, but the eclectic compromise that followed does not provide much guidance to new trainees or others in the field. Many clinicians, especially new trainees, are seeking another ideology, and a reified DSM-III can be such an ideology. What these clinicians need to realize is that there is another alternative, a pluralistic model of psychiatry that provides guidance, like the ideologies, but which is not itself an ideology. Since this pluralistic approach is not well understood in psychiatry and rarely implemented, many clinicians lapse into dogmatism. The reification of DSM-III and beyond is perhaps the most prominent indication of the bankruptcy of eclecticism and the resurgence of dogmatism.

Another factor, also important though less difficult to establish, is cultural. It probably was not inconsequential that DSM-III was proposed by the American Psychiatric Association and that this nosology was implemented in 1980. A similar nosology proposed in Australia, or East Asia, or Latin America likely would not have had such an impact. The last few decades have been a period of Pax Americana politically, and American culture has undoubtedly influenced the world, not only in the categories of movies and clothes but also in science and medicine. This impact has not been avoided in psychiatry. Many clinicians, such as those I mentioned in Quebec, who were previously influenced by the French tradition, assume that American approaches are especially valid. It has been my experience in the Middle East, even in countries like Iran, where American culture is ambivalently viewed, that American views in medicine and psychiatry are taken almost too seriously. The standard texts (such as Kaplan and Sadock's *Textbook of Psychiatry* [Sadock and Sadock 2000]) are studied with an almost religious devotion, and the DSM nosology is considered the first and last word, meant to be memorized and implemented. Even if the American nosologists did not intend it, DSM-III and beyond have indeed become a reified system, rather than a flexible nosology.

8.

In summary, the diagnostic changes marked by DSM-III in 1980 constituted, in large part, an advance over the psychoanalytic dogmatisms of the past. However, despite this progress, further revisions of DSM-IV have not progressed with as much empirical validation as was initially hoped. Further, the DSM-III and later nosologies have not proved capable of supporting as much progress in biological and genetic research as was expected. Lastly, an unfortunate consequence of the advantages of DSM-III, and its acceptance in the U.S. psychiatric establishment, is that DSM-IV has become reified by many clinicians and in many countries as the final diagnostic word, rather than as an early set of hypotheses. At the same time, the number of psychiatric diagnoses has ballooned, probably partly because of the multiple purposes of different groups who wish to use a diagnostic label. I suggest that the limitations of the current DSM-IV nosology can be best handled by a stronger adherence to an avowedly pluralistic model of psychiatry (rather than the attempt to be eclectically "atheoretical"). Multiple nosologies for multiple purposes make sense, and clinicians and new trainees need to be carefully instructed in the rationale for treating DSM-IV as a set of testable hypotheses, always a work in progress, rather than as a closed system of validated entities. To emphasize this last point, I think it can also be useful to think of the classic DSM-IV categories as what Jaspers, following Weber, called ideal types; I will flesh out this idea in the next chapter.

CHAPTER 12

A Theory of DSM-IV

Ideal Types

> Kraepelin's manic-depressive insanity and dementia praecox are very important groups of cases, which do not, however, exhaust the material that presents itself to us. His types had best be used as paradigms.
>
> —ADOLF MEYER, 1906

1.

The DSM system in psychiatry is a convenient straw man for all sides of the diagnostic discussion. Even by its name, DSM-IV seems like the kind of arid cookbook approach to human beings that produces shudders in our collective humanistic spines. Why should we categorize the richness of humanity into these labels? And on what basis?

On the face of it, the whole enterprise appears questionable to many. A committee of psychiatrists, bureaucrats, and academics who belong to a guild (the American Psychiatric Association) get together behind closed doors and decide which symptoms, and how many, are to define the various diagnoses. *Schizophrenia* is a label given to someone with a certain number of psychotic symptoms; *depression* is the diagnosis for a person who displays four out of eight mood symptoms for two weeks; it is *mania* if the patient has three out of seven symptoms for one week. Why those numbers of symptoms? Why those durations? Why those specific symptoms?

The suspicion exists among some critics that the process is arbitrary. The thought is that these members of an elite are defining illness for their own social, economic, or political purposes. This all seems a far cry from "real" medicine, where a scalpel and a microscope are expected to define a disease, rather than a committee of a medical society.

These suspicions are unfounded, as I discussed in the previous chapter, insofar as they commit the essentialist fallacy in psychiatric nosology. Diagnoses in medicine are not really different from diagnoses in psychiatry. Hence, although there are some ways in which the DSM system is indefensible, I will defend it as necessary, largely accurate, and basically scientific. And I will do so knowing that it is ridden with limitations and imperfections. Its strident critics seem to misinterpret its whole purpose and its underlying logic.

At the outset, it is important to clarify what the DSM system is not.

2.

DSM is not a method of discovering or divining illnesses among psychiatric patients. The psychiatrist Manfred Spitzer has made this point in distinguishing between "contexts of discovery" and "contexts of justification." As he points out, quoting the British scientist Peter Medawar, this is an old distinction in medicine: "First, there is a clear distinction between the acts of mind involved in discovery and in proof. The generative or elementary act in discovery is 'having ideas' or proposing a hypothesis. Although one can put oneself in the right frame of mind for having ideas and can abet the process, the process itself is outside logic and cannot be made the subject of logical rules" (1994, 174). Spitzer goes on:

> However, what is of interest in science is not the peculiar way in which a scientist arrived at a hypothesis but rather, very simply, whether this hypothesis is true. In other words, what is of interest is the justification of the hypothesis, not its discovery. . . . Diagnostic manuals are important when it comes to the question of why patient X suffers from disorder Y, that is to say, when it comes to the justification of a diagnosis. Sets of necessary and sufficient criteria provide a basis for answers to such questions and are indispensable as long as medicine is a science. Hence, a useful answer to the question of why patient Z suffers from, for example, schizophrenia, is not that the psychiatrist had that peculiar praecox feeling, but instead consists of a list of criteria met by the patient. It is equally as ridiculous to answer the question, "How did we get at the correct diagnosis of schizophrenia in this patient?" by stating, "We checked all criteria we found in the entire DSM-III-R, and ended up with the ones for schizophrenia being met." (174–75)

I believe that this touches on one of the main misconceptions that leads to unjustified criticism of the DSM system of nosology. The DSM criteria are often seen as a cookbook; patients and clinicians are forced to simply run down this checklist, answer yes or no, and accept the resulting diagnosis. All of this occurs in place of a presumably more nuanced and humane interaction, such as occurred in the not-too-distant pre-DSM past. But the DSM system is not meant to tell clinicians *how* to obtain the information used to diagnose patients; it is simply meant to organize how those data are utilized in the last instance to define diagnoses. In other words, clinicians can use whatever means they wish to obtain the relevant information, and, as discussed in chapter 22, this can and should entail the use of sophisticated interviewing techniques and complex psychotherapeutic methods that are a far cry from a cookbook or checklist. But in the end, this information needs to be organized along the lines of the DSM criteria.

The point of all this is to allow clinicians and researchers to communicate using the same language. When one person uses the term *schizophrenia,* another person knows what is meant according to the DSM criteria. If no criteria are agreed upon, one man's schizophrenia might be another man's mania, and this was indeed the case before the adoption of DSM-III in 1980. In that setting, research comes to a halt, because diverse definitions of patients' conditions will not allow for studies to be compared to each other or to build upon each other. The results of those studies could not be translated to clinical practice for the same reasons. That was the whole impetus for DSM-III, which is the basis for the current nosological system in psychiatry.

In summary, DSM is not meant to be a way of telling psychiatrists and patients how to assess signs and symptoms. It simply is a way of organizing what they find or discover into a consistent common language.

3.

This relates to the issue of reliability. The DSM system ensures that we all speak the same language: diagnoses are "reliable." But are they valid? Do they correspond to any real entities, any diseases? Or are they just made-up labels?

This is the deeper criticism of the DSM system. I agree with the criticism that the diagnostic labels in DSM are just that, labels, and they do not necessarily correlate with underlying "real" disease entities. This is not unique to DSM, however, and as I discussed in chapter 7, something like this occurred in Darwin's definitions of species. Nevertheless, I also agree with the view of defenders of DSM that those labels are important for research and allow closer and closer approximation of true disease entities. One connecting idea, which allows us to surpass this dichotomy, is the concept of ideal types, derived from

Max Weber. I will argue that the diagnoses in DSM essentially function as ideal types, rather than as pure fictions or as true disease entities.

4.

Weber developed the concept of ideal types to explain the underlying method of his work in sociology.[1] He borrowed the idea from its historical background in German intellectual circles in the late nineteenth century. At that time, influenced by Kant, German thinkers were trying to conceptualize the role of newly emerging science in human society. Was science something special, completely different from the humanities? If so, how? Was science in some way more important or accurate than the humanities? Today, our culture is still suffused with some of these antinomies. Two of the great neo-Kantian thinkers of the nineteenth century, Wilhelm Windelband and Karl Rickert, had a major influence on Weber. They argued that the *natural sciences* (what we would call science, meaning the empirical and logical sciences of biology, chemistry, physics, and mathematics) were indeed different in principle from the *cultural sciences* (termed today the humanities, particularly social science disciplines, history, economics, sociology, psychology, and the like). I will use *science* and *the humanities* to modernize these terms. Windelband and Rickert argued that science dealt with quantitative knowledge, which could be universalized to general, abstract laws. The humanities, in contrast, involved qualitative knowledge, which was by nature concrete and particular because it involved the choice and action of human beings. Since human beings possess free will, these actions can never be completely universalized to general laws. Today, many social scientists would object; they would say that many of the laws of economics, for instance, seem to be general laws that take into account the aggregate of many individual human actions. The German thinkers might respond that they did not intend to state that the humanities are *never* quantitatively accessible, or subject to general laws, but that *in principle* these two disciplines are best seen as being different in the ways mentioned.

As touched on previously, another of these thinkers, Wilhelm Dilthey, argued that these two disciplines of knowledge entailed two different ways of knowing.[2] Science was knowable through the method of *Erklaren,* which means causal explanation; in this method, empirical access to observation is required, and external events are linked with each other as cause and effect. The humanities, by contrast, are most knowable through the method of *Verstehen,* or meaningful understanding, in which one focuses on the internal subjective meaning of events or facts for specific individuals. Thus, the causal explanation approach to Napoleon's invasion of Russia would focus on the social class strata of each society, their military capabilities, their economic states, and so on. The meaningful explanation would include Napoleon's state of mind, his character, the influence of his advisers, his impressions of the Russians, and all these aspects of the czar's mind and his thinking. Although the causal explanation approach is useful, Dilthey would argue that the understanding of the phenomenon is not complete in the humanities until the meaningful understanding method is also employed.

Weber would agree with this. He wished to implement an "interpretive sociology" that employed meaningful explanation to go beyond the strict causal approach that had already begun to become popular at the turn of the century. However, Weber and his predecessors were faced with the apparent problem that the method of the humanities seemed less trustworthy and less likely to be useful than the method of science. At least with science, there seems to be less controversy about its laws. Anyone can verify them by experiment, and the whole process seems public, sober, and careful. In the humanities, everyone is capable of an opinion about the meaning of almost any historical event or figure. Consensus seems difficult to reach and is founded on vague insights rather than easily reproducible facts or experience.

Weber found this state of affairs unsatisfactory. He wanted to show that the humanities, though different from the natural and physical sciences, possessed a method of knowledge that had value and was accurate and effective. The method these thinkers devised, and which Weber most powerfully advanced, was the method of ideal types. This was seen as the method of the humanities that would bring it near the method of science in accuracy and utility.

5.

The concept of the ideal type is meant as a standard, or simplified version, of reality. Let us take Weber's example of the historian, because this is where the concept was developed, but everything that is said here can apply to the psychologist or the psychiatrist when faced with clinical aspects of treating patients. The historian observes certain aspects of a historical event. He then abstracts from the rest of the details of the event those aspects that are the most striking, those that are the most unique or interesting to him. Out of those special features, connected in the abstract and limited to the most salient aspects of the historical reality, the historian creates the ideal type for that event.

The point of the ideal type is not to directly correspond to reality but to highlight certain aspects of reality that might otherwise get lost in the varying details of concrete reality. The ideal type is not seen as a general theory, either, changing as more and more information on the empirical details of concrete reality is gathered. The ideal type is itself the standard to which concrete reality is compared.

By using the word *ideal*, Weber did not mean that the ideal type is the best type or that it is better than concrete reality; he meant to emphasize that it is an abstraction, a conceptualization created from concrete reality.

A conceptual analogy for the ideal type is a ruler, an instrument by which objects are measured. The ruler is not made based on empirical comparisons to reality. It simply is created by us, by humans, stipulated to be a certain length, and then used to measure real objects. Similarly, ideal types are concepts that are created by historians, and the facts of history are measured against them. The point of ideal types is to help us understand the meaning of those facts of history.

Weber applied the ideal-type method most famously in his book *The Protestant Ethic and the Spirit of Capitalism* ([1904] 1993).[3] There he wanted to understand why capitalism arose specifically in Western countries in the post-medieval era. Economic and political forces existed that allowed it to happen, but they also existed at other times in other parts of the world. Weber wanted to know why capitalism actually happened where it did in the West. His main answer was the effect of Protestantism.

He created the ideal type of the Protestant Spirit: the industrious, frugal, God-fearing Christian who believed that hard work was not simply necessary for worldly success but also divinely ordained. Of course, in some ways, this ideal type does not correspond to the reality of many Protestants, but it captures the essence of the influence of Protestantism on the subjective consciousness of early-capitalist-era Westerners. It was this consciousness that uniquely led to the birth and growth of capitalism in the West.

6.

This is Weber's approach to history and sociology with the ideal-type method. I wish to suggest here that the DSM system of nosology in psychiatry utilizes the same method. The diagnoses in DSM-IV are not "real" entities; they are abstractions. No single patient exactly meets the specific criteria of any diagnosis; every patient is uniquely different in some way. This reflects the concrete uniqueness of human existence, the aspect of human cultural reality that Weber and Jaspers so emphasized. Thus, the DSM diagnoses are not meant to directly and completely correspond to clinical reality. Nor are they meant to represent general theories of diagnoses, which are to be changed as more and more empirical evidence is gathered. In fact, this can happen, as noted previously, because the humanities can utilize the methods of the sciences to a certain degree. But in principle, at root, the DSM criteria are stipulated by psychiatrists based on a consensus of their clinical experience, to best pick out various clinical situations, so as to best facilitate communication and research in a common language. This is an ideal-type approach.

Thus, it is vain to criticize the DSM nosology for not corresponding to clinical reality. That is not its goal. The nosology is used to *understand* clinical reality, not to copy it. Nor is it useful to criticize it for being abstract or for not being based completely on empirical evidence. Diagnoses cannot be established in psychiatry completely on the basis of empirical evidence, for the same reason that history cannot be understood using the methods of physics. Abstraction is unavoidable, unless one limits psychiatry to nothing but observation of the details of each clinical case, with little attempt at a more general level of understanding (which was Adolf Meyer's eclectic error).

Ultimately, the DSM nosology may lead to the recognition of specific diseases, quantitatively defined in demonstrable abnormalities in brain structure or function or in genetic coding. At that point, the humanities-oriented ideal-type approach will give way more completely to the science-oriented empirical approach. However, given the uniqueness of human action, there will always be a role for some kind of ideal-type approach in psychiatry.

7.

It is worth mentioning that if ideal types are relevant, then psychiatry differs from other medical disciplines. This is so on the assumption that human beings are free. If we have free will, then human action will always be at some level unique and concretely particular. To that extent, it will resist complete subsumption under universal scientific laws. Since psychiatry deals with human behavior as the core of its symptoms, it necessarily will always run up against this limitation. Free human action will limit the accuracy of causal explanation through empirical scientific methods. Again, this is unlike other medical disciplines, because in those cases the signs and symptoms observed are not subject to human will. Chest pain, nausea, blurred vision—these all happen to the patient and cannot be altered voluntarily. It is true that certain psychiatric symptoms happen to the patient and are not voluntary (depressed mood, loss of appetite, increased energy), but their expression in behaviors has at least some element of voluntariness that might have resulted in different behaviors. The depressed patient attempts suicide because she is alone, whereas she might not have done it if someone close to her had been present. The manic patient engages in sex with a prostitute, whereas he might not have done so if he lived somewhere with less access to prostitution. Or perhaps he decided to engage in that behavior on a certain night, whereas he might just as well have waited until the next night.

In essence, these counterfactual scenarios are not avoidable, because of human freedom. Humans can always do things at least slightly differently, even under the influence of a psychiatric illness. And it is this wiggle room, however slight, that makes psychiatric reality always unique, always concrete, and always particular. Since those behaviors are the actual symptoms and signs used for diagnoses in psychiatry, diagnoses will always have to deal with unique, concrete, particular reality. That is, they will deal with a reality that is more similar to a historical event, like Napoleon's invasion of Russia, than to a set of empirical facts, like the fever, chills, and night sweats of an infection.

Does this mean, then, that psychiatric conditions are not medical diseases, as Thomas Szasz has argued (1974)? This may be the case only if we define science as solely causal explanation, excluding the method of meaningful understanding. But, as I pointed out in chapter 6, there is no need to do so.

8.

In the interest of making it clear that I am not arguing against a scientific basis for psychiatry, let me clarify again what I mean by the term *science*. As I said in chapter 6, I believe that psychiatry can and does utilize the scientific method. This method is not limited to the causal explanation based on empirical evidence that Weber associated with the traditional sciences (biology, chemistry, physics, mathematics). Weber pointed out that these methods can also apply to a great extent to the humanities. Thus, there is overlap. But beyond that, I would define science, in the spirit of Weber, as that method which most accurately and completely captures knowledge about its subject. Since psychiatry and psychology involve, at their roots, concrete, unique human reality, the purely empirical method of knowledge, though necessary, is not sufficient. The added aspect required is the ideal-type method, which provides a consistent, useful way to understand the meaning of the concrete, particular aspects of psychiatric reality. Thus, scientific method in psychiatry, as Karl Jaspers argued, is a combination of these two methods—empirical observation and ideal types, or, more generally, the use of both causal explanation and meaningful understanding. In *General Psychopathology,* Jaspers alluded to the utility of the ideal-type method in the nosology of personality. I am extending that perspective to all of psychiatric nosology.[4]

I think Weber's important contribution is in making the ideal-type method a structured approach to improving our ability to engage in meaningful understanding. Indeed, the main criticism of Weber, which will likely be on the minds of readers of this chapter, is this: if we allow for meaningful understanding in psychiatry, what will keep everything from being vague and idiosyncratic, as each psychiatrist puts her own spin on what is going on with each patient? Weber's ideal-type method is meant to limit this idiosyncrasy: we are enjoined to ignore certain aspects of the concrete realities of psychiatric phenomena for the moment, while we attempt to understand certain salient aspects of those phenomena highlighted in the ideal types. Hence, when we are seeking to apply DSM criteria to make a diagnosis in a patient, we temporarily suspend interest in certain aspects of that patient's reality that are not captured in the diagnostic criteria we are seeking to elucidate. For instance, in seeking to determine whether a depressed patient has bipolar or unipolar depression, I will not inquire into his early childhood relationships, because those are not part of the ideal-type criteria for those diagnoses. Those early life relationships may later turn out to be relevant to understanding certain aspects of that person's life or condition, but at the moment they are not relevant to determining which diagnosis seems most applicable to his depression. This has practical implications, given the empirical evidence that if he meets the criteria for one of those diagnoses, he may respond well to antidepressants in the one case or to mood stabilizers in the other. Had his early childhood relationships distracted us from looking for those diagnoses, those treatments would not have been given, and empirical evidence exists that he would likely have had a poor prognosis if he indeed had bipolar or unipolar depression.

Thus, although ideal types are limited, can be misinterpreted, and do not have the general reproducibility and ease of validation of the empirical method, they are useful nonetheless and can go hand in hand with empirical research in helping understand and treat individuals with psychiatric conditions.

The DSM nosology is best understood in this context, in my opinion, and it has proven its practical utility in improving many patients' lives and in promoting diagnostic and treatment research, albeit with many limitations.

9.

If we accept that psychiatric diagnoses can be reliably made and that they are not entirely arbitrary, then we can discuss the relative merits of different types of classification systems. Two basic types are the categorical and the dimensional approaches, which I discuss in the next chapter.

CHAPTER 13

Dimensions versus Categories

The follow-up is the great exposer of truth, the rock on which many fine theories are wrecked and upon which better ones can be built. It is to the psychiatrist what the postmortem is to the physician. —P. D. SCOTT

Mood and Psychotic Disorders

1.

Categorical knowledge involves all-or-nothing qualitative phenomena; that is, something either belongs to category X or to category Y. An example is pregnancy; one either is or is not pregnant. Dimensional knowledge is continuous and is characterized by possessing or experiencing more or less of something. An example is blood pressure. Every living human has blood pressure; in some it is high, in some low, and in most in between. One of the criticisms that has been made of the evolution of psychiatric nosology after DSM-III is that diagnosis has become hypercategorical. It has been suggested that we have gone too far in trying to categorize psychiatric diagnoses. There are too many diagnoses now, it is alleged, practically one for every mental symptom. This is an exaggeration, but it may hide a deeper truth. Historically, before the shift in nosology that occurred in mainstream psychiatry with DSM-III in 1980, mainstream psychiatry went to an extreme in the dimensional direction. Influenced by certain psychoanalytic doctrines, many individuals in the field held that the only partial dichotomy in diagnosis was between neurosis and psychosis. Everyone was a little bit neurotic, and only more severe forms seemed problematic. Some people, such as Harry Stack Sullivan, even held that psychosis was not an all-or-none phenomenon and that psychotic-like thinking was not unusual in normal (i.e., mildly neurotic) persons (1953). Another view was that everyone is somewhat depressed and that depression thus is not a categorically abnormal phenomenon. (Freud once said that he simply wanted to replace the abnormal misery of mankind with normal unhappiness.) I will discuss the useful aspects of some of these psychoanalytic ideas, but the disadvantages should be obvious. DSM-III was a reaction to this hyperdimensionalism, which prevented psychiatrists from diagnosing individuals who might be treated with newly emerging antidepressant and antipsychotic medications. Has DSM gone too far? Probably. But a reversion to pre-DSM-III hyperdimensionalism is not the solution.

2.

Some argue that the major mental illnesses (schizophrenia and manic-depressive illness) are not categorical. The straw man that these opponents of the current nosology prefer to battle is Kraepelin's nosology. Kraepelin, it may be recalled, designated schizophrenia and manic-depressive illness as the two main disorders in psychiatry. He felt that the concept of manic-depressive illness subsumed all affective disorders (what we might call today bipolar disorder, unipolar depression, cyclothymia, and dysthymia), and he believed that the concept of schizophrenia subsumed all cases of chronic psychosis in which there were no affective symptoms at all (nonaffective psychosis). The Kraepelinian straw man is the view that all psychiatric conditions should be divisible into one of these two categories: schizophrenia (nonaffective psychosis) and manic-depressive illness (affective illness). The reason this is a straw man is that Kraepelin, being an astute clinician, realized that borderline cases existed.

He presaged later views of a spectrum of affective illness, for example, in which mild versions of mood disorders (like hypomania) merged with personality traits of mood instability (like cyclothymia). He also recognized mild versions of schizophrenia, which also merged with personality traits (such as, in today's terminology, schizotypal personality disorder). Another reason a pure dichotomy is a conceptual straw man is that we know that most individuals fall somewhere on a normal curve when diagnostic criteria are applied to their psychiatric symptoms. This is common in some other medical conditions as well, such as hypertension. For instance, most patients who have nonaffective psychosis will not have symptoms of their illness or features of the course of their illness in common with most patients who have affective disorders. But as in a normal curve, there will be overlap at the extremes (see fig. 13.1).

The fact that there is overlap at the extremes does not invalidate the concept that in general these two peaks of symptom and course characteristics differ from each other. In this respect, this difference is similar to the situation

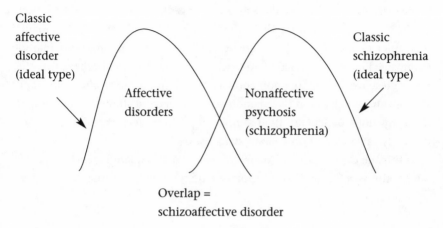

Fig. 13.1. Overlap of populations of diagnoses

with populations of individuals that form species (see chapter 7). From a Darwinian perspective, those populations are different, even though they are always in flux and there will be overlap. Only an essentialist perspective would insist on no overlap at all.

Further, if we accept the idea of ideal types in nosology, then our classic categories (the ideal types) really may represent the extremes of the natural distribution of the diagnosis. The cases of patients who have some features of the other illness (which is the majority) might be seen as the psychotic spectrum (fig. 13.1), that is, those features of psychosis held in common between affective disorders and schizophrenia. A similar approach to differentiating unipolar and bipolar mood disorders, within the affective disorder distribution, also can be taken (see below).

With the features of this straw man in view, I am skeptical of the view of a group of contemporary psychiatrists who believe that the Kraepelinian system is completely wrongheaded (Crow 1998, 1990; Kendell and Brockington 1980). The argument of these anti-Kraepelinians is basically that a few inconvenient facts invalidate the Kraepelinian structure, pointing instead to a "unitary psychosis" model, meaning that there is no dichotomy among psychiatric diagnoses, at least with psychotic disorders: they are all part of one overarching psychotic illness.

The first inconvenient fact, which these thinkers seem to view as a counterexample practically sufficient to invalidate the entire Kraepelinian nosology, is the existence of schizoaffective disorder. This diagnostic concept dates back to 1933, when J. J. Kasanin ([1933] 1994) published a case series of six patients who appeared to have characteristics of both schizophrenia and manic-depressive illness, as defined by Kraepelin. Crow and Kendell believe that the mere presence of this phenomenon is sufficient to refute Kraepelin, and Kendell and Brockington have conducted an empirical study that found that most psychotic patients in their sample, like schizoaffective patients, cannot be neatly categorized into separate diagnoses.

Is this the case? Does schizoaffective disorder invalidate Kraepelin's nosology? If this is the case, then psychiatry requires a major overhaul of its ideas once more.

3.

I will return to the question of schizoaffective disorder in a moment. But first, I want to point out that similar criticisms have been made *within* each broad Kraepelinian diagnostic category. For instance, some claim that the broad category of schizophrenia is too heterogeneous and can be broken down into a number of subtypes (hebephrenic type, catatonic type, paranoid type, disorganized type, and others). Kraepelin himself was inclined to recognize some of these distinctions. Others claim that the broad category of manic-depressive illness should be divided into at least two subcategories, unipolar depression and bipolar disorder. Since the unipolar-bipolar distinction is codified in DSM-III and IV, and since it is widely used today, I will discuss this issue in detail here (as well as somewhat in chapter 16).

Another question, therefore, is this: is there basically one broad spectrum of affective illness (this is essentially Kraepelin's view in his definition of "manic-depressive insanity"), or are there two or more mood diseases (this is the current DSM-IV view, with its separate diagnoses of unipolar depression and bipolar disorder, the latter being further subdivided into Type I and Type II based on the presence of mania or hypomania, respectively)?

Kraepelin's view was attacked almost from the outset, as chapter 11 indicates. Many clinicians do not realize that Kraepelin's key criterion for diagnosing manic-depressive illness was recurrence, not polarity (Goodwin and Jamison 1990).[1] By this I mean that Kraepelin was not interested in whether the patient was experiencing a manic or a depressive episode; what mattered was how many mood episodes the patient had experienced. If the patient experienced only one depressive episode, Kraepelin viewed that condition as melancholia, which he called a "clinical picture," not really a diagnosis with an underlying basis in biological disease. If the patient experienced numerous mood episodes, whether depressive or manic, then the patient was diagnosed by Kraepelin as having manic-depressive insanity. What mattered was recurrence of mood episodes, not the nature of the episodes (i.e., mania versus depression). Thus, a patient with a manic episode followed by three depressive episodes would be diagnosed with manic-depressive insanity. Someone with five depressive episodes would also be diagnosed with manic-depressive insanity.

This approach was attacked by Hoche and others as being too broad. Yet it was not until genetic studies were conducted in the 1960s that serious criticism was given to Kraepelin's broad view of what had come to be called manic-depressive illness. Jules Angst (1998) and Carlo Perris (1966), two European psychiatrists, observed that manic episodes were found mainly in families of persons with manic episodes, whereas manic episodes were absent in families of persons with only depressive episodes. Hence the unipolar-bipolar distinction, which had been proposed earlier by Karl Leonhard and others (Baldessarini 2000b), received some genetic validation. If a patient had unipolar depression (only depression without mania, regardless of recurrence), then her family members tended to have unipolar depression but not bipolar disorder (characterized by the presence of at least one manic episode). If a patient had bipolar disorder, then his family members tended to have both bipolar and unipolar disorders. These findings were confirmed in other studies and also supported by treatment studies that found that tricyclic antidepressants were effective in unipolar depression but appeared to cause mania in bipolar disorder, whereas lithium was quite effective in bipolar disorder. The course of bipolar disorder also seemed somewhat worse than the course of unipolar depression, and psychotic symptoms were more frequent in mania than in depression. These differences led to the distinction between bipolar disorder and (unipolar) major depressive disorder in DSM-III in 1980. The category manic-depressive illness was dropped and split into these two subtypes.

Recently, however, there has been a rebirth of the original broad Kraepelinian notion, renamed as the concept of a "bipolar spectrum" (Akiskal 1996).[2] This has occurred because the original distinguishing features of unipolar depression and bipolar disorder have proved to be less clear-cut than they seemed initially. Again, we are faced with a likely distribution in the real world of patients who do not share all the same characteristics but who have a good

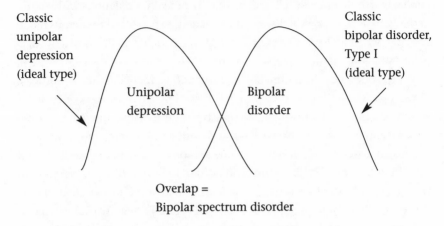

Manic-depressive illness (Kraepelin's view)

Classic
unipolar
depression
(ideal type)

Unipolar
depression

Bipolar
disorder

Classic
bipolar disorder,
Type I
(ideal type)

Overlap =
Bipolar spectrum disorder

Fig. 13.2. Manic-depressive illness versus the bipolar-unipolar distinction

deal of overlap (see fig. 13.2). Bipolar disorder, Type I (classic mania alternating with depression), represents one extreme of the natural distribution of bipolar disorder (again, it can be seen as an ideal type), and classic unipolar depression represents the other extreme. The overlap area can be considered the bipolar spectrum. If the overlap area proves to be quite large, then one might have a rationale for dropping the whole distinction and returning to Kraepelin's broad definition of manic-depressive illness. This is an empirical question that needs to be evaluated in research. For now, I would simply say that the bipolar-unipolar distinction, like the larger affective disorders–schizophrenia distinction, is one of degree, with areas of overlap that do not necessarily invalidate the overall categorical ideal types. Nonetheless, in the case of the bipolar-unipolar distinction, I believe there is some utility for a middle dimensional diagnosis, which Frederick Goodwin and I have suggested calling "bipolar spectrum disorder," as opposed to the term *Cade's disease,* which one might use to identify the ideal type: bipolar disorder, Type I (Ghaemi, Ko, and Goodwin 2002).[3]

4.

We should step back for a moment. I am trying to address the dialectic between a categorical and a dimensional approach to major psychiatric illnesses. At a basic level, Kraepelin was a categorical advocate, separating schizophrenia from affective disorders, whereas his critics advocate dimensionalism (a single psychotic spectrum of illness). At the next level, Kraepelin had dimensional sympathies, especially in his attempt to characterize manic-depressive illness broadly on recurrent mood episodes, whereas later critics (and today's DSM-IV nosology) are categorical (dividing unipolar and bipolar subgroups).

I will now focus on the schizophrenia–affective disorders distinction, since that is the distinction at the root of all of Kraepelin's nosology. If it falls, then everything else falls. As Karl Jaspers might ask, What are the assumptions underlying the views of the critics of Kraepelin's nosology? There appears to be a major philosophical assumption behind their opinions. Stemming from the philosopher Karl Popper, this is the view that scientific theories can be refuted, but they cannot be proved. The opposite view, that repeated confirmations at best lead to an approximation of truth for a scientific theory, is an *inductive* philosophy of science, best enunciated by the philosopher Charles S. Peirce.[4] The anti-Kraepelinians are engaging in a deductive attempt to refute Kraepelin— one good refutation of a prediction of Kraepelin's nosology would suffice. Schizoaffective disorder appears to be that refutation, since it strikes at the very core concept of Kraepelin's nosology, that psychoses can be differentiated into two categories.

So the next question is, What is the empirical evidence for the validity of the concept of schizoaffective disorder? Assessing diagnostic validity is a process that in modern medicine derives from certain accepted principles first established by the English physician Thomas Sydenham in the eighteenth century. These principles were extended in medicine by the nineteenth-century German pathologist Rudolph Virchow and his French contemporary the physiologist Claude Bernard.[5] Given that these principles underlie the major advances in medical science in the past century, one might not be faulted for accepting them as first principles with a certain strength of conviction. The basic conviction that Sydenham introduced was that medical diagnoses should be based on recurring syndromes, consisting of consistent groups of symptoms, and these syndromes should be distinct from the syndromes that underlie other medical diagnoses. Virchow and Bernard added that the syndromes should then be confirmed in the pathological and physiological analyses of the bodily organs that produce the disease. Thus, the syndrome of jaundice, fever, and chills, with a recurring course, when combined with a pathological examination of the liver that produces a typical histological pattern associated with those symptoms, results in the diagnosis of the disease hepatitis. Research aimed at finding the pathogens in the liver that produce the disease would then identify the virus, in this case, that is responsible. Research on that virus in laboratories would produce treatments that kill it. Then these treatments, given to humans, would resolve the symptoms of the hepatitis syndrome. This is how medical science basically continues to function today. Sydenham and others also noted that certain syndromes seemed to run in families, so they added a family history of a syndrome as one of the features of proposed syndromes.

This perspective on medical practice is codified today in the ClinicoPathological Conference (CPC), the most famous of which, at the Massachusetts General Hospital, has been publicized weekly in the *New England Journal of Medicine* for decades. An attendee at the weekly CPC at Massachusetts General Hospital is impressed with the stereotypy of the process. The clinicians describe the complicated signs and symptoms that the patients suffered, the vagaries of treatment, and the inevitable failure to respond to treatments for the initial diagnoses. A specimen is obtained for pathological analysis, and the pathologist, almost regularly appearing as the omniscient savior of the day, pronounces the correct diagnosis. In those cases in which the pathological specimen was obtained while the patient was alive, the clinicians are able to save the patient's life, with treatments aimed at the now-known diagnosis.

It is clear that psychiatry suffers from a major problem in this CPC model of medical practice. We do not have the omniscient pathologist to help us. Like neurologists, we think we know where the pathology is in major mental illnesses: in the brain. But unlike neurologists, we do not know exactly where and how this pathology manifests itself in a regular manner.

5.

To face this dilemma, Eli Robins and Samuel Guze at Washington University in St. Louis proposed a psychiatric version of the medical process of diagnosis that they hoped would validate a more scientific psychiatric nosology (Robins and Guze 1970).[6] Since we cannot rely on pathology as a primary means of validating diagnosis, Robins and Guze argued that we should rely on data obtained from a number of different methods of validation. If many different types of data seemed to converge on a single diagnosis, then we could judge that diagnosis to be valid. They identified four factors that could serve to validate a psychiatric diagnosis. First, the phenomenology of the syndrome in terms of cross-sectional symptoms: the presence of delusions and hallucinations characterizes a psychotic disorder, and the presence of a sad mood with changes in appetite, sleep, interest, and energy characterizes a depressive syndrome. Second, the course of the illness: as Kraepelin emphasized, schizophrenia displays a chronic worsening course, whereas affective illness may not. Third, a family history of illness, or a genetic basis for a syndrome: patients with schizophrenia tend to have family histories of schizophrenia, but patients with manic-depressive illness tend not to have family histories of schizophrenia. Fourth, biological markers or laboratory tests: this gets at the underlying pathology or physiology of the illness; in psychiatry we have no such markers or tests at present. Since the fourth validator is not available yet in psychiatry, a fifth variable, treatment response, has been suggested for use in the validating process: patients with schizophrenia tend to respond to antipsychotic agents but not antidepressant agents, and patients with the depressive syndrome tend to respond to antidepressant agents but not antipsychotic agents.

As Robins and Guze admitted, no one of these factors is sufficient by itself to validate a syndrome. Often there is syndromal overlap, as with schizoaffective disorder. Or the genetic data from research is sometimes conflicting; some studies, for instance, suggest that patients with schizophrenia have relatives with manic-depressive illness. Treatment response can overlap as well: antipsychotic agents also work for the manic phase of bipolar illness. And so on. But this was the point of this approach: the more validators we have that point in the same direction, the more likely we are to identify a true diagnosis. The underlying philosophy of science in this approach, it should be clear, is Peirce's inductive method of approximate confirmation of a theory, rather than Popper's deductive method of falsifying a theory.

With this background, where does the argument regarding schizoaffective disorder fall? Clearly, the argument is partially a disagreement on underlying philosophy of science. The anti-Kraepelinians view schizoaffective disorder as a sufficient falsification of the current nosology. The Kraepelinians, following the Robins and Guze model of nosological validation, view the clinical overlap of the schizoaffective syndrome as just the first factor that needs to be considered in assessing the validity of schizoaffective disorder as a separate diagnosis that would invalidate the Kraepelinian nosology. They ask, instead, How does schizoaffective disorder fare on the other criteria?

The answer is, Not so well. In terms of course of illness, schizoaffective disorder does not truly seem to fall into a separate category: the bipolar type of schizoaffective illness—those patients who have manic symptoms along with chronic psychosis—seems to have a course like bipolar disorder; the unipolar type—those with depressive symptoms along with chronic psychosis—follows the same course as classic schizophrenia. Similarly, in genetic studies, the bipolar type of schizoaffective illness frequently segregates with bipolar illness, whereas the unipolar depressed type of schizoaffective disorder segregates with classic schizophrenia in families. In treatment response, the bipolar type requires mood stabilizers, like bipolar disorder, and the unipolar type requires antidepressants, like unipolar depression. In other words, the various factors do not separate out schizoaffective disorder as a validated diagnosis that can be demarcated from schizophrenia, bipolar disorder, and unipolar depression. In fact, it seems to be divisible, based on whether it is unipolar or bipolar type, into a variant of either bipolar illness or schizophrenia. Some genetic data even support the likelihood that schizoaffective disorder is the phenotype of the comorbidity of having, by chance, both schizophrenia and affective illness at the same time. Thus, the Kraepelinian view is that the majority of the research data argues that schizoaffective disorder is not a separate condition that invalidates the Kraepelinian nosology, but either a variant of the two main illnesses of that nosology, or the phenotypic result of the comorbidity of those two major mental illnesses.

6.

One can see, then, two different approaches to science here. The anti-Kraepelinians take an all-or-nothing view. A theory is either completely true, in which case it allows of no exceptions, or it is false. The Kraepelinians take an approximate view, one that is more like the practical decisions of the law and the judicial system than the abstractions of philosophy of science. This view holds that we should accept a theory if the preponderance of the evidence supports its validity, in the absence of the definitive validations provided by pathology and physiology.

I lean toward the Kraepelinian view, which is closer to the accepted canons of modern medical science. As discussed in chapter 4, although Popper's absolutism looks good on paper and works in the realm of abstract physics, it runs into a lot of trouble with biology and medicine. Furthermore, there must be something to be said for the pragmatic benefits of modern medical science, functioning under the inductive principles described here. Ultimately, though, medical science is also Popperian when it comes to pathology. If a pathological result disagrees with a syndrome, then the pathology trumps the syndrome. The problem is that this is not yet the case in psychiatry. And schizoaffective illness has only syndromal evidence going for it; it lacks genetic, course, and treatment response data that would subvert the Kraepelinian system. Thus, with purely syndromal evidence, it does not trump the other diagnostic evidence that supports the Kraepelinian system.

7.

In some sense, since all natural distributions of persons with features of a diagnosis are dimensional, all categorical distinctions are based on cutoffs on a dimensional scale (as in figs. 13.1 and 13.2). This is simply a biological reality. We need to be open to categorical distinctions where, as ideal types, they usefully capture differences between two populations as a whole. But there will also be overlap areas, where we need to be willing to also broaden our classic categories into concepts of spectra in which patients will share many nonclassical features of two illnesses (as in schizoaffective disorder, or as in the bipolar spectrum). In this sense, the major mood and psychotic disorders are somewhat similar to diagnoses of mental retardation, where cutoffs based on dimensional IQ scores are used to categorically define mental retardation.

This distinction between categorical and dimensional thinking was also at the root of part of Adolf Meyer's opposition to Kraepelin's nosology. Meyer felt that Kraepelin was purely categorical and that he did not appreciate the underlying dimensionality of patients' symptoms, which Meyer viewed mainly as reactions to life stresses. Yet Kraepelin was both a categorical advocate and a dimensionally oriented nosologist (this flexibility in his approach is often underrecognized). We can allow for dimensionality in psychiatric diagnosis without giving up on categories altogether, at least as they apply to major mood and psychotic illnesses. I think, however, that the issue of personality disorders raises many more doubts about the utility of any categorical approach to diagnosis.

Personality Disorders

8.

Where do dimensional approaches to psychiatric syndromes make sense in the current nosology? Probably the most important area involves personality. It seems to make sense that one either experiences delusions or not—or mania, or panic attacks, or compulsive rituals. Thus, these diagnoses (schizophrenia, manic-depressive illness, panic disorder, obsessive-compulsive disorder) seem categorical, and a good deal of excellent research supports this view. But what about personality? In the DSM system, a second axis is set aside to record personality disorders. The use of different axes (placing the above categorical disorders on Axis I and placing personality disorders on Axis II and pertinent medical conditions on Axis III) is supposed to remind clinicians to assess something on each axis for each patient. So, whereas we may or may not have schizophrenia, everyone has a personality of some kind or another, and everyone has a physical medical state of health. It is on Axis II, the assessment of personality, where the DSM reliance on categorical diagnoses is least supported by the research literature.

Historically, the DSM descriptions of personality disorders, such as the narcissistic, antisocial, or borderline personality types, are directly based on mostly psychoanalytic notions dating from the 1970s and earlier. Psychoanalysts noted, in the 1950s and 1960s in particular, that many of their patients who appeared to possess run-of-the-mill levels of neurosis were actually more ill than at first glance. When these neurotic persons were placed on the couch in psychoanalysis, all sorts of unusual things occurred that did not happen with most of the "worried well" patients whom analysts treated. Major conflicts occurred between analysts and these unusual patients, such that the analysts actually began to experience marked rage *(countertransference hate)* toward these patients; the patients frequently terminated therapy and would go through analyst after analyst without success; sometimes the patients even became psychotic, leading some to label their condition "pseudoneurotic schizophrenia" because they appeared merely neurotic but actually became psychotic under the microscope of psychoanalysis. After a while, it was determined that these patients were on the borderline between neurosis and psychosis and that their problems tended to be a lifelong aspect of their personalities, not merely symptoms of the typical conflicts that most people experience with their normal (mildly to moderately neurotic) personalities. The name *borderline personality* therefore became common to describe these individuals and remains in use as the main type of personality disorder diagnosed in modern psychiatry.[7]

Yet is this categorical approach to diagnosis of personality disorders valid?

9.

I suggest that the categorical approach to personality disorders is clinically useful at times but that these patients are better understood dimensionally in

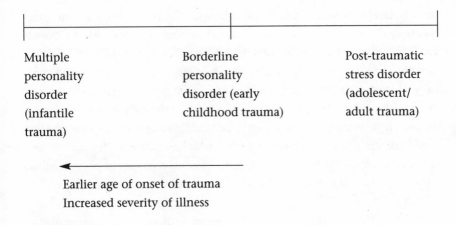

Fig. 13.3. Dissociative spectrum disorder

terms of extremes of personality traits. Let us take multiple personality disorder, borderline personality disorder, and post-traumatic stress disorder as examples. I suggest that these three categories are better understood as varieties of a single dissociative spectrum disorder (fig. 13.3). This may be the case because the underlying psychopathology in all three conditions is the phenomenon of dissociation, where a person is out of contact with the world surrounding her for a while. This hypothesis is supported by research using the Dissociative Experiences Scale, which indicates increasing symptoms as one moves to the left of the figure (toward multiple personality disorder) (Kirby, Chu, and Dill 1993). During these periods, patients can experience fugue states, periods of being spaced-out, loss of memory, panic attacks, and flashbacks to traumatic episodes. They are emotionally frozen, as it were, during these episodes. In multiple personality disorder, one sees earlier and more severe history of sexual trauma, whereas in borderline personality disorder, the trauma history is slightly later in childhood and sometimes less severe, and in post-traumatic stress disorder, the trauma occurs later in adolescence or in adulthood. This conceptualization will also explain how patients can go back and forth between these diagnoses, or have them "comorbidly," possibly as a reflection of how severe their symptoms might be at a particular period in their lives.

10.

The two other main types of personality disorder often diagnosed, narcissism and antisocial personality disorder, have similar roots. Narcissistic symptoms were also common among persons with the borderline characteristics mentioned above and were often more prominent in males with the overall syndrome than in females. There is indeed a good deal of overlap between narcissistic and borderline personality disorders when they are diagnosed clinically. Historically, different schools of psychoanalytic thought have favored one or the other diagnosis, and both have been preserved in the DSM system. Antisocial personality disorder used to be called *psychopathy,* and the term was used to describe individuals (mostly men) who had numerous legal problems, tended to commit crimes, and seemed to have no remorse (or conscience, or superego). Many individuals in jails are diagnosed with this condition if DSM criteria are applied.

Unlike better-established categorical diagnoses (like schizophrenia or manic-depressive illness), clinical studies of the personality disorders reveal a good deal of overlap. That is, many, if not most, people diagnosed with borderline personality disorder also meet the criteria for narcissistic personality or antisocial personality disorders, or often other diagnoses. There is some empirical evidence in favor of the categorical diagnoses of these three conditions in some people. Yet the other personality disorders listed in DSM (histrionic, avoidant, obsessive-compulsive, schizoid, and schizotypal personalities) have little support to stand on as true valid diagnoses. Histrionic personality practically always occurs only with borderline or narcissistic personality. Avoidant personality seems to be a generalized version of a true categorical anxiety disorder, social phobia, and thus not a personality condition at all. Schizotypal personality appears to be a mild subtype of schizophrenia, with a similar genetic inheritance and with latent psychotic symptoms that respond to the same medications.[8]

11.

Although we all possess thoughts and emotions, schizophrenia and manic-depressive illness demonstrate a constellation of symptoms that helps to distinguish them reasonably well from normal persons without those illnesses. Personality disorders are more subtle. We all have personalities, but only some of us have personality disorders. Where do you draw the line? It is my view, based on my understanding of the available empirical research (see below), that personality disorders are inherently dimensional, in a way that is difficult to categorize even at the extremes, unlike the major mood and psychotic illnesses.

To understand this view, we need to examine research in experimental psychology on normal personality. Probably one of the first pathbreakers in this regard was Hans Eysenck (1953), the great British psychologist. Eysenck validated the famous personality dimension of extroversion versus introversion, which he derived clinically from the work of C. G. Jung. Later Eysenck added the personality dimension of neuroticism (high versus low anxiety), based on further empirical research. And lastly, he introduced the dimension of psychoticism (abnormal thinking). These three dimensions were the first empirically validated approaches to carving up human personality. Later research suggested altering the psychoticism dimension to reflect the willingness to engage in new behaviors, termed *openness to experience.* Those three dimensions (neuroticism, extroversion, and openness to experience) underlie perhaps the most commonly used personality test, the NEO. Each person's personality can be plotted on a grid with these three axes, and most people fall somewhere near the middle on each; that is, most people are not too extroverted and not too introverted, somewhat anxious at times but not excessive worriers, and interested in new experiences but not reckless or too timid. Alternatively, a person might fall more toward the extreme on one or more axes. C. Robert Cloninger, a psychiatrist who has done much research on the dimensions of personality as well as on categorical personality disorders, has provided strong empirical evidence that the two approaches (dimensional versus categorical) can be reconciled (Cloninger, Svrakic, and Przybeck 1993). Those who are on the extreme of one or more of the axes of personality tend to have characteristics similar to the categorical DSM personality disorder descriptions. Thus, persons who are high on extroversion, high on openness to experience, and high on neuroticism would tend to meet the criteria for borderline or narcissistic personality disorder; and those with the same profile but low on neuroticism would tend to be diagnosed with antisocial personality disorder.

Cloninger (1999) has provided a separate way of dimensionally assessing personality, based on three to five dimensions. He also makes a distinction between temperament and character, which may prove to be a useful way of further refining our dimensional understanding of personality. In place of Eysenck's NEO, Cloninger has validated three other (but related) primary dimensions of personality: harm avoidance (anxiety-proneness versus risk-taking), novelty seeking (impulsiveness versus rigidity), and persistence (determination versus fickleness). He considers these three basic dimensions of personality to represent one's biologically endowed temperament, which is genetically based. Based on animal studies, some have also related specific neurotransmitter systems to these temperamental dimensions: dopamine to novelty seeking, serotonin to harm avoidance, and norepinephrine to persistence. Cloninger then adds three other dimensions: self-directedness, cooperativeness, and self-transcendence, and he calls these dimensions of character, which are acquired mainly from culture and family. Personality is the result of temperament plus character and thus comprises these six dimensions. Cloninger goes on to suggest that the various personality disorders can be explained and best understood as various combinations of extremes on these dimensions of personality. He extends his analysis to all psychiatric diagnoses, but, for my purposes, I want to ally myself with his approach as it relates at least to personality disorders.

I believe the empirical evidence at this point is sufficient for psychiatry to reorganize its thinking regarding personality disorders and recognize that they are based at root on fundamental dimensions of personality.

12.

In summary, I suggest that the different perspectives of categorical versus dimensional thinking do not apply arbitrarily to any psychiatric condition. Nor does one or the other perspective accurately describe all psychiatric conditions. Some conditions (many of the Axis I conditions of psychotic, mood, and anxiety disorders) are best described with a largely categorical approach, whereas other conditions (mainly the Axis II personality disorders) are better described with a largely dimensional approach.

13.

Finally, in going back and forth between dimensional and categorical constructs, I think it is important to clearly explain the issue of the underlying biology of psychiatric illnesses, as well as the role of life events.

The biology of psychiatric illnesses can be viewed a few different ways (fig. 13.4). The original hope of Kraepelin and others was that the biology of psychiatric illnesses would follow the infectious disease model, that single powerful etiologies would be discovered by working backward from diagnoses that reflected underlying diseases specific to those etiologies. One hundred years of biological research by brilliant minds have proved that this hope was not based on reality. Unfortunately, most psychiatric illnesses are influenced by multiple genes of small effect and multiple environmental etiologies, which converge on a few shared pathophysiological final common pathways. It also appears

The infectious disease model

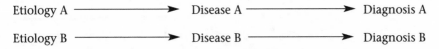

The diabetes model

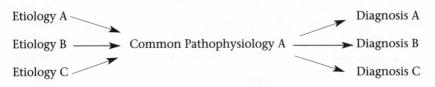

Fig. 13.4. The biology of psychiatric illnesses

that our diagnostic entities are not specific to any unique pathophysiology or any single etiology. This is much more like the model of diabetes as currently understood than like that of infectious diseases. Elevated cholesterol and hypertension are other illnesses in a similar state of lack of understanding.

If we accept the diabetes model as the basis for the biology of psychiatric illnesses, we are likely to be faced with a stress-diathesis model of that biology (fig. 13.5). This model tries to explain the interaction between genetics and environment in influencing the biology and course of an illness. In the case of most major psychiatric illnesses, genetic influences combined with unshared environmental influences (those not shared by siblings in a family) produce the baseline biological susceptibility to the psychiatric illness (e.g., bipolar disorder). Later life events serve as triggers for the occurrence of the mood episodes. The later life events do not cause the illness in a general sense; they only determine how frequently and when the illness reveals itself in mood or psychotic episodes. The episodes are part of the illness, not the entire illness. In fact, without the underlying biological susceptibility, the illness would not occur. Hence, the biological susceptibility is the necessary component of the illness, whereas the life events are the later circumstances that create the sufficient conditions for the illness to manifest itself. Both life events and underlying biological susceptibility are legitimate targets of interventions, with psychotherapies and medications, respectively. It should be noted, however, as discussed in chapter 23, that the biological susceptibility is not static. The brain is plastic: it changes with further life events. Thus, life events can increase or,

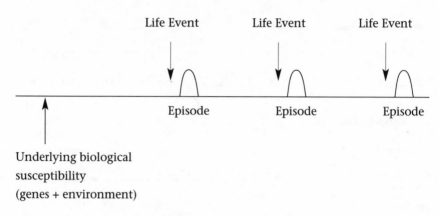

Fig. 13.5. The stress-diathesis model of psychiatric illnesses

potentially, decrease the underlying susceptibility to the illness. Where the underlying susceptibility to illness increases over time, fewer and fewer life events are required for episodes of the illness to become manifest (this is sometimes called the kindling model).

In terms of nosology, the relevance of this discussion is that we often go back and forth between our diagnoses and the underlying diseases or biologies of the illnesses at hand. We wish that each diagnosis, at its simplest level, reflected an underlying disease entity. This does not appear to be the case. The next issue is whether our diagnoses can reflect the underlying biologies of the relevant illnesses. This also does not appear to be the case, partly because our diagnoses may not be valid enough and partly also because the biology of psychiatric illnesses may more closely reflect psychopathological states (as van Praag suggested) than diagnostic constructs (see chapter 11). If this is true, it does not invalidate the utility of diagnostic constructs, but it may suggest the need to augment our clinical nosologies with other nosologies more closely tied to the underlying biology or genetics of these illnesses. Those other nosologies might also be more closely tied to the underlying environmental or psychosocial etiologies of the relevant illnesses. I have suggested, for instance, that the concept of a dissociative spectrum disorder may better reflect the underlying psychopathology and etiology of three apparently unrelated categorical diagnoses. Cloninger suggests that the dimensions of personality may better explain personality disorders in general, and these dimensions may be more directly linked to the relevant biological systems that influence those personality disorders.

14.

In general, I think the categorical versus dimensional distinction is not an either-or in psychiatry. Psychiatrists have tended to go to one extreme or the other. My inclination, based on these considerations, would be to support categorical approaches to major mood and psychotic disorders, allow for dimensional spectra for overlap areas, and at the same time support primarily dimensional approaches to personality disorders. As stated in previous chapters, I hold these views against a backdrop of a pluralistic approach to psychiatric nosology, being willing to allow for multiple nosologies for different purposes, as well as viewing classic categories as ideal types rather than as pure disease entities. I think this approach to psychiatric nosology avoids dogmatism, while staking specific claims for specific conditions based on the strengths and weakness of our methods. This is the pluralistic model in action.

15.

In chapters 14–17, rather than focusing on diagnoses, I want to assess a few specific important clinical phenomena in psychiatric practice, the psychopathology of major clinical pictures seen in mental illnesses.

CHAPTER 14

The Perils of Belief

Psychosis

> The term delusion is vaguely applied to all false judgments that share the following characteristics. . . . (1) they are held with an *extraordinary conviction,* with an incomparable, *subjective certainty;* (2) there is an *imperviousness* to other experiences and to compelling counter-argument; (3) their content is *impossible.* —KARL JASPERS, 1913

1.

The definition of psychosis is tendentious. This can be disheartening: if, after all, we cannot agree on what psychosis means, how can we claim to diagnose it, much less treat it? Superficially, one would expect psychosis to be the simplest thing to diagnose. Even the unversed, when faced with the "crazy" person who talks to himself on a street corner, seem to be able to recognize the psychotic symptom of probable hallucinations. Psychosis appears utterly at odds with "normal" psychological experience, and thus it should be easy to recognize as different from normal experience. All this is not the case with mood, since depression and happiness are part of normal human experience.

Yet psychosis remains controversial. Part of this controversy may reflect the penchant of psychiatrists to argue. Part of it may reflect some real problems.

The standard view is that psychosis is defined by the presence of delusions or hallucinations. Hallucinations are described as the experience of sensory phenomena in the absence of an appropriate stimulus. Delusions are said to be fixed false beliefs. Hallucinations are not purely sensory experiences, however, because the individual experiencing them needs to believe, according to the classic definition, that they are true, when they are not. If someone hears a voice, for instance, and knows that the voice is not "real," this is not technically a true hallucination, according to standard accounts in psychopathology texts. This experience, when the person has insight into a hallucination, is sometimes referred to as a pseudo-hallucination. Although these terms are somewhat arbitrary, the general concept holds that there is a cognitive component to a hallucination. One experiences something sensory and *believes* it to be real, when it is not real. This leads to the conclusion that delusions, the psychotic symptom expressed in thought, are necessary for hallucinations and that therefore all psychosis at bottom rests on the presence of delusion.

2.

So let me now turn to delusion. I said that the standard current view is that a delusion is a fixed false belief. Sometimes it is added that this fixed false belief is held against incontrovertible evidence to the contrary, and sometimes that it also lies outside of the bounds of beliefs that are accepted as true within the culture of the individual involved.

So it appears that the standard view of delusion has at least four properties: it is fixed, false, held against incontrovertible evidence, and culturally atypical. But all of these properties are subject to doubt.

First, are delusions fixed? Not always. Obviously, they can resolve with medications, and sometimes they are amenable to some psychotherapeutic techniques (such as the counterprojective techniques of Harry Stack Sullivan). Also, the same individual can be seen to hold a delusion with varying intensity over the course of a number of days. Second, are delusions false? Not always. The classic example is the Othello Syndrome, in which a person has the delusion that her spouse is cheating on her, based, say, on the constellation of the stars that day; suppose that, for reasons totally unknown to that person, her spouse in fact is cheating on her. We still might say she has a delusion. The conclusion is not false, but we sense that her thinking is not right because it is illogical, or it follows from false premises. Third, are delusions always held against incontrovertible evidence to the contrary? Usually, a clinician does not possess incontrovertible evidence, and yet delusions are diagnosed. Much evidence might be available to show that someone's delusion is false, but rarely is that evidence incontrovertible. I am reminded of the manic patient admitted to the hospital who told us on her arrival that if the Cardinal of Boston called, we should please transfer him to her room. She had delusions regarding many subjects, and we felt that this was one more. The Cardinal called later that night. Fourth, are delusions culturally atypical? This would seem to water down the concept of delusion almost beyond recognition. It is frequently difficult to draw the lines between culturally acceptable and unacceptable ideas; who is to make those judgments? Besides, if some psychoses are mainly biological, why should they differ from culture to culture?

3.

These are the standard objections to the standard definitions of delusion. If we applied a Popperian standard of scientific truth, any one of these objections would be sufficient to refute the whole concept of psychosis, never mind the controversies between a unitary psychosis model and the Kraepelinian dichotomy. This is in fact what the "antipsychiatrists," such as R. D. Laing and Thomas Szasz, preach. But this is too easy. Have we missed something in our descriptions of delusion that gets closer to the mark?

We noted that one aspect of delusion appeared to relate to the logic of the thinking process, as in the Othello Syndrome. It seems not only relevant that the *content* of a thought might be false; it seems relevant also that thought *processes* might be illogical. But is there something about thought processes in delusions that separates them from normal thought processes? Apparently not. Neuropsychological studies of "normal" logical thought processes suggest occasional "abnormal" illogical thinking similar to that which occurs in patients with schizophrenia (Maher 1990). The quality of the logic of thought processes does not appear to differ between normal individuals and those with schizophrenia.

Rather, the frequency and severity of illogical thought processes that are used in a train of thought appear to be increased in schizophrenia. So again, we are left with a continuous dimensional difference rather than a qualitative, categorical one. And this goes against our intuition that psychosis seems categorically quite unlike "normal" human experience.

Others have focused on another aspect of thought processes in schizophrenia that might explain delusions: "looseness of associations." It appears that patients with schizophrenia pay too much attention to all the thoughts and stimuli they experience; they are unable to "filter" those thoughts and stimuli, they become overwhelmed, and they stumble into delusional systems in an attempt to make sense of a crowded jumble of ideas (Andreasen, Paradiso, and O'Leary 1998). This explanation might help with schizophrenia, but it does not seem to apply to all psychosis. In psychotic depression, for instance, this kind of inadequate filtering of associations has not been demonstrated in neuropsychological studies, nor is it prominent clinically.

4.

So, where are we with delusions? If we step back, we can reconstruct how we came to the current impasse. In *General Psychopathology*, Karl Jaspers most clearly described the reasoning behind the standard view about delusions (see chapter 5). Jaspers noted that delusions are generally fixed and false beliefs. He also emphasized that the clinician, trying to understand the patient, hits a major obstacle with delusions: they are "incomprehensible"; the clinician is unable to make heads or tails of them.

The clinician can empathize with many things a patient describes or believes, but this empathy stops when a delusional idea comes forth. The clinician just cannot understand or agree with a delusion for the various reasons described: it may fly in the face of logic or be demonstrably false, among other reasons. In fact, Jaspers believed that this was the hallmark of delusions: the inability to empathize with them. But this seems to place the essential aspect of delusions in someone other than the patient (namely, the doctor). Moreover, this Jasperian intuition, though it agrees with the common feeling that delusions are qualitatively different from normal experience ("This is crazy!"), has not been borne out by neuropsychological research.

So we might lay many of our ideas regarding delusions, along with their problems, at the feet of Karl Jaspers. Can we improve on Jaspers? The philosopher and psychiatrist Manfred Spitzer (1990) has attempted to do so. Reviewing Jaspers's ideas analytically, Spitzer concludes that the key feature of delusions is not that they are beyond our capacity for empathy but that they involve a set of ideas that has no possible objective referent in the real world. The words used to express a delusional idea refer to a state of affairs that is logically and metaphysically *impossible*. Thus, rather than searching the evidence, or assessing the patient's logical processes, or evaluating one's own internal state of empathy, one must search the world to see if the delusional idea could possibly be.

This view could explain bizarre delusions, but it still falls short for nonbizarre delusions. Bizarre delusions are those that are logically impossible: for example, I may believe that the world will end tomorrow because I believe Martians have begun to eat my intestines from the inside out. Nonbizarre delusions are not impossible, though they may be false: the FBI may not be out to get me, but the FBI does "get" people from time to time.

5.

For most delusions, which are nonbizarre, we seem to be in a quandary. Let us return to Jaspers's admonition to assess our philosophic presuppositions. What are we assuming in the above discussion? At bottom, we seem to be presuming, once again, the Popperian view of science, that if a certain definition of delusion is falsified, the definition is false. What if we take here, as we did in our chapters on nosology, the alternative view, fashioned by Peirce: *Let us accept a theory if multiple routes of evidence support it, in the absence of definitive contradictions to the theory, as long as we have no better alternative theory to explain the data.* If we do this with the concept of delusion, we see again that we have a number of routes to assessing whether or not a certain thought is a delusion: first, is it demonstrably false? Second, is it fixed? Third, is it held against overwhelming evidence to the contrary? Fourth, is it not culturally acceptable? Fifth, is it based on illogical thought processes? Sixth, is it logically or metaphysically impossible? The more a belief meets these criteria, the more likely it is to be a delusion. This approach does not give us absolute certainty, but again, it provides a degree of approximate certainty that works for our clinical needs.

6.

If psychosis is so difficult to understand, we might be forgiven for breathing with relief upon turning to something more familiar: mood. After all, most of us are never psychotic, but everyone experiences moods. So this topic should at least be more familiar to us. Does contemporary psychiatry have a good handle on depression and mania?

CHAPTER 15

The Slings and Arrows of Outrageous Fortune

Depression

> [Some] worry that therapeutic approaches to depression undermine explorations of values, as if prescribing Prozac to Mill would have impeded the history of ethics. —MICHAEL MARTIN, 1999

He was an immaculately dressed thirty-three-year-old man. He shook hands firmly and quietly rebuked me for being late. He eventually described going from job to job, being either underqualified or overqualified. Graduating with an M.B.A., he found that "the market" had no room for him. He could not marry his girlfriend, he felt sincerely, because he had a "financial responsibility" to her. Too much pressure on himself—it all ended up in his returning to live with his family, and doing some consulting here and there, and depression. "I'm just not comfortable in my own skin," he said with tears welling up in his eyes. The tears never fell.

1.

Neurologists are sometimes criticized for admiring disease rather than treating it. Psychiatrists have never been subject to similar indictment. If anything, psychiatrists have gone to the other extreme, downplaying diagnosis for years and seeking "great and desperate cures" (Valenstein 1986) for that one illness: insanity.

The philosopher Michael Martin (1999) has provided a nuanced discussion of whether depression should be treated aggressively, as is common practice today, or respected for its moral value, as many suggest. In so doing, he raises a number of important questions that bear on how we understand depression and how we view ourselves as moral agents.

2.

John Stuart Mill serves both as a model and as a warning to philosophers and psychiatrists. He read Homer in the original Greek at the age when children today might just be entering kindergarten. He wrote a major philosophical treatise, "On Utilitarianism," at about the age of college sophomores today. And yet, by that same age, he appears to have experienced a clinical depression of noteworthy severity. He attributed it to an overweening intellectual development, which worked to the detriment of the nourishment and guidance of his emotional life. Whether that is the case or not is unclear. Michael Martin pays a good deal of attention to the lessons of John Stuart Mill's crisis; he suffered severe depression, yet he seemed to learn some important things about himself and humanity. Is there something special about depression, something we should cherish rather than treat? Would society suffer without its shy, studious types—its cautious, deliberative citizens? Excluded would be persons like George Washington, whose thinking Thomas Jefferson described as "slow in operation but sure in conclusion." Jefferson added that "in all aspects of his life, [Washington] was inclined to gloomy apprehensions" (Flexner 1974, 45). Would an extroverted, backslapping president have done as well in trying times as did the brooding Lincoln?[1]

3.

Lincoln's well-known melancholia is just one example out of many that might be cited in defense of admiring rather than treating certain types of depression. The moral value of depression also translates into concrete political and cultural value. The American Civil War may best demonstrate this fact.

The historian T. Harry Williams once compared the three greatest Northern generals (George McClellan, William Sherman, and Ulysses S. Grant) and concluded that the secret of their generalship lay in their character. The greater generals (Grant being better than Sherman, who was more effective than McClellan) were slow to make decisions but unwavering after they were made; thus, their subordinates could rely on their support. This translated into character traits of courage and persistence that paid off in battle. Strikingly, these qualities were penalized in civilian life as much as they were rewarded in war. McClellan had been a golden boy before the war, so successful in school, business, and social life that at age thirty-five, without any prior battle experience, he was given absolute control over a vast army by acclamation. He had never suffered failure, dejection, or doubt; yet his simple untried character unraveled under the pressure of war. Sherman experienced severe depressions and, in my opinion and that of some historians, likely suffered from manic-depressive illness (Ambrose 1967). He was mostly a failure before the war and became paranoid and depressed when commanding by himself during the war ("Wm. T. Sherman Insane," declared a contemporary news clipping); but when supported by and subordinated to Grant, he functioned well and channeled his rage and fury into effective new battlefield tactics. Grant, the ultimate victor, had been an abject failure in civilian life, forced to live with his parents as an adult, a probable alcoholic, shy and reticent to the extreme. In war, he was calm, careful, wise, persistent, and bold; his courage marked him for success.

It is notable that different times (for example, civil war) call for different talents, and success in life does not rest with a single set of psychological skills. Are we treating such skills away when we write prescriptions for depressed individuals?

4.

Depression seems simple. What psychiatrists add to the common conception of depression is the presence of "neurovegetative symptoms." Clinical depression is characterized not only by saddened mood, but also by a constellation of physical symptoms that have in common a general slowing and deadening of bodily functions. One sleeps less, and nighttime becomes a dreaded period. Or one never leaves the bed; better to sleep, if one can, since nothing else can be accomplished. Interest in life and activities declines; what previously engendered motivated effort now produces only listless memories. Thinking itself is difficult; concentration is shot; it is hard enough to focus on three related thoughts, much less read a book. Energy is sapped; constant tiredness, inexplicable and unyielding, wears one down further. Food loses its taste; the pleasures of meals go the way of other lost enjoyments. Or, in an attempt to feel better, one might eat more, perhaps also staving off boredom. The body moves slowly, falling to the declining rhythm of one's thoughts. Or one paces agitatedly, unable to be calm or relaxed, if anxiety pervades the gloomy mood state. One reviews one's life; it seems that everything is the fault of the depressed person; guilt and ceaseless remorse control one's waking thoughts, recurring over and over again. Ultimately, suicide seems like the only action that can put an end to it all; if nothing else prevents it—God, children, family, a loving pet—the reaper's hand falls. About 10 percent or more of these individuals will feel that hand (Goodwin and Jamison 1990).

5.

Freud made his only definitive statement on this subject in his paper "Mourning and Melancholia," which was later published as a book (1917).[2] He held that depression is phenomenologically similar to mourning and that psychologically, what happens in mourning may provide the key to depression. When we mourn the death of a loved one, we often feel a set of ambivalent feelings, Freud argued. We love the person who died; but we are also angry at him, for dying or for things he did while living. If part of our feelings toward that person while alive involved anger toward him, we also feel guilty about this anger once he has died. We irrationally fear that our hatred somehow contributed to the person's demise. Sad at our loved one's death, guilty about our anger toward him, we turn our anger inward, repressing its outward expression, and become even sadder. Freud hypothesized that pathological depression also involved these kinds of ambivalent feelings toward others, repressed by an anger turned inward and directed at oneself.

For decades, Freud's view on this, like his perspective on most other psychiatric syndromes, prevailed. This hypothesis, unlike many of Freud's ideas, is empirically testable, however. Do depressed patients possess a great deal of hostility that is directed toward themselves? This has not been confirmed empirically. In fact, although anger and irritability are present in up to about one-half of individuals with major depression, the other half do not experience any significant anger, either toward others or toward themselves (Nierenberg et al. 1996).

Another idea regarding the explanation of depression stems from research on animal models of depression. One of the most popular paradigms here is the "learned helplessness" model (Huesmann 1978). In this paradigm, it is shown that animals that are shocked or otherwise injured but are not allowed any escape eventually appear afraid and cower; they retain these feelings even when escape routes are later offered. The animals have learned to be helpless, and they remain so. This theory, with roots in behaviorism, suggests that individuals develop depression in adulthood based on experiences earlier in life in which they suffered but had no means of escaping their suffering. A child, for instance, would typically be largely helpless in the face of abusive adults and might develop chronic depression as a result. This evolution of depression does seem relatively common in clinical practice in those individuals with abusive or particularly unstable childhood environments. But many persons appear to have childhoods that are more or less in the normal range of others' experience, and yet they develop depression in adulthood.

Whereas the learned-helplessness model entails a certain cognitive distortion of reality ("I am helpless; life is hopeless; I am sad"), another model involves a very different situation. This view, the "depressive realism" model (Alloy and Abramson 1988), derives from empirical studies of college students, in which depressive symptoms were correlated with responses to special experimental tests of the students' realistic assessments of the world. In these tests, students were exposed to various experiments, in some of which they could control the outcome and in others of which they could not. Depressive symptoms were *more* likely in those students who correctly figured out when the tests were rigged so that they could not affect the outcome of the tests by their own actions. Those who felt they were in control, even when they were not, tended to experience fewer depressive symptoms. The proponents of this model conclude that depression results from seeing the world too much as it is, with all its pain and mortality and with all our weakness and cosmic insignificance as individuals.

6.

The depressive realism model has an important implication. One might conclude that "normal" nondepressed persons have some lacunae of insight, some psychological blind spots, which are necessary for normal emotional functioning. The philosopher Daniel Dennett (1991) has discussed this subject in reference to the neglect syndrome, a severe type of absence of insight in which individuals do not realize that paralysis has occurred after a parietal lobe stroke. Dennett sets up the neglect syndrome as a type of clinical counterpart of the normal phenomenon of the visual blind spot, where the optic nerve enters the retina and thus where no rods or cones exist for vision. This small area of the retina corresponds with a spot in the visual field that, technically, we cannot "see." However, normally, we do not notice this blind spot. Only visual field testing can confirm its existence. Current research in cognitive science is seeking to understand how it is that the brain compensates for the retinal blind spot, either by "filling in" through interpretation from the surrounding retinal regions or through some other mechanisms. Dennett explains the absence of recognition of the blind spot in the visual field through the idea that this empty spot is not missed by the mind because it does not feel a need for it. In other words, the mind does not expect something to be there, so it does not become concerned when nothing is there. It lacks "epistemic hunger" for the blind spot. Similarly, Dennett suggests, parietal lobe injury may lead to a loss of the normal epistemic hunger one possesses for the opposite visual field, leading to a similar lack of awareness and unconcern for the results.

This idea may be extended to lack of insight in psychiatric syndromes. There is a certain attraction to this view. Common sense suggests that we go about our lives ignoring certain painful realities that tend to make us sad, such as the ultimate reality of death. Existentialists, in fact, emphasize that this way of living is inauthentic, "routine" life, and they contrast it with the angst engendered by recognition of the limits of life. We will discuss the topic of insight, denial, and illusion in more detail in chapter 18.

7.

The two explanations of depression seem contradictory. However, comprehending them in terms of the role of insight may clarify matters. Normally, everyone experiences mild depressive symptoms that follow the ups and downs of life: Shakespeare's "slings and arrows of outrageous fortune." In these cases, a certain lack of awareness, a mild psychological denial, may serve a useful purpose. On the one hand, the slings and arrows of life bounce off us, rather than penetrating, if we do not attend to them too closely. On the other hand, we might perceive them as larger and more dangerous than they truly are; they then become mortars and missiles, and we crumble under their perceived power. This may be what happens in the cognitive distortions of severe depression: we are overly aware of evils that we do not truly face. Where insight only incites pain, one needs to learn how to ignore, avoid, and forget.

One theory, then, argues that depression is associated with more insight, and the other that it is associated with less. In part, Martin makes a conceptual argument for the former perspective, holding that even severe pathological depressions can be "insight-provoking." Is there any empirical evidence on this subject? In principle, it should be testable: is depression associated with more or less insight? In studies conducted by my colleagues and others, it appears that in milder types of depression, such as seasonal affective disorder, more depression may be associated with more insight. But severe depressions tend to be associated with some impairment of insight, though modest in comparison with other psychiatric conditions, such as mania or psychosis (Ghaemi 1997).

8.

So what can we conclude? I would agree with Martin that there is no simple distinction between pathological depression, to which a medical perspective applies, and "healthy" depression, to which a moral perspective applies. His discussion of the moral dimensions of therapy is apt. But I would not agree that *most* depression is not a sickness; that too should be empirically testable, and my hunch is that only *some* depression is not sickness. The depressive realism model applies best to that kind of mild depressive syndrome that does not usually quite meet clinically diagnosable parameters of severity. In most cases of clinical depressive illness, severe enough to interfere with one's life and require some intervention, the cognitive distortion model appears to be the rule.

Martin argues against the clean distinction between a type of depression that is healthy, associated with new insights and important thoughts, and one that is pathological and simply needs to be treated. He holds that some pathological depressions can be "insight-provoking" and some healthy depressions can undermine moral autonomy. I would argue that clinical depressions, those that are severe and require some kind of intervention, almost always interfere with the free, rational exercise of moral agency as a result of cognitive distortions and rarely are associated with new important insights, at least during the depressive episode. What Martin may be noticing is that once depressive periods are over, individuals often assimilate those experiences into their worldviews, and the episodes can then exercise an important influence on their values and beliefs. Besides Mill, Martin could have described the seminal depressive experience of William James, which was *followed* by his pragmatic philosophy of life. The temporal sequence is important. James himself believed that his new insights in some way allowed his depression to lift. But the possibility equally exists that his depressive period resolved spontaneously, as is the natural course of any depression, and he then came to terms with what it meant for him. The psychiatrist and anthropologist Arthur Kleinman (1988) has applied this type of interpretation in his distinction between the concept of "disease," or the actual medical condition, and "illness," the individual's interpretation of the impact of a disease on her beliefs, values, and worldview.

9.

If some depressions are pathological, what are their etiologies? The Freudian theory seems too unsubstantiated to help. One hypothesis might be that these individuals, much as is the case with mania, simply suffer from mood states that cannot be understood psychologically. They have a pathology of some kind in the limbic system of the brain, which leads to depressive symptoms. And this neuropathology is the sole explanation for their depressions, despite the phenomenological similarities their clinical symptoms may have to more "psychological" depressions, such as those related to depressive realism or learned helplessness.

Even those "psychological" depressions, if repeated, become biological, however. The learned helplessness studies, for instance, showed that repeated helpless experiences produce certain physiological changes, which then become permanent. The adrenal glands secrete more steroids, the thyroid gland is less responsive to declines in circulating thyroid hormone, and the brain may be altered in its neurotransmitter production or activities. Indeed, repeated major depressive episodes appear to be associated with atrophy of part of the hippocampus, which can be permanent (Brown, Rush, and McEwen 1999). So, although the etiology of the depression may be psychological in some cases, its final common pathway involves brain and hormonal physiological changes.

An important point here is to distinguish between etiology and pathogenesis, to which I also alluded in chapter 13 (see fig. 15.1).[3]

The etiology of an individual's depressive syndrome, based on twin studies (Eaves, Eysenck, and Martin 1989), is typically equally weighted between genetic and environmental factors. The genetic factors are additive and not categorical. Thus, they are not like traditional Mendelian inheritance, where certain genes are dominant and always lead to an illness or trait, while others are recessive and can lead to an illness if two recessive genes occur together. Genes influencing most psychiatric syndromes, as with other medical conditions such as diabetes and hypertension, are additive. Each gene contributes only a little to the risk of developing the illness, and many genes are required to develop

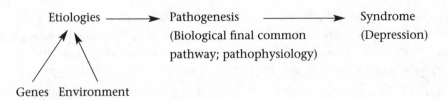

Fig. 15.1. Etiology, pathogenesis, and syndrome

the illness. Even then, the genes confer only susceptibility in many cases, not the illness. That is, they only increase the likelihood that fewer or less severe environmental factors are required for the illness to develop, compared with someone who has fewer disease-related genes. The environmental factors identified are specific rather than shared. That is, they do not reflect the shared family environment; they are specific to each twin. Thus, these may be "the slings and arrows of outrageous fortune" that no one can predict, but they might also be ubiquitous: most of us experience certain types of events—we leave home, we may go away to school, we experience the end of love relationships, we lose jobs, we lose money, we get ill. Two other possible explanations for specific environmental influences exist: the first is birth order, and the second is nonfamily peer relationships. Birth order results in a different family environment for an older versus a younger sibling; the historian of science Frank Sulloway (1996) has marshaled some impressive data showing that birth order can influence many personality traits, with older children generally being more powerful than their younger siblings and tending toward being responsible, conservative, and parental; younger siblings are often more rebellious and nonconformist. Peer relationships are nonfamilial and differ for each sibling, and others have held that much of personality development is related to the influence of peers (Harris 1998). Which one of these factors is related to the environmental aspect of the etiology of depression is unclear. One or all may be relevant. In any case, genetics and environmental effects may explain the etiology of a depressive illness, but still they are mediated by the brain and changes in the physiology of brain and bodily function, resulting in the biological aspects of depressive syndromes. These changes in the brain, such as hypothalamically mediated loss of pleasure and sex drive and changes in appetite, can produce the stereotypic clinical syndrome of depression. This may be why diverse etiologies for depression produce the same clinical syndrome:

the final common pathway in the brain follows the same contours and produces similar symptoms. One can imagine that if the genetic susceptibility to depression is strong enough, very little or practically no environmental precipitant might be required to lead to recurrent depressive illness; this might explain those unexplainable severe depressive illnesses for which no psychological or social factors of significance appear to be implicated in their etiologies.

10.

In summary, depression is not best understood as either psychological or biological, nor as exogenous versus endogenous, nor as reactive versus manic-depressive. All of these distinctions are based on a dualistic view regarding the mind-brain relationship, the limitations of which I discussed in chapter 2. Viewed pluralistically, depression can be caused by many variations of additive genes and specific environmental effects, but these etiologies are always mediated by a biological final common pathway. Clinically, this biological mechanism is demonstrated in neurovegetative symptoms, which differentiate depression as an illness from normal depressive mood. Whatever benefits may accrue from the experience of depression generally follow recovery and do not argue against the need for treatment.

CHAPTER 16

Life's Roller Coaster

Mania

A doctor told me during a counseling session early in my diagnosis that [bipolar disorder] was a garbage-can like diagnosis. I thought to myself: if it's a garbage can diagnosis, I don't want to be bothered with it. I'm not taking medications for a garbage can diagnosis. . . . The best thing about mania is the confidence it gives you—a little bit is great, too much is disastrous. —ANONYMOUS PATIENT

1.

He was thin, a bit too thin for health. He looked bedraggled by life, pulled from Kansas to Washington, D.C., leaving his wife and children behind. "I left it all because I was manic," he said, with an air of disgust. Who was he disgusted with? "I wish someone would have just grabbed me by the scruff of the neck and said, Hey, don't make any life decisions; you've lost your judgment." Life decisions—making too many and/or making them too easily is as dangerous as not making them at all. How clearly mania and depression outline the extremes of the dilemma of us all before the terrible fact of choice: indecisiveness in depression—nothing can be done; overdecisiveness in mania—everything is to be done and nothing gets done. We are doomed to choose, Sartre said, yet we don't know when to choose and when not to choose. "I denied the illness until I discovered that my biological mother was hospitalized for a mental illness; then, I finally realized that it could be true." He was adopted, a perfect setup for ignoring biology. Why did he not accept it despite those facts? Many people know of a family history of mental illness but still won't accept it. For all his disgust at himself, he was an aware man, an unhappy, depressed, dejected man, but an aware man. He fulfilled Socrates' dictum—Know thyself—yet his knowledge gave him neither joy nor power to change things, at least not without taking the step of allowing medicine and science to intervene. He was a podiatrist; now he is a temporary worker. He shook my hands firmly when he left, looking into my eyes as if trying to drain some of my confidence in his recovery into himself. I hoped I was right.

2.

If the nuances of depression seem confusing, one might hope that the opposite mood state, the condition called *mania,* would be more straightforward. However, mania, too, is a complicated phenomenon. Here the mood is classically elated, although usually one alternates between elation and irritability, and sometimes one is purely irritable and not euphoric at all. There often is a sense of giddiness. Time seems to be sped up; the world is slowed down. One does not need to sleep much; everything is going twice as fast. Four hours can do it. While the rest of the world is sleeping, one's energy is running as if it were eleven A.M. on a Wednesday: why not clean the entire house at three A.M.? Things need to get done, even if they don't. Redecorate the house; do it again; buy a third car. Work two hours longer daily: the boss loves it. One's thoughts pour forth; the brain seems to be a many times more efficient organ than the mouth. Trying to keep up with those rapid thoughts, one speaks quickly, interrupting others, running a conversation from only one end. Friends and coworkers get annoyed that they cannot get a word in edgewise. This may produce more irritability; why can't everyone else get up to speed? "Depression is a curse to oneself," Robert Lowell remarked; "mania, to one's friends." Sex becomes even more appealing; one's spouse may like it, or might tire of it. The urge is so strong that one might look to satisfy it elsewhere; affairs are common; divorce is the rule; HIV rates are high. Self-esteem rises; sometimes, it leads to great successes, where one's skills are up to the task; too frequently, it leads to equally grand failures, where circumstances overwhelm one. But there is no past; there is hardly today; only the future counts, and there, anything is possible. Decisions become easy to make; no guilt, no doubt, just do it. The trouble is not in starting things, but in ending them; so much to do, so little time, it's easy to get distracted. Ultimately, bad decisions might get made; too impulsive, they stereotypically fall into four categories: sexual indiscretions, spending sprees, reckless driving, and impulsive traveling. The car becomes a dangerous extension of one's sense of power; accidents, poor driving records, and lethal risks are not uncommon. Traveling is a preferred mode of life; it seems decisive, and things must be better somewhere else. Living in numerous places in a year is typical. Or simply visiting someplace with no plans seems reasonable. Divorce, debt, sexually transmitted diseases, occupational instability: mania is the perfect antipode of the cherished simple goals of most persons: a family, a home, a job, a stable life.

In depression, one takes one's life; in mania, one ruins one's life. In manic-depressive illness, one suffers from both tragic risks.

3.

Theories of mania do not abound.[1] It is as if this condition were too superficial to require deep reasons.

The psychoanalytic view is the most coherent but probably the most wrong-headed. This view sees mania as a defense against depression (Janowsky, Leff, and Epstein 1970). Since patients with bipolar disorder or manic-depressive illness tend to experience both mania and depression, and since mania sometimes follows depression (though usually the reverse is more common, i.e., depression usually follows mania), this view has a certain superficial appeal. I sometimes hear patients spontaneously imagine the same explanation. "Sometimes I think I make myself become manic to ward off a depression," one patient told me. "I make myself be happy about everything and I do a lot of things and I stop sleeping because I know if I don't do this, I'll become depressed." Psychoanalysts used to speak of a "flight into mania," as if the could (albeit presumably unconsciously) decide to become euphoric rather than deal with the important psychological work that the anguish of depression forced him to face. For psychoanalysts, depression was respectable, mania was not. This is why there is so little written about mania in the psychoanalytic literature. Freud at least was honest about this: he wrote practically nothing about mania, and he admitted that psychoanalysis had no role in the understanding or treatment of manic-depressive illness. His followers, as always, spoke where he was silent. They blamed the manic patients for being too childish to face their depressions. When antidepressants and antipsychotic agents began to be used in the 1960s, many psychoanalysts reacted by opposing their use. There was much fretting about how such medications would remove the anxiety and the dysphoric mood that give impetus to patients to enter into psychoanalysis and engage in the difficult work that psychoanalytic therapy involved.

The problem here is that the vast majority of patients describe mania as completely uncontrollable. It comes on involuntarily, sometimes quite rapidly, and, in most cases, it takes charge of one's life no matter how hard one tries to stave it off. Ascribing the motivation to become manic as an unconscious one is a cop-out at best. This psychoanalytic piece of dogma also misunderstands mania: it assumes mania simply to be pleasurable, but most manic patients are irritable or dysphoric rather than euphoric. Thus, clinically, most manic patients do not want to become manic. But many want to be hypomanic: a little bit of mania is often "addictive," as some patients put it. The psychoanalysts may have hit on something. Yet the involuntary nature of mania still makes it hard to conceive of it as in any way motivated by an individual's wishes (without assuming the unknowable unconscious forces, as always).

Finally, about 10 percent of manic patients never experience depression, so it is unclear how they could be fleeing from experiences of depression into mania.

If mania is not a defense against depression, then what is it?

4.

Mania is incredibly difficult to conceptualize. Seeing patients with bipolar disorder day in and day out, I find that they also have a hard time describing their understanding of themselves when they experience mania. The main thing they focus on is the aspect of manic symptoms that they think may be a part of their basic personality: those who are artistic, in particular, feel that their creativity is part of their personality. Frequently their creativity is enhanced during hypomanic or manic episodes, and they value those episodes for making them more creative. So they see mania as, in some way, an enhancement of some of the best aspects of their personality. Others, especially those who are not in the arts but may work in more regimented occupations like business or accounting, see mania as an enhancement of their physical energy, allowing them to spend more time at work and accomplish more. For them, mania is an enhancement of their basic biological energy level. Others, who are usually introverted, become much more outgoing and extroverted when they are manic. Mania becomes a temporary "personality transplant," turning them into the "life of the party" type of character that our society rewards. But most people see negative sides to their manic periods too: there is the calm, friendly fellow who becomes irritable and insufferable when manic. There is the loving husband whose sexual energies go out of control when he is manic, resulting in visits to prostitutes, irrational affairs, and intolerable pain inflicted on his spouse. (Not being divorced is exceptional.) And there are the impulsive business deals, and the years of work needed to recover from debts.

5.

Mania is a double-edged sword. In Freudian terms, one might say that it enhances the id, for better or for worse. All energies, sexual and otherwise, overwhelm the usual controls that we learn over a lifetime. Recent research suggests that impulsivity is the key factor that is increased in mania (Swann et al. 2002). That is the one consistent characteristic of patients with mania: they may be euphoric or depressed, irritable or not, have racing thoughts or not, be distractible or not; but they almost always are more impulsive than when they are not manic. One would be tempted to describe this in neurological terms as did John Hughlings Jackson (1958), the pioneer of English neurology, who argued that the higher centers of the brain (i.e., the neocortex) are more evolutionarily advanced areas whose role is to curb the impulses of the lower centers of the brain (our "animal" natures). The frontal neocortex, in particular, has been shown to exert this control. We know too little about the specific pathways involved to describe the exact mechanism by which frontal lobe dysfunction may be involved in underlying the impulsivity that characterizes mania. Suffice it to say that phenomenologically the key feature of mania is impulsivity, tied to euphoria/irritability and sped-up thinking.

If to be manic means to be impulsive, mania may be best described by saying that the civilized veneer that holds our lives together is stretched. If it is stretched only a little, we may function fine and actually be rewarded for our creativity and extroversion. If it is stretched too much, society disapproves, and we ourselves tend to disapprove when we see the consequences of our lack of control.

6.

Besides the irrefutable necessity to use mood-stabilizing medications, I think it is an underappreciated reality that the therapeutic alliance between clinician and patient is a mood stabilizer.[2] By this I mean that the relationship between the clinician and the patient is an important aspect of stabilizing the moods of a person with bipolar disorder. When the patient is becoming manic, it is mood-stabilizing if he or a family member knows that a phone call to the clinician can result in an immediate discussion and also a face-to-face visit within days. When the patient is becoming depressed, it is mood-stabilizing if he can call the clinician and perhaps be reassured that there is no need to make changes in his medications unless the depressive symptoms persist another week. At that time, when he comes for a newly made appointment, he and his clinician may decide to begin antidepressant medication, or may not. In any case, at every point of the inevitable ups and downs of this condition, the patient's mood is stabilized by knowing that the clinician is there for him, easily accessible, able to make medication changes or not on short notice.

Once, when I described this concept of the therapeutic alliance as a mood stabilizer to a group of psychiatrists in Quebec, one of them came up to me and asked, "What is the dose of the therapeutic alliance as mood stabilizer?" I thought he was joking, but he was serious. And then I realized that there was a dose. The dose was how much time and effort I spent in the treatment focusing on developing, maintaining, and expanding the therapeutic alliance. I often use existential psychotherapy techniques, such as those described by Havens, to establish a better alliance with new patients with bipolar disorder. I prefer to have a 30-minute psychopharmacology session, rather than 15 or 20 minutes, because I need 10–15 minutes for the existential psychotherapeutic work that propagates the therapeutic alliance. In other words, I split the psychopharmacology session into 15–20 minutes in which we talk about the mood-stabilizing medications and 10–15 minutes in which we foster the mood-stabilizing therapeutic alliance. As I spoke more with my colleague, I realized that I had in fact developed my own habit in this regard. Usually, as I walk with my patient from the waiting room to the office, we discuss the weather or some other innocuous topic. Again, Havens (1986) has seriously discussed the relevance of talking about the weather in psychotherapy. This kind of benign topic allows one to establish an initial nonthreatening rapport with the patient on that visit. (One of the few benefits of the rapidly changing weather in Boston is that it makes for a constant topic of conversation.) When we reach the office, I say nothing; either I simply listen, or I prod patients to tell me how they are, what they are doing in their lives, or whatever else they may wish to discuss. Sometimes patients come with an agenda, and we discuss their wishes; sometimes they come unprepared, and we discuss whatever comes to mind. We do this for 5–10 minutes, and then I segue into a discussion of symptoms, medications, and side effects (some of which might have been mentioned spontaneously earlier). After 15–20 minutes, I end with another 5 minutes of unstructured conversation about whatever else might be on the patient's mind, or a discussion of another benign topic (like sports, or other personal interests of the patient).

Hence, attention to psychotherapeutic methods is also important in the treatment of bipolar disorder. By enhancing the therapeutic alliance, the clinician himself can exert an important mood-stabilizing effect.

7.

Underlying all our attempts to understand psychopathology is the basic phenomenon of self-consciousness, of awareness of our existence and of our mental states. Self-awareness is itself a topic of importance and some complexity.

CHAPTER 17

Being Self-Aware

Insight

> Psychic illness looks different to the medical observer from what it looks
> like to the patient who is reflecting on himself. —KARL JASPERS, 1913

1.

Thus far I have surveyed the traditional subject matters of psychiatry: psychosis, depression, mania, personality, nosology. One phenomenon has been touched on that underlies all those discussions; it is, to my mind, the central phenomenon of psychiatry: *insight.* The term here refers to the perspective that an individual maintains toward her own psychological state. If one knew, from a God's-eye perspective, so to speak, that certain individuals suffered from certain psychopathologies (depression, mania, psychosis), then those persons would have insight if they were aware of experiencing those mental states. For physical conditions, nonpsychiatric medical illnesses, this is usually not a problem. I have a pain *here;* the patient is aware of the pathological physical state of a part of the body. With rare but important exceptions in certain neurological diseases, most nonpsychiatric conditions are not, by nature, associated with impairment of insight. Psychiatric conditions, however, often entail impaired insight. Is this something special about psychiatric illnesses? Does this argue decisively against the psychiatric belief that mental illnesses are disease states like physical illnesses? In other words, is impaired insight merely disagreement between doctor and patient? And when the doctor is a psychiatrist, with his poor diagnostic methods and lack of laboratory tests, who is to say who is right?

The problem of insight is a central conundrum for psychiatry. At one level, it simply raises the question, How can we know that someone else's mental states are pathological? How can we know that a person is mentally ill? How can we know anything about anyone else? Indeed, at its extreme, the question is, How can we know anything about any mental states, our own or those of others?

A popular belief about psychiatrists is that they actually possess this power. They can know the mental states of others; they almost seem to read the minds of others. The ubiquity of this view is amazing. A minority hold the opposite view. Psychiatrists are quacks, understand nothing, and are nothing but pretenders to science. One wonders how many of those who attack psychiatrists actually fear shrinks because they secretly are believers in psychiatric omniscience. But to say this would be to act the part of a psychiatrist. Psychiatrists do not tend to vehemently argue with those who believe in their powers; instead they dispute with those who attack the field wholesale. But when honestly speaking among themselves, psychiatrists focus on how little they know about other human beings, how unpredictable patients are, how difficult it is to diagnose, how haphazard success at healing is. In more philosophical moments, they may applaud human unpredictability; after all, that is freedom. If psychiatrists could know everything about anyone, what would stop such knowledge from leading to a police state? Did not Hitler's men exercise such rudimentary knowledge ("the big lie")? But practically speaking, for psychiatrists, some knowledge must be possible if patients are to be helped. We must be able to understand our patients' minds, sometimes better than they do, in order to help them. But can we really do this? How do we get inside someone else's head?

At a very basic level, we don't. Everything in psychiatry is inference. Sometimes those inferences are correct. And we are correct with certain matters frequently enough to become rather confident in those inferences. But this is a probabilistic matter. In any one instance, we cannot be sure we have divined someone else's mental state correctly.

2.

But can we really know anything about another person's mental states? Some hold that we cannot even know what is in our own heads, much less those of others. And some argue that we know everything in our own heads but nothing in those of others. I have alluded to these philosophical arguments in the first part of this book. Here I want to emphasize the clinical syndromes in which insight into oneself is impaired and try to conceptualize what these syndromes mean.

There is a set of psychological syndromes characterized by a relative lack of awareness of oneself or of one's surroundings. Knowledge about these syndromes is advancing only gradually, but it is touching upon important aspects of human psychology and philosophy. In this chapter these "awareness syndromes" will be explored.

The awareness syndromes involve some degree of impairment of subjective awareness of mental phenomena. What they hold in common is the phenomenological property of some degree of lack of awareness. Given this conception, they can be outlined as follows: denial is the mildest of the awareness syndromes, with a small degree of impairment of subjective phenomena of consciousness; it occurs in everyone and is normal to that extent. Lack of insight represents a moderate amount of impairment of awareness; it occurs mainly in psychiatric disorders of moderate to severe intensity, such as manic-depressive illness or schizophrenia, and is thus to that extent abnormal. Anosognosia is more dense and more noticeably abnormal than lack of insight, occurring mainly in neurological conditions such as stroke or Alzheimer's disease.

3.

The first and most important thing to note about denial is that it is normal. Everyone engages in denial in some circumstances and to some degree. Followers of Freud have discussed it as one of the defense mechanisms, among which it is one of the more commonly used. Compared to other defense mechanisms, it is intermediate in terms of the degree to which it can be harmfully or excessively used.

The idea of defense mechanisms probably represents one of the core of ideas derived from Freud that have evolved some empirical backing and have maintained their usefulness in clinical practice today despite the decline of other psychoanalytic doctrines. The basic idea follows from Freud's division of the functioning of the mind into three parts: the id, which represents the unconscious source of emotions; the superego, which represents the unconscious source of conscience and parental influence; and the ego, which represents the mostly conscious source of our feelings and behavior. The defense mechanisms are, in a way, the constituents of the boundaries between the ego and its unconscious surroundings, the id and the superego.

The defense mechanisms defend the ego against these unconscious sources of influence. Freud's earlier topography of the mind, in which the mind was divided into conscious and unconscious processes, would also be sufficient to allow for an understanding of the role of defense mechanisms. Defense mechanisms essentially guard the border between unconscious and conscious mental processes; they protect the conscious mind as best they can from disturbing unconscious directives. One could make a reasonable argument today that there is both experimental and clinical evidence for at least this first Freudian division of the mind, into conscious and unconscious mental processes. Experimentally, numerous neuropsychological studies have shown that much mental processing occurs without any awareness; for instance, the well-known phenomenon of *blindsight,* in which the subject who has experienced a stroke involving certain visual cortical fibers claims not to be able to see at all but is able to locate objects in the visual field at better than chance levels under conditions of forced-choice guessing.[1] This type of unconscious mental processing should not be surprising to those who subscribe to a version of the identity theory of mind, which holds that the mind and the brain are identical; this is because it is clear from basic neuroanatomy that most neural functioning occurs at a level preceding that which involves awareness of conscious mentation or behavior.

But this type of experimental processing, though it supports the existence of certain *nonconscious* mental phenomena, does not directly confirm Freud's notion of *unconscious* mental phenomena, with the specific connotation Freud gave to the unconscious, that is, the suppression of anxiety-inducing emotional drives. Here one must rely on clinical evidence, which fails many of the tests of experimental science, for it cannot control for many variables and because there is no blinding of the observer, thus allowing for multiple sources of bias. Despite these shortcomings, one is still struck by the stereotypic manner in which many psychotherapy patients will demonstrate behavior that resembles unconscious mental phenomena to the observing psychotherapist. Young psychotherapists, no matter how skeptical of such matters, will soon experience many times the unaccountable hatred of their patients, which later seems to follow a pattern of a certain anger directed toward someone else. And when this anger toward this other person is revealed or otherwise allowed to direct itself toward that person, the anger toward the therapist ceases. Or the therapists, despite their best intentions, will suddenly discover that they have hated a patient secretly and have behaved as if they hated that patient, all the time not realizing that the patient has elicited such hatred. These patterns of unrecognized emotions occur over and over again so stereotypically that it becomes hard not to suspect that not everything that happens in the human mind is clear and visible to the mind's owner. Again, this is not scientific proof. The only proof in such matters could be a clear refutation, as Popper has suggested. But in the absence of clear refutation, such evidence should allow a cautious limited recognition of the likelihood of the existence of unconscious mental processes.

Proceeding from there, similar lines of evidence may be drawn for the existence of defense mechanisms. Empirical evidence has been collected in a number of different studies. One of the best examples is the impressive work of George Vaillant (Vaillant, Bond, and Vaillant 1986). He described "an empirically validated hierarchy of defense mechanisms" based on a forty-year follow-up of 307 men, recruited during college and followed into adulthood with a number of psychological evaluations and outcome measures. They were interviewed extensively again at age forty-seven, and conclusions were made regarding different types of defense mechanisms used by these men. These defense mechanisms, derived from mainly Freudian origins, were compared with actual social and psychological outcomes, measured objectively by such characteristics as career success, incidence of divorce, and physical health, as well as with more subjective measures of perceived satisfaction with work, family, and relationships. In a remarkably consistent manner, more "mature" defense mechanisms such as altruism, sublimation, and humor were highly correlated with success in psychological outcome measures, whereas less mature defense mechanisms, including denial, correlated poorly with good psychological outcome. This study is one of the few research studies that has been able to apply accepted scientific standards of objective measurement and statistical significance to carefully assessed psychological characteristics like defense mechanisms over a lifetime in normal subjects. This type of research, daunting in its difficulty, is what has been missing in getting beyond mere theoretical debate in psychology.

Clinical evidence for defense mechanisms is tied up with clinical evidence of unconscious mental processes in general. The experience of being hated by a psychotherapy patient because of a transfer of feelings of hatred held toward someone else is the experience that psychoanalysts subsume under the name *projection*. Similarly, a therapist may not recognize that he has a certain feeling about his patient which (he sees clearly in retrospect) he must have had to explain his behavior—that is, he had been in denial. Again, Popperian certainty is not achieved, because such evidence does not refute some putative "antidenial" phenomenon, but the preponderance of the clinical evidence lends weight to the assertion that defense mechanisms are one manifestation of the functioning of the mind.

Denial as a clinical phenomenon is also recognized in medical illnesses, such as smoking or cardiac illness. It is a commonplace of medical practice that the cigarette smoker will ignore the harmful effects of smoking, engaging in clear-cut (to others) denial of the risk. Many persons with cardiac illness will deny that they have symptoms of such illness, ascribing chest pain and other typical symptoms to varied noncardiac illnesses, such as the flu.

Hence denial, a normal defense mechanism, can be wrongly or excessively used in circumstances in which it may interfere with necessary awareness.

4.

Lack of insight is an awareness syndrome of greater severity than denial. It tends to be characteristic of psychiatric conditions such as schizophrenia or manic-depressive illness, in which most patients are unaware of having their illness or needing treatment. This lack of awareness is more severe than denial in that it cannot be considered normal. Many patients possess insight into their symptoms of schizophrenia, for instance, and they tend to have a better prognosis. The rational faculty of those patients who do not have such insight, although they are often quite capable in other arenas, seems to stop short at the line where their diagnosis is made.

The British psychiatrist Aubrey Lewis (1934) held that lack of insight was an aspect of certain psychiatric illnesses, as much a part of their presentation as any other symptom. For Karl Jaspers, in contrast, insight depended on one's personality and intelligence. Freud initially seemed to think that gaining insight was tantamount to cure, but later in his life, he downplayed insight and focused on the impact of the transference relationship between doctor and patient (1910). More recently, the psychiatrist Anthony David (1990) resurrected the problem of insight and threw new light on it by making an important distinction between psychosis and lack of insight. Traditionally, the two often were vaguely deemed equivalent, and psychosis, following Jaspers, was tersely defined as "fixed, false belief." In other words, a thought was delusional if it was false and held rigidly despite "incontrovertible evidence to the contrary." Persons with delusions obviously would seem to lack insight into the unreality of their thoughts. But the psychiatrist Kenneth Kendler and colleagues

(1983) showed that there are dimensions to delusions, and they argued that rather than simply having "fixed, false beliefs," "often deluded patients do not have absolute conviction." Delusions, rather than simply existing or not, thus have gradations of severity. Thus, insight may be completely absent in some delusions and partially present in others; insight may even be completely present in some delusions (which are then labeled ego-dystonic: "I hear my dead grandmother's voice, but I know it can't be her.") Lack of insight and psychosis are not equivalent. Interestingly, neither are delusions necessarily false; delusions of jealousy in which a spouse is deemed unfaithful, for instance, are sometimes true, their delusional character resulting from the poor logical grounds on which the belief is based rather than on the verity of its content. Two studies support the distinction between lack of insight and psychosis. First, David found no correlation between "the ability to reinterpret psychotic experiences and amenability to contradiction" and his overall insight measure, suggesting that lack of insight and delusions are unrelated phenomena (1990). Also, the psychologist Xavier Amador and his colleagues found that no measure of delusions correlated with any score on their insight scale, which included measurements of degree of insight into "delusions," "thought disorder," and "hallucinations," again suggesting that insight is not a proxy for severity of delusions (Amador et al. 1991). Amador and colleagues added that insight was "modality-specific" in that it might exist in relation to one set of symptoms and not another. They also suggested that insight be phenomenologically divided in two: one aspect representing "awareness" or "recognition of signs or symptoms of illness," and another representing "attribution" or "explanations about the cause or source of signs or symptoms."

Many empirical studies now exist in both schizophrenia and manic-depressive illness, using scales developed by some of the above-mentioned researchers, showing that around 60–70 percent of these patients have some impairment in their capacity for insight. These studies confirm that such a dimensional approach to lack of insight does seem to identify a psychopathological phenomenon at work in these illnesses.

5.

Anosognosia is the awareness syndrome that has been identified most clearly. Being the most extreme and severe of the awareness syndromes, its phenomenology is impressive. It mainly consists of the neglect of certain parts of one's body or of the presence of one's physical incapacities as a result of certain neurological conditions.

The paradigmatic case of anosognosia is the parietal lobe syndrome, usually resulting from cerebrovascular disease, or stroke, affecting the nondominant parietal lobe (Heilman, Valenstein, and Watson 1985). In this condition, if a person is presented with an affected limb, such as the left hand, she would deny that the hand belongs to herself. She may pay no attention to the left side of her visual field. All the relevant stimuli, visual and auditory and otherwise, are present; the patient simply does not *attend* to them in the usual manner.

Recently, the neurologist V. S. Ramachandran has demonstrated a curious phenomenon whereby contralateral vestibular stimulation causes a temporary cure of the neglect syndrome, with the parietal stroke patient recognizing and attending to the affected side for a few hours after cold calorics testing (Ramachandran and Blakeslee 1998). This finding may suggest the possibility that the neglect syndrome reflects altered subcortical function, which is temporarily reversed by vestibular system activity, rather than permanent cortical neuronal death, as in typical motor-sensory stroke syndromes.

A second major example of anosognosia occurs in Alzheimer's disease. In this case, patients do not realize that they have lost their memory and are unable to function normally. Thus patients will attempt to drive although they are not able to handle a car. Or they might seek to handle their finances although they are unable to do simple calculations. Or they may insist that their memory is perfectly intact, when they cannot remember a family member's name from one moment to the next. This type of lack of awareness of severe cognitive deficits occurs in 15–25 percent of persons with Alzheimer's disease. Recently it has been suggested that this anosognosia of Alzheimer's disease is associated with abnormalities of the right frontal lobe (Starkstein et al. 1995). Such patients did not have other neuropsychological deficits (such as memory, attention, or abstract reasoning), compared with Alzheimer's patients who did not have anosognosia. Thus, unlike hemineglect, where the nondominant parietal lobe is thought to be injured, in this case the source of anosognosia may be the nondominant frontal lobe.

6.

As noted earlier, the philosopher Daniel Dennett (1991) has discussed the neglect syndrome in terms of his theory of mind by reference to the concept of "epistemic hunger," as a clinical counterpart of the normal phenomenon of the visual blind spot, which we do not notice. Similarly, the awareness syndromes in general may all possess lack of epistemic hunger as their unifying phenomenological feature. Lack of insight in psychiatric syndromes and denial in normal psychology are simply more subtle expressions of the dense anosognosia of stroke and dementia.

If this suggestion is true, then a few conclusions may follow.

First, lack of epistemic hunger would be normal. The psychological correlate of the retinal blind spot may be the normal psychological defense mechanism of denial. A certain amount of unawareness of what we do not know psychologically may be adaptive, useful, and thus "normal" for human beings.

Second, lack of epistemic hunger may be abnormal when it is extreme, as in stroke and dementia, or when it is somewhat less severe, as in schizophrenia and bipolar disorder.

Third, philosophical speculation about the relevance of the limits of thought, as suggested by some philosophers (McGinn 1990), may be supplemented by a discussion of the limits of awareness. In other words, our understanding of the mind or of nature or of any other field of inquiry may not be limited so much by the fact that we possess minds, or are part of nature, or have some structural defect of human reason that limits its capability of knowing. Rather, we may simply be unable to be *aware* of some things, in the perceptual sense implied by the difference between awareness and thinking, and this lack of awareness that is hardwired in us prevents us from recognizing certain aspects of ourselves or of things around us.

Fourth, if this is the case, if a certain (possibly small) lack of awareness is a fundamental datum of human consciousness, then theories of consciousness and self-consciousness should include attempts to understand and take into account the facts of the awareness syndromes.

7.

The psychoanalyst Donald W. Winnicott's theories may support the philosophical implication that lack of awareness may be a fundamental datum of human consciousness (Winnicott 1958). Working a few decades after Freud, Winnicott emphasized the positive role that illusion plays in the life of the mind. He held, unlike Freud, that certain normal psychological phenomena are "illusions" that are unreal or misunderstood by the subject in some way.

This not only is unavoidable, Winnicott added, but it is good. We need illusions for our psychological health. His classic example was the "transitional object," the endowment of subjective powers to an inanimate object, such as a stuffed animal or a blanket, which occurs almost universally in preschool children. Winnicott described this phase of a child's development as involving the belief in a necessary psychological illusion that allows the child to gradually move toward mature "object relations" in which the child can distinguish the self from outside persons.

In the temporary phase of the transitional object, the child uses the illusion of the existence of a subjective being in the object to practice learning object relations. Thus, as a psychological illusion, the transitional object is useful and healthy.

Later writers have expanded on Winnicott's concept of illusion and applied it to other phenomena such as religion, intending to indicate the positive psychological effects of such illusory phenomena. This thinking has roots as far back as William James, but fleshed out by Winnicott's psychological work, it may hold some promise.

Another source of support for Winnicott's line of thinking may come from the awareness syndromes. If it is true that a certain amount of lack of awareness, manifested as the defense mechanism of denial, is normally present in a healthy mind, then this denial may produce a certain amount of illusory psychological phenomena. Again, if this normal reliance on illusion is similar to the retinal blind spot in the functional role it plays psychologically, it may simply reflect a certain lack of epistemic hunger. Maybe we do not need to know that which we deny, at least temporarily or in certain stages of normal psychological development.

8.

Readers of psychoanalytic theory may wonder why so much is made of Winnicott with only a passing reference to Freud. Freud, of course, famously argued that religion is basically one big illusion ([1927] 1953–74). He did not consider illusions to be good or to serve any positive purpose, as Winnicott did.

Some of Freud's successors have not been as antireligious in their interpretation of illusion. Often building on Winnicott, many psychoanalysts have worked hard to reconcile psychoanalysis and religion. But they have not cleared up the question of the role of illusion: is it good or is it bad?

Freud held concretely that illusion is completely bad. Early in his work, he felt that once illusory beliefs were revealed to be what they are, the truth would set people free from their neuroses. In one of his last works, the ever-revealing "Analysis Terminable and Interminable," he took almost the opposite view ([1937] 1953–74). Brooding on the difficulties of convincing patients of the accuracy of psychoanalytic interpretations, the vexing problem of "resistance," Freud more or less threw his hands up in the air. He basically stated that analysis takes a long time, and sometimes it works and sometimes it doesn't, and it is unclear why certain analytic "truths" seem accepted and helpful for the patient and others do not.

Again, the awareness syndromes may provide a new perspective. It may be that the resistance Freud encountered had little to do with the truth of the psychoanalytic interpretations, or even with a patient's transference (or unconscious psychological reaction) to the analyst. Rather, certain interpretations, even if true, may have been resisted because they transgressed the bounds of normal illusion, of healthy denial. No patient wants this level of analysis. When patients come for medicines, they will not accept surgery.

When interpretations seem to be helpful to a patient, or seem to advance the analysis well, it may be because they break through negative illusions, unhealthy denial, whether because this denial is occurring at an inappropriate stage of psychological development or because it is encroaching upon areas of psychological functioning where insight is necessary. When lack of awareness becomes pathological, in excessive denial or in lack of insight, it may be true, as Freud held, that the illusions it fosters are unhealthy. It is these illusions that psychoanalytic technique can strip and throw away, leaving patients unburdened and free to vest themselves with truth. But, as is admitted by many clinicians, by delving into a core of illusion that should not be touched, psychoanalysis can make a patient's condition worse (even sometimes precipitating psychosis in a vulnerable person). In those cases, the stripping work of analysis leaves patients bare and helpless to ward off certain emotions or aspects of their psyche that they need to keep at bay.

It may be, then, that Freud and Winnicott are best understood as describing aspects of psychological life that are touched upon by different levels of awareness, Winnicott describing the normal illusions that protect an untouchable core of the self, and Freud revealing the need for insight into parts of mental life that are ignored at one's peril.

9.

Certain common psychiatric conditions, such as clinical depression, may be better understood in terms of the relevance of awareness syndromes.

Two perspectives on the psychological mechanisms underlying depression, which have evolved along separate lines, are the cognitive-behavioral and the social psychology schools. The cognitive-behavioral school, which has gained much stature among clinicians, has compiled evidence suggesting that a major psychological mechanism behind clinical depression is the tendency of patients to distort reality through inaccurate cognitive mind-sets. In other words, what they think about the world is consistently wrong, and wrong in such a way that it makes them sad. Their mood is depressed because their cognition is depressing. A good deal of success has been achieved with cognitive-behavioral psychotherapy that aims at altering depressive cognitive styles.

An approach that was noted earlier, termed *depressive realism,* is based on research in the social psychology literature. This line of thought has grown out of research done with normal subjects: the subjects were given certain tests of cognitive functioning, in some of which their errors were due to their own decisions, and in others of which errors were introduced randomly outside of the subjects' control. Subjects were asked to describe to what extent they felt they were causing the errors produced. Those who had some depressive symptoms based on self-report rating scales were more accurate than those without depressive symptoms in correctly attributing error to themselves as opposed to random error beyond their control. Conversely, the "normal," nondepressed subjects had a sense of greater control than they really possessed. Therefore, researchers suggested that these mildly depressed (but not clinically depressed and thus "normal") subjects were more realistic than their completely nondepressed counterparts.

These two explanations of depression seem contradictory. However, comprehending them in terms of the awareness syndromes may show how they might converge. As discussed in chapter 15, everyone experiences mild depressive symptoms that follow the ups and downs of life, and a mild denial is usually helpful in relation to these life events. However, in clinical depression, we may exaggerate these life events, thereby worsening our mood state through our own cognitive distortions (excessive insight).

10.

The awareness syndromes are a set of psychological conditions that range from normal to abnormal and can be divided into three types, with increasing severity of abnormality: denial, lack of insight, and anosognosia. Until now, anosognosia has been the most studied and discussed awareness syndrome. Denial and lack of insight are beginning to be studied more carefully, and they too may possess important implications for human psychology and philosophy. The most important implication may come from the recognition that a certain amount of lack of awareness is psychologically normal. This implies that lack of awareness (albeit perhaps small, like the retinal blind spot) may be a fundamental datum for human consciousness, a putative fact with potentially large implications. This fact may be incorporated into Dennett's concept of epistemic hunger, or it may reflect an aspect of the natural limits of human knowledge, based on perceptual and psychological rather than cognitive foundations. Winnicott and Freud have provided clinical evidence for the relevance of illusion, in some cases, and insight, in other cases, to different aspects of mental life. Also, clinical depression can be understood, from one perspective, in terms of an excess of awareness of life's slings and arrows. In all these cases, the awareness syndromes throw new light on human psychology and suggest novel implications for the philosophy of mind.

11.

Impairment of insight, as a form of psychopathology, leads us directly to an ethical problem touched on earlier: can someone who is mentally ill, who lacks insight into his illness, be coerced into treatment and thus *forced* to become well?

There are those who insist that mental illness is a chimera. They point to the difficulties in establishing what is "normal," and thus in differentiating the abnormal from the normal, and they conclude that there is no such thing as mental illness. These persons justifiably oppose any attempt to treat purported mental illness coercively. Others who oppose forcible psychiatric treatment include civil libertarians. Traditionally, activists for civil liberties have tended to focus on physical rights. Thus, proponents of civil rights would oppose the legal jailing of someone's body. It is not surprising that such civil rights activists would be even more opposed to the imprisonment of someone's mind. Psychiatry as a profession has, in the past, also overstepped its bounds. Physicians have sometimes hospitalized patients excessively or given patients treatments without obtaining fair informed consent. Thus, over the years, patients and their families also have tended to grant too much power to psychiatrists and hospitals.

However, although it is true that sometimes it is difficult to distinguish psychiatric illness from normality, strict civil libertarianism seems too extreme a reaction. The strongest argument against such extreme civil libertarianism is the problem of lack of insight. If it is true, as it seems to be, that in some of the more severe mental conditions, patients do not recognize that something is going wrong with them, their ability to make decisions for themselves might be impaired.

In recent times, this issue has come to the fore when individuals diagnosed with severe mental illness, often schizophrenia, went untreated and then hurt others. In one case in New York, a person with schizophrenia pushed another person in front of a subway car.

I believe that careful attention to the two underlying concepts here will help clarify a fair-minded approach to public policy on this subject. On the one hand, subtle forms of mental illness are hard to distinguish from normality, and in fact the general concept of mental illness, conceived broadly, is subject to real philosophical debate. On the other hand, severe mental conditions like schizophrenia and mania are associated with impairment of insight on the part of the person who possesses those conditions. Further, research and evidence indicate that those conditions have the marks of true illness and thus represent abnormal states of mind.

Taken together, these views might support coercive treatment in the case of those severe illnesses only, and only when associated with documented impairment of insight (which can be rather objectively assessed with standardized interview rating scales). However, it would seem reasonable to avoid coercion in any but those circumstances. Further, coercive treatment ideally would best occur when guardianship of some kind could be legally established with a family member or court-appointed individual.

Mental illness is a broad and vague concept. Impaired insight in mania and schizophrenia is more precise. Policymakers could do well to recognize that distinction.

CHAPTER 18

Psychopharmacology

Calvinism or Hedonism?

> Today's high-tech capitalism values a very different temperament: Confidence, flexibility, quickness, and energy—the positive aspects of hyperthymia—are at a premium. —PETER KRAMER, 1993

1.

She was a timid young woman; nervously, and at odd intervals, she sucked at her water bottle, as if it could provide the comfort that the rest of the world denied her. She was slightly chubby, pale, and had an air of innocence about her; she looked like she came from a place where the air was pure and the terrain expansive. She did; North Dakota, however, was too boring. So she left home at eighteen and came to Boston; she worked as a nanny, spent money on clothes rather than school, and has been seeking an end to her boredom ever since. "I'm disconnected from everyone else," she complained, her boyfriend and the forty girls who live with her in a rooming house notwithstanding. As far as she was concerned, she lived alone in a crowd of strangers. So, when she saw a friend taking Prozac, she decided to try it. One a day for a month; she didn't need a doctor to tell her how to do it. And it worked. "How did Prozac affect you?" I asked. "It was like putting on glasses for the first time," she replied. "Everything suddenly became clear." But without a doctor, her friend's supply ran out, and she sank down again into her pure, innocent, disconnected world.

The advent of relatively safe and effective medications has transformed psychiatry. But, instead of simply treating diseases, will we try to "improve" normality in the future? One of the issues that have become prominent with the availability of many new and well-tolerated antidepressant medications is the question, Who should be treated?

The treatment-enhancement distinction is a problem of health care ethics that involves devising the right approach to therapeutic intervention for a particular disease, in this case, depression. Depending on one's definition of what it means to have depression, the therapeutic approaches fall into these two main categories, treatment and enhancement. I will argue that defining the problem this way clarifies many of the controversies about the use of medications and psychotherapy in depression, both from the standpoint of health care policy and from that of ethics.

2.

The concept of *treatment* is based on a biomedical model of disease. In this model, illness represents a breakdown of the physical constituents of the body, leading to a functional loss of a capacity to perform typical activities of the organism. Ethicist Norman Daniels refers to this as "impairments of normal species-functioning" that lead to a "reduction in the range of opportunity open to an individual" (1985, 27). Daniels adapts the philosopher John Rawls's concept of "the good life," defined as the ability of the individual to construct certain "goals and projects" and to pursue the means by which they may be achieved. Applying the biomedical model, depression represents an abnormality of the brain leading to a restriction in the ability of the individual to pursue those activities which will allow the achievement of the individual's goals in life. A proponent of this approach would hold that treatment is needed to heal the brain and permit a resumption of normal functioning compared to one's peers.

The proponent of the *enhancement* approach to the therapy of depression comes at the problem from other disease models. In one, advocated by the World Health Organization, there is an explicit rejection of the biomedical conception: "Health is a state of complete physical, mental, and social well-being, and not merely the absence of disease or infirmity" (Daniels 1985, 29). This approach invokes, as Daniels puts it, an equivalence between health and happiness. Another model of enhancement holds that disease represents some deviation from a statistical norm; for example, hypertension is defined as a diastolic blood pressure above or equal to 95; thus a person with a diastolic blood pressure of 94 does not have disease. Similarly, depression might be defined as a mood state outside of the usual range of individuals in the relevant society. Another model that seeks to avoid the biomedical approach is a values-oriented or normative approach, where one defines disease by certain value-based judgments that rest on moral intuitions or beliefs and are thus relative to one's ethical theories. Hence, depression may represent a mood state that is deemed unacceptable or harmful from an ethical perspective, because it is thought to interfere with certain accepted virtues or certain necessary ethical criteria for good living.

Any of the alternative nonbiomedical models imply the conclusion that therapeutic interventions in depression should seek to enhance the functioning of the individual, rather than simply to permit redress of loss of functioning.

3.

Traditionally, physicians have supported the biomedical model of disease and the consequent treatment approach to depression. In terms of mental health policy, this means that insurance coverage for mental health treatment should be limited to mental disease or disability, which also includes long-term treatment aimed at improving functioning. It should not include enhancement of functioning when unrelated to a mental disease and disability.

This argument could be stated as follows. Psychiatric diagnosis limits the definition of depression to a small number of persons. The societal cost of depression, defined as severe disease or disability, far outweighs the expense of its treatment. Therefore, mental health services in depression should be limited to treatment of severe disease or disability.

The two premises of this argument are empirical statements. Diagnostic methods in psychiatry have undergone a major revision in the past two decades, becoming restrictive in their definitions of illnesses such as major depression, and, if applied strictly, would not apply to large segments of the population. For the major adult psychiatric illnesses, only 5–10 percent of persons at any time in their life will be diagnosed with major depression, only 2–5 persons with bipolar disorder, and only 1 percent with schizophrenia. These diagnostic rates compare favorably with other medical illnesses, some of which are much more ubiquitous and thus more costly to treat in the aggregate, such as gastritis, hypercholesterolemia, or hypertension. Also, data exist to show that inadequate treatment of depression results in more expense eventually, both in terms of the consumption of other medical services and the effect of depressive morbidity on lost economic productivity.

Turning to the alternative enhancement approaches, many objections could be made to their underlying definitions of disease from the public health perspective. One approach might be the following. All medications are (at least potentially) toxic; they have some side effects. Assuming that if the risks outweigh the benefits, a treatment should not be given, medication treatment should not routinely be given for depressive symptoms that do not meet criteria for a diagnosis of major depression.

The first premise merely reflects a medical fact. Every pill, no matter what it is, can exert harmful effects in the human body. Even apparently innocuous medications, like aspirin, can harm patients (in aspirin's case, ulcers or Reye's Syndrome can result). Thus, no treatment is risk-free, although some may be riskier than others. Stated bluntly, all medications are directly harmful, as Oliver Wendell Holmes ([1860] 1911) put it; the question is whether they are indirectly beneficial. Medications should therefore be given only when the benefits outweigh the risks, which is usually the case when significant major depression (with its mortality risk from suicide and high morbidity) is present. The argument could be made, however, that some medications carry so little risk that they should be used more freely for minor depressive symptoms that are not diagnostic of disease.

This thesis, most famously put forward in relation to the medication fluoxetine (Prozac), is not self-contradictory, but it is potentially hazardous. Part of the medical establishment's hesitation in this regard may reflect an outmoded "psychopharmacological Calvinism." Yet, if one accepts the Hippocratic ethical maxim "primum non nocere" (first, do no harm) as a primary medical standard for moral practice, the adoption of an enhancement model ought to be a rare exception rather than the rule. Certainly, with Prozac, certain risks exist, such as a controversial association with suicidality and adverse interactions with other medications.

4.

In their description of the logic of clinical judgment, medical ethicists Edmund Pellegrino and David Thomasma (1981) suggest ideas that could undermine the mainstream biomedically oriented argument. They state that clinical decision-making in medicine consists of three phases: First, there is observation and the collection of information; this is the art of medicine. Second, the collected data is understood on the basis of knowledge about syndromes, diseases, prognosis, and effectiveness of treatments; this is the science of medicine. Third, a treatment decision occurs on the basis of value judgments, made by the patient and the physician, which are in turn dependent on a number of factors (cultural, economic, interpersonal, ethical, and religious); this is the ethics of medicine. It is this last step, they suggest, that makes medicine what it is and not some other activity. What characterizes medicine as opposed to pure science or pure humanities, according to them, is that its goal is not knowledge for knowledge's sake, or art for art's sake, but the right *action* in the interest of the patient. This final end, action, is what stamps the ethical on medicine. And it is this last step that could trip up the attempt to apply the treatment-enhancement distinction in depression. The distinction, it could be argued, is one of values, not data; ethics, not science; personal decisions, not health policy. If one were to adjudicate the treatment-enhancement distinction in depression on a case-by-case basis, one could make a good argument for enhancement, as follows: If I am unhappy, I will seek to become happy. If there is a medication that can make me happy, I will take it, as long as the degree of subjective unhappiness I am feeling seems worse to me than the possible side effects or risks of medication.

Economic issues do not come up in this argument because it is approached as an individual ethical decision-making process, not as a larger moral decision with social implications. Assuming I can afford the medication, or that my insurance will pay for it, the financial aspects do not enter the decision-making process. Further, arguments against enhancement that rely on a lack of scientific effectiveness for the proposed treatments hold little weight; even if something has not been *proved* to work, it *may* still work *for me*.

Thus, in any individual case, once the values of the participants become part of the decision-making process, enhancement may seem to be a viable therapeutic option.

5.

It might be proposed that the above arguments fail to refute each other clearly because they hold incompatible underlying theories of health and disease. The main reason why the treatment-enhancement distinction represents a philosophical dilemma rests on this problem. Since there is the added complexity of the mind-body problem in psychiatric disorders, it is small wonder that these different perspectives rarely meet.

Although the biomedical model appears more scientifically valid to many clinicians, philosophers have more often noted its many weaknesses. It is largely accepted, for example, that a purely biological approach to psychiatric illness is rather limited. There are psychological and social dimensions to psychiatric (and indeed all medical) illness. As noted earlier, George Engel proposed the now-famous biopsychosocial model for the understanding of illness, and this model has become the status quo in contemporary psychiatry. If we accept this model, we might then seek to improve "normal" psychosocial states, which indeed we might consider normal only relative to certain historical epochs. Perhaps we could prevent depression, for instance, if everyone took the benign drug X, just as we accept vaccines today to prevent certain infectious illnesses.

Indeed, this prospect has alternately exorcised and stimulated thinkers on this topic for at least two generations. A symposium in 1961, with the slightly sinister title *Control of the Mind,* brought together figures as respected and as disparate as the writers Aldous Huxley and Arthur Koestler, the political scientists Harold Lasswell and Seymour Martin Lipset, the intellectual historian H. Stuart Hughes, the neurosurgeon Wilder Penfield, and the psychiatrists Seymour Kety and Jonathan Cole (Farber and Wilson 1961). This symposium's proceedings make for informative reading as one looks back from the early twenty-first century. The participants generally fretted about the possibility that psychiatric drugs would ultimately control the human mind, to the detriment of freedom. The main consolation they possessed was that it seemed unlikely that psychiatric science would ever reach that level of sophistication.

In 1993, when Peter Kramer published his *Listening to Prozac,* the public response indicated that we had reached that point. Are we now where Huxley, Kety, and colleagues hoped we would never be? Do these drugs free us, or do they control us?

6.

Instead of arguing the merits of different models of health and disease, we may be better off to look carefully at the practical limitations imposed on the enhancement model by empirical data with even the latest and most sophisticated psychiatric medications. Would Prozac, for instance, really enhance functioning for most nonclinically depressed persons, defined by the biomedical model? Would it be safe to prescribe as a public health measure, much like a polio vaccine?

I suggest that the answer is no. Prozac, in fact, may enhance the function of personality in certain individuals. But the larger public health question concerns how safe it is. I will put aside for the moment the specific pharmacological risks of the medication (sexual dysfunction, drug interactions), because these can be fine-tuned with similar but slightly different pharmacological compounds. The larger issue, I believe, is that antidepressants, including Prozac, can be clinically risky even in the treatment of depression.

It should be noted, first, that there are two kinds of depression: unipolar (depression alternating with euthymic, or normal, mood) and bipolar (depression alternating with mood elevation, such as mania or hypomania; also known as manic-depression). A great many depressions are of the bipolar variety: there is controversy still about how many, but some good epidemiological studies put the figure of bipolar depression at about 2–5 percent of the population (Angst 1998). The standard unipolar depression rate is 5–10 percent of the population. If we combine the two percentages and compare the bipolar rate with the total, this would suggest that one out of every two or three individuals with depression actually has bipolar rather than unipolar depression (Ghaemi, Ko, and Goodwin 2002).

The problem here is that antidepressants are less effective in bipolar than in unipolar depression, can cause immediate mania in about 30–50 percent of persons with bipolar depression, and can cause a long-term worsening of the illness (more manias and more depressions) in about 25 percent of persons with bipolar depression (Ghaemi, Ko, and Goodwin 2002). Thus, perhaps 25 percent of individuals with depression (bipolar) may get worse with antidepressant medications. In the hands of a competent clinician, these persons can improve with mood stabilizers and the occasional use of antidepressant medications. But the risks should be clear if we were to propose that all these individuals were to receive antidepressant agents as a public health measure, or if they all went to their local health food store to buy herbal antidepressants like St. John's Wort. (Indeed, cases of mania with St. John's Wort have already been reported.)

So there is an immense practical problem: antidepressants are effective and safe only in some depressed individuals. We still need the careful assessments of clinicians to determine who should receive antidepressants and who should not.

7.

Still there is a question, which might be delayed but cannot be ignored, the ethical and philosophical question: if some future drug does enhance functioning or mood in the majority of nonbiomedically depressed persons, and if it is not addictive or does not have other significant risks, then what is the principled ethical stance that one should take?

I believe that now we can repeat the statement of the San Francisco symposium four decades ago: We are not at that point. But soon we very well could be. If all those conditions are met, we might have to admit that many of the objections to enhancement fall away.

I feel that the future has something else in store. We may never need to develop those ideal drugs. Genetic prevention is more likely to do the work for us. Something similar happened with infectious disease, that great paradigm of modern medicine. Even though vaccines and antibiotics have been developed and are essential, and new ones continue to be produced, the vast majority of infectious diseases have been eradicated by public health measures of prevention. The environmental circumstances that spawned the infections (overcrowding for tuberculosis and the plague, absence of sewage systems for cholera) have been identified and ameliorated, at least in developed countries. Psychiatric illness involves genetic and environmental causation; while research continues on identifying and ameliorating the environmental aspects of psychiatric illness, it will also proceed on their genetic aspects. As the human genome project progresses, the potential may exist to identify the important genetic factors that underlie susceptibility to psychiatric illness. In those cases where the genetic risks for psychiatric illness are identified, prospective parents would have the possible option of not proceeding to birth, or potentially of genetic therapies.

The ethical questions that arise with genetic enhancement are, I believe, of the same ilk as those related to psychopharmacologic enhancement. We still have some time to prepare ourselves to answer them. I think there is no doubt we need to, if not now, then soon.

8.

In general, unease with psychopharmacology often has to do with unease about biologizing the mind. Fears that the mind may be reduced to the brain have a living target in clinical psychopharmacology. A major danger in attacks on biologically oriented psychiatry, however, is that suffering may be ignored. The philosopher Michael Martin refers to this when he notes that some writers "worry that therapeutic approaches to depression undermine explorations of values, as if prescribing Prozac to Mill would have impeded the history of ethics" (1999, 280). Indeed. It is worthwhile to dust off some out-of-print psychiatric books from the 1960s, where one frequently finds antibiological psychoanalysts and others weighing in against the use of medications for psychiatric conditions.[1]

A common argument was that such treatments might reduce anxiety, depression, and psychosis, thereby removing the kind of painful impetus that alone could push patients to discover the "true" underlying causes of their misfortunes. A kernel of truth notwithstanding, such a perspective reeks of the sacrifice of human beings to abstractions. Contemporary objections to the "medicalization" of depression share a similar fault, though less obviously subservient to specific dogmas.

This does not mean, however, that we should go to the other extreme, using medications indiscriminately as we engage in the "pathologizing of everyday depression." But let us first note that no one worries about pathologizing everyday mania, or pathologizing everyday psychosis. Some mental states seem more clearly pathological, and we mostly agree that they should be treated. I believe that the bigger problem today, from the perspective of public health, is not overtreatment of depression but undertreatment of mania and psychosis (witness recent episodes of untreated mentally ill individuals harming bystanders in New York's subways). I would make this case even though I also have argued that antidepressants are probably overutilized in patients with bipolar disorder, who tend to get misdiagnosed as having uncomplicated depression. But I also agree with Martin and others about the dangers of "cosmetic psychopharmacology," as Peter Kramer has called it: the urge to use psychotropic medications to alter parts of our personalities or ways of being that may appear socially or morally undesirable to ourselves or others. At the risk of being labeled a psychopharmacological Calvinist (which, by the way, is an injustice to Calvin), I maintain that there are too many risks in such a practice, beginning with how we would know when to treat.

Martin (1999) argues that neither the medical establishment nor social norms should establish what is healthy versus what is unhealthy. The individual must exert some effective agency in "reasonably" making such assessments. The problem is that in some psychiatric conditions, as discussed in chapter 17, individuals are not able to make such assessments. Determining what is healthy for oneself may be distorted by conditions in which insight is absent, such as manic depression. Some persons seek a diagnosis in order to obtain certain pleasurable pharmacological effects, such as those whose attention deficit symptoms are intended to lead to amphetamine use and those who express anxiety or panic symptoms to obtain benzodiazepines (which have alcohol-like properties).

9.

Also, it is worth noting, as Baldessarini does, that many of us are influenced by a "pharmacocentric" view of the world (2000a, 392). In Western society today, drugs have become both metaphors and mechanisms by which we understand and interpret our lives. Valium calmed the anxiety of the 1960s, Prozac spurred the acquisitiveness of the 1990s, and Viagra may unleash a new sexuality in this millennium. All of these drugs are also promoted and supported by a vast industrial enterprise, the pharmaceutical industry, which advertises their value heavily in mass markets. When one takes this factor into account, one wonders to what extent an individual's value judgment is influenced by the manufacturing of desires that such advertising produces. This possibility has been discussed in other settings by social critics such as Herbert Marcuse (1968) and John Kenneth Galbraith (1973);[2] it exists today, in my opinion, in psychiatry as well.

Thus, although it is attractive to postulate in theory the individual's role in determining the border between health and illness, in practice this approach not only grants privileged access but also assumes Cartesian infallibility regarding our own mental states. Beginning with Freud, and ending with modern cognitive science, we know that we have no such infallibility. Yet we cannot disprove the veracity of an individual's self-report of a mental state in any specific case. So the individual's input is necessary, but it is not a sufficient criterion for assessing health and illness; medical science and social norms are needed as well. We can only conclude, with Martin, that assessments of health are not "wholly subjective." This returns us to the need for an open attitude toward the value of medical science in psychiatry as well as a recognition of the social and political aspects of our worldviews.

10.

In summary, we might conclude that although at present a treatment approach for depression is better supported by current empirical knowledge in psychiatry than the enhancement approaches, enhancement may become appropriate if sufficiently powerful yet benign medications or genetic methods were to become available. We are not quite at that point, but we may soon be.

Today, though, enhancement approaches seem most relevant to altering personality traits rather than affecting clinical syndromes like depression. Serotonergic antidepressants, such as Prozac, seem to shift personality traits up or down the normal curve that characterizes humankind. Thus, for instance, a less extroverted person becomes more extroverted, or a more anxious or neurotic person becomes less anxious or neurotic. These kinds of personality changes are sometimes quite notable and, not infrequently, are independent of any effects on depressive symptoms per se. In this sense, the apparent conflict between treatment and enhancement may represent a confusion about what is being affected: an illness or a personality trait.[3]

CHAPTER 19

Truth and Statistics

Problems of Empirical Psychiatry

> In medicine everybody tends to vaunt the results of his own experience and to quote only the facts which support it. But if experience is to provide an authentic and conclusive basis for any method of treatment, then it must be derived from a large number of patients, on whom observations have been made with extreme care, according to a fixed and regular plan, and repeated for some years on exactly the same lines: favorable and unfavorable results must both be reported equally and the respective numbers of each given. In other words, it must depend on an application of the theory of probability. —PHILIPPE PINEL, 1806

Many of us, as clinicians and as citizens, have an uneasy relationship with statistics. As clinicians we may not understand the more complicated methods: multiple logistic regressions and Bonferroni corrections sound as foreign to us as medical lingo does to statisticians. We also fear, perhaps, that statistical truths may not translate into clinical truths (with some justification, as we shall see). As citizens, we may feel that statistics are too cold for us to trust our rights to them. Statistical polls and focus groups are roundly condemned, by voters and politicians alike, yet, with the odd exception, their pronouncements are just as assiduously noted by voters and politicians.

Yet statistical methods in psychiatry have been part of the revolution that has moved the field in the last few decades closer and closer to its medical brethren. Psychiatry seems more scientific; the psychopharmacology revolution has occurred; we now have clinical trials with double-blind placebo-controlled methods that match any study of a cardiac medication or any research on treatments for the kidney. In sum, psychiatry has finally appeared to accept those scientific standards that doctors and patients expect from a medical specialty. In practical terms, the many new effective medications for psychiatric treatments seem to exemplify the success of these methods.

This optimistic interpretation of the current state of things has its justifications, but certain doubts remain.

1.

I have already pointed out that at a very basic level there are limitations to
a purely objective empirical approach to psychiatry. Psychiatry is a discipline
that deals with subjective syndromes: the mind, mental phenomena, thoughts
and feelings. And these mental phenomena are not yet amenable to complete
explanation by means of mathematics, statistics, biology, or physics. I have
suggested other perspectives and methods that can be useful to assess and understand those aspects of psychiatry that are not explained by straightforward
empirical science. I have further recommended Jaspers's views as providing perhaps the most complete description of a nuanced scientific method for psychiatry that takes into account objective-descriptive approaches as well as the
search for meaning in mental phenomena.

There is, however, another way to emphasize the need for perspectives other
than simple biological empiricism in psychiatry. Besides the limitations imposed by the nature of the subject matter (minds, persons, meaning), there are
the limitations of the methods of empirical science itself. For psychiatry, perhaps the most important empirical method that needs to be critiqued is statistics. This is because psychiatry cannot yet rely on laboratory science: there
are few clear pathologies of the brain, biochemical abnormalities, or physiological dysfunctions that can consistently be shown to occur in psychiatric
conditions. Besides, most of this kind of research is laboratory research, which,
though useful, still needs to be linked to living human beings, to clinical research. And clinical research relies on statistics.

This reliance on statistics in psychiatric clinical research is most clear in psychopharmacology studies. Research on medications in psychiatry now relies
on the statistical methods of clinical trials. This refers to the need for standardized valid methods of assessing whether or not a medication works in a
particular condition. In the last half-century, psychiatry has followed every
other medical specialty in accepting the need for clinical trial methods in
pharmacology research. Similar methods are used sometimes to assess the efficacy of psychotherapies. And statistics are also used in experimental psychology to evaluate an array of potential findings with psychological tests or
survey results.

Much of empirical research in psychiatry therefore comes down to clinical trials and statistics. How reliable and accurate are these empirical methods?

2.

When one hears a phrase like "Scientists have shown that . . ." one might expect that the word *shown* reflects some kind of empirical proof. These days, in medicine, adequate clinical trial methods are thought to represent such proof. The most rigorous clinical trial method is the randomized, double-blind, placebo-controlled trial. *Randomized* means that patients receive treatments at random, without any choice on the part of either treater or patient. *Double-blind* means that neither the treater nor the patient knows what medication the patient is getting. And *placebo-controlled* refers to the fact that one of the treatments may be inert, a "sugar pill" that has no pharmacologic effect at all. Thus, one would expect that the findings of such a trial would be definitive: assuming sample sizes adequate to detect a difference, a "yes" would mean yes and a "no" would mean no. The clinical trial would prove whether something was so or not. I will show that this is not the case, that even the most rigorous clinical trial methods can still be wrong, and that the empirical methods of statistical research in clinical psychiatry are inherently limited by the boundaries of statistical accuracy.

3.

It is important to remember that the systematic use of statistics in medicine and psychiatry is a recent phenomenon. I do not share the opposition expressed by many to the introduction of statistical methods in medicine. In his book *The Antidepressant Era,* David Healy (1998) provides an excellent description of this history. The principle of randomization was controversial as far back as the mid–nineteenth century. The concept was that patients should not be chosen to receive a certain medication for specific reasons in research studies because this could bias the results for or against a certain treatment option. The samples receiving two treatments would differ based on many characteristics because the treaters might choose to use one treatment in a certain group of people and another treatment in another group. The simplest way to understand this is to think about a new drug that might be given to more severely ill patients in a certain study in comparison to an old drug that might be given to less severely ill patients. The old drug would probably do better, not because it is better but because those who took it were more likely to respond to any treatment. Thus, the principle of randomization holds that treatment samples should randomly receive one treatment or another. Many physicians initially opposed this idea in the nineteenth century, sometimes on grounds such as the belief that random treatment might obscure real efficacy in specific chosen subgroups of patients. But on the whole, randomization has become a standard feature of any empirical treatment study that can claim to be somewhat rigorously scientific. The placebo and the double-blind go together. It can safely be said that before the introduction of penicillin in the 1940s, medicine had very few truly effective treatments. In fact, most of nineteenth-century medicine consisted either of nonpharmacological treatment (that is, the psychological effects of a sympathetic physician, a psychotherapeutic benefit) or homeopathic treatment (minidoses of drugs that probably mainly functioned as placebos, with no chemical grounds for their efficacy). Thus, the benefits, and the limits, of essentially placebo treatment did not go unnoticed by astute physicians of the premodern era. On this subject, the reader may benefit from reference to the famous argument of Oliver Wendell Holmes, the great Boston physician and author (and father of the Supreme Court Justice):

> Presumptions are of vast importance in medicine, as in law. A man is presumed innocent until he is proved guilty. A medicine . . . should always be presumed to be hurtful. It always is directly hurtful; it may sometimes be indirectly beneficial. If this presumption were established . . . we should not so frequently hear . . . that, on the whole, more harm than good is done with medication. Throw out opium, which the Creator himself seems to prescribe, for we often see the scarlet poppy growing in the cornfields, as if it were foreseen that wherever there is hunger to be fed there must also be pain to be soothed; throw out a few specifics which our art did not discover, and is hardly needed to apply; throw out wine, which is a food, and the vapors which produce the miracle of anesthesia, and I firmly believe that if the whole materia medica, *as now used,* could be sunk to the bottom of the sea, it would be all the better for mankind,—and all the worse for the fishes. ([1860] 1911, 202–3)[1]

Holmes's influence on the use of empirical methods in medicine deserves further discussion.

4.

It must have been a dark and damp day—that May 30, 1860—a typical wet Boston spring day, when Oliver Wendell Holmes addressed his medical colleagues at the Massachusetts Medical Society. Maybe Holmes was in something of an irascible mood that day, when he made the above statement. I can imagine that many in his audience were more preoccupied with the great issues of the day—civil war, slavery, abolition, a vital presidential election—than with seemingly harmless potions. But Holmes, the famous physician and writer and Harvard Medical School professor (later eclipsed in fame by his son the Supreme Court Justice), did not toss off those words as a mere peripheral opinion. That day, at the medical society, he gave a lecture that built up to the argument he made, a considered examination of the nature of medication treatments, and his conclusion that aside from certain specific treatments, most medications were worthless, or worse, harmful. Maybe he meant to provoke. And indeed, his lecture stimulated a great deal of discussion about the topic that continued long afterward. Holmes's statement is still not infrequently quoted in many contexts.

Holmes was a judicious man, well respected by senior physicians. He did not offer his judgment lightly. He felt that the profession of medicine, as well as the public, was harmed by use, and overuse, of inadequately proven medications. In 1860 Holmes went after pharmacology in general, not to mention polypharmacy.

In fact, I might hazard to state that medical care before the 1950s consisted of polypharmacy if it consisted of anything at all. This is because physicians rarely prescribed just one treatment; they usually prescribed multiple medications at once. There are many reasons for this, but one major factor might have been, as Holmes claimed, that almost all medications did not work, and thus physicians tended to use many medications, hoping to elicit benefits that were not present when medications were used singly. Anton Chekhov, the Russian writer who practiced medicine all his life, once commented that if many medications are used, then the disease is incurable. In Holmes's view, nineteenth-century medicine simply possessed ineffective medications; disease might be curable, but treatments needed to be proved to cure disease before being used.

Oliver Wendell Holmes's credo became that of modern medicine. He and William Osler,[2] two giants of medicine, led the field away from a symptom- and treatment-oriented approach toward today's disease- and diagnosis-oriented approach. That famous speech by Holmes has been referenced by FDA officials in justification of the need for clinical trials in psychiatry (Yolles 1966; Leber 2000). In his efforts against homeopathy, Holmes even anticipated the need for placebo-controlled trials, which he saw as little more than pill-based suggestion.

Holmes quite rightly realized that placebo treatments in medicine, though somewhat beneficial, hardly contributed to advancing science. For those who, like him, wished to make medicine scientific, the use of the placebo was needed as a comparison to drug treatments so as to prove that a drug actually worked, that its benefits went beyond what would happen naturally, and thus that its benefits would outweigh its risks.

5.

The placebo-controlled study thus eventually became justified on the grounds that it was the only way to definitively know whether any treatment works and what its side effects are. For a while, in psychiatry, some researchers argued that new drugs should be compared to already proven effective treatments. If new drugs were as effective as previously proven treatments, then presumably the new agents would also be effective. In fact, the need to use an active proven treatment as a control comparison, rather than a placebo, was enshrined in the Helsinki agreement on human rights, written after World War II to protect the rights of research subjects (partly the consequence of the excesses of Nazi medicine in Germany). This debate continues, but the U.S. Food and Drug Administration came down on the side of placebo treatment in the late 1970s, requiring that all new treatments in psychiatry be compared to a placebo rather than an active control. The scientific argument for this view is partly based on the problem of statistical power, or sample size. Statistical power reflects the ability of a study to detect a real difference. For instance, if the issue of interest is whether one drug is better than another drug, then there would be a difference in percent improved between two groups of patients treated by those drugs. This difference is what the study needs to be designed to detect. The smaller the difference, the larger the sample size needs to be to detect it. The larger the difference, the smaller the sample size can be and still detect the difference. Thus, in the case of comparing a new drug to an old proven treatment, one would think that if no difference could be detected, then the two drugs would likely both be effective. However, the same finding could be the result of too small a sample size. If the sample size is not large enough, the two treatments would not be proved to be different, even though they might have been proved to be different with a large enough sample. (Think of an extreme example: Suppose I treat only four persons; two get drug A, two get drug B. One person with drug B improves, while both persons with drug A do not. Running statistical tests would be far from ever showing that this difference was statistically significant). The same problem holds with placebos: a drug might not differ from a placebo in its effects because the sample might be too small. However, the chances of running into this problem should be lower with placebo treatments, because placebo response rates should be lower than already proven active treatments. Thus, a smaller sample size would be needed to prove that a drug is better than a placebo than to prove that it is as effective as (or better than) another already proven drug. Hence, by insisting on placebo controls, the FDA wished to banish any lingering doubt about whether absence of a difference between two drugs is due to no difference or due to small sample size.

Of course this insistence on placebo-controlled studies on the part of the FDA is ethically double edged, since it sometimes conflicts with the Helsinki accords; in addition, from the standpoint of individual research subjects, it seems less protective of individual rights than always being given an active treatment.

6.

Another phrase deserves definition before I move on to pointing out how, despite all these careful constraints, these rigorous clinical trials can still be wrong and are thus limited in their utility as a scientific method for psychiatry. That phrase is *statistical significance*. This concept goes hand in hand with the idea of statistical power. Power reflects sample size, the ability to detect a difference between two groups. Once a difference is detected, assuming a large enough sample size, the next step is to say whether or not that difference is real (as opposed to random). By *real* one means statistically significant, which means that the difference is not likely to have occurred by chance alone. The standard definition of this criterion is that something is statistically significant if it could have occurred by chance alone in less than 1 of 20 occasions ($p < 0.05$). In statistical parlance, p stands for the probability that a detected difference might have occurred by chance alone, consistent with the *null hypothesis,* meaning that there really is no difference. Thus, in clinical research in psychiatry, one says that the difference in treatment response between a drug and a placebo is statistically significant if the statistical analysis follows these outlines, which implies that the difference is real, that is, that the drug is effective. All this work underlies the general statement one might make when one says that "Scientists have proved that Drug X is effective for Disease Y."

One of the problems with statistical significance is that it does not necessarily translate to clinical significance. Thus, if one uses complicated statistics, one can often find some way or another in which a particular data set can be analyzed to find some kind of difference between two treatments. Among adepts in clinical trials, this is referred to (with some hint of irony) as "massaging the data." Also, if one has an extremely large sample size, then very small differences in magnitude can still be shown to be statistically significant. Thus, in a rating scale of depression, for instance, where most nondepressed persons rate a score of 0 and a moderately but clinically depressed individual might score 20, a difference of 0.5 points in magnitude is clinically meaningless. However, a large enough sample size can force any difference, even that small, to meet the criterion of statistical significance. By using fancy methods or assessing too large samples, random or unimportant results can be found. This is another reason why one should not be overly impressed by huge samples, such as studies of tens of thousands of persons, because in such samples, anything and everything might be statistically significant but, in reality, meaningless.

7.

Statisticians have devised means of limiting such problems. One approach, still controversial, is to use Bayesian methods. One interpretation of Bayesian statistics is the idea that a single study is not definitive. One always needs to weigh the findings of a study against the backdrop of other studies. This is an important intuition often lost on laypersons, doctors, and statistical extremists alike. I think the use of Bayesian methods may become more frequent and better understood in medical research in the future.[3] But in the meantime, the medical research community is focusing on other approaches to dealing with the limitations of standard statistics.

Perhaps the main viewpoint today is to emphasize the importance of randomized clinical trials. Clinical trials are supposed to predict, before the study begins, what specific statistical analyses they plan to employ, so as to avoid the temptation of "post-hoc" (after-the-fact) massaging of the data. Also, before the study, the researchers need to conduct a power analysis, based on available pilot information, indicating what amount of difference they plan to detect and showing that the sample sizes are the right size to detect such a difference (not too small, and not too large).

Let us assume that all of these precautions are in place. We are going to conduct a double-blind, placebo-controlled, randomized clinical trial. We have chosen, before the study, to do a specific statistical analysis of a certain rating scale for a new drug compared to a placebo. We have conducted a power analysis and have shown that two samples of a certain size (say, eighty patients each) are sufficient to detect a clinically meaningful difference suggested by earlier research (say, a 20% difference in depression rating scale scores between the two groups). Adherents of the strict empirical approach to psychiatry, one might think, would hope to say that if the study showed the drug to be superior to the placebo, then it would have proved that that drug was superior to the placebo. And vice versa.

Yet this is not the case. And at one level, even strict empiricists would admit that things are not this simple. Such careful clinical trials can fail for a number of reasons. One reason might be that, although randomly picked for the study, the individuals in both treatment groups are too severely ill for any treatment to work. Or they might not be ill enough, and the placebo would prove too effective. The latter scenario is frequently the case, since research studies require informed consent. This is especially a problem with severe illnesses like schizophrenia and acute mania, which often impair the ability of persons to make judgments; when patients are carefully chosen who fully understand the risks and benefits of a study and are thus able to give informed consent, the more severely ill patients are excluded. Because of the vagaries of sample selection, therefore, any single clinical trial might fail to find a drug to be effective, even though the drug may well be effective. Furthermore, certain illnesses have relatively high placebo response rates: for anxiety disorders, the placebo response tends to be about 50 percent, for depression, about 40 percent. Drugs need to be, in general, 20 percent more effective than the placebo to be shown to be statistically significantly better (in usual sample size ranges of one hundred to two hundred patients). Thus, if a certain sample for some reason has a slightly better placebo response in a particular study, a drug might not be able to differentiate itself from the placebo. It should also be noted that many researchers think that placebo responses in clinical trials are higher than in the real world of clinical practice. This may occur for a number of reasons. Frequently patients get paid to participate in clinical trials, an obvious motivator to stay in them and perhaps an agent in making patients feel better. Research patients get much attention from research staff, often more attention than they receive from clinical staff in nonresearch clinical practice. This is partly because research groups depend on treating research patients for their income, they treat far fewer research patients than are treated in standard clinical settings, and thus they expend a great deal of time and energy on making sure their research patients are satisfied. Beyond these economic factors, when placebos and double-blinds are used, researchers have ethical and legal obligations to carefully follow their patients, and they therefore see the research patients more frequently and scrutinize their clinical state in more detail than is the case in standard clinical practice. All of these factors may tend to inflate the placebo response rate in clinical trials.

Given this picture, it is well known among statisticians and researchers that any one clinical trial may fail to find a difference between a drug and a placebo, even though such a difference may exist. This is part of the reason why the U.S. FDA requires that two placebo-controlled studies show psychotropic medications to be effective, without limiting the number of such studies that might have been attempted with negative results. It is frequently the case that an antidepressant will be indicated by the FDA as effective in treating depression based on two positive studies, despite numerous other placebo-controlled studies that do not show effectiveness (frequently four to eight other studies are negative).

8.

As a result, even strict randomized clinical trials can be wrong when they fail to find a difference between two treatments, or between a drug and a placebo. For various reasons, one negative study (e.g., one study that finds that a drug could not be shown to be effective compared to a placebo) could be wrong. But it would seem at least that a positive study, a study that asserts that a drug is effective, is likely to be right. This may be the case in a placebo-controlled study, but in a clinical trial that compares two different medications (without a placebo), such convictions of certainty are not well founded.

Here we run into the next layer of problems. Even if one ensures the double-blind, randomized design; even if one has a large enough sample and one finds a positive result between two treatments on a predetermined rating scale analysis; still this difference might not be real. The problem lies in the fact that one can design a randomized clinical trial in such a way as to be to the advantage of one treatment and to the disadvantage of another. For instance, one drug might be dosed in a proven effective dose, whereas another drug might be dosed somewhat lower than its likely effective dose. This kind of subtle tinkering with the design of a clinical trial is sometimes a problem with studies organized by a specific pharmaceutical company seeking to show an advantage over a competitor. Unfortunately, this approach often is marketing under the guise of research, and it serves only to confuse clinicians and patients, many of whom become skeptical of any pharmaceutically sponsored research.

9.

The problem of pharmaceutically sponsored research is an important topic. David Healy (1998) has discussed the role of the pharmaceutical industry in research and clinical practice. In this chapter, I want to focus on the question of the integrity of pharmaceutically sponsored research. I often find that such research is met with a great deal of skepticism, particularly by psychiatric residents, as well as many practitioners. My experience is that those with the greatest skepticism are also those with the least research experience. I do not think this is a coincidence. The problem is superficially obvious. Most published studies are to the benefit of the sponsoring pharmaceutical company. The implication seems to be that such research is biased. And many clinicians therefore conclude that they will ignore such research.

But despite my comments above, I consider such extreme skepticism to be a grave mistake; it is usually a reflection of a certain amount of ignorance about research. I find that many such clinicians want to read the results of a study and believe them. To some extent, this attitude is inevitable. It is partly the job of scientific journals and scientific editors to weed out unscientific studies or poorly analyzed results. But only partly. It is also essential that clinicians be able to understand and analyze research studies published in medical journals. Reading the results section is just not enough. Often different studies differ in their results. If the studies are sponsored by pharmaceutical companies, and the differing results correlate with the sponsoring company, then the results-reading clinician will be totally confused. Indeed, he would seem to have no option but to ignore all such studies. Yet this, again, does not necessarily reflect the nefarious ways of pharmaceutical companies; it equally reflects the sorry state of the scientific knowledge of many clinicians.

Not all studies are equally false. And there are many reasons why one study of a topic might be positive and another negative, unrelated to the funding sponsor. It is important for clinicians to be able to interpret such studies and make their own reasoned judgments based on simple statistical knowledge such as that reviewed in this chapter.

The reality is that the superficial appearance of bias in pharmaceutically sponsored studies is not straightforward. Such research occurs in two basic forms; in the first, an academic researcher designs and conducts the study, with or without pharmaceutical funding; in the second, the pharmaceutical company designs the study and then hires numerous researchers to conduct it. In the first kind (called investigator-initiated studies), the data belong to the researchers; most universities have contracts with pharmaceutical companies permitting the researchers to solely analyze and publish the data. In the second kind, usually large multicenter clinical trials designed for FDA submissions, the data belong to and are analyzed and published by the pharmaceutical company. In investigator-initiated studies (IITs), two scenarios exist. The study might not have been funded by any source initially. If the results are to the benefit of a company, then the company may assist the researcher in presenting the results in research meetings as well as in analyzing and publishing the data. When the study is published, it will be positive and will be cited as sponsored by a pharmaceutical company (even though it initially was not sponsored by anyone). In the second scenario of an IIT, the study will have been funded from the start by a pharmaceutical company, and, whether positive or negative, the results will be published as supported by the pharmaceutical company. In the large multicenter clinical trials, if the results are positive, the pharmaceutical company will publish them. If the results are negative, as I stated earlier, the pharmaceutical company may ignore them and never even present them at a research meeting, much less publish them.

Consequently, regarding the impression that all studies conducted by pharmaceutical companies are positive for those companies, it is not the case that this result is due to biased methods; rather, it is due to systematic suppression of negative studies (except those conducted by academic researchers in IITs). It is not that the researchers cook the data to make them positive; the negative data just never get into print. Even academic researchers can have trouble persuading editors and peer reviewers in scientific journals to publish their negative studies. This is a well-known bias in research. Negative studies are less interesting and less likely to be published. All of these factors contribute to the suppression of negative studies and to the resultant impression that pharmaceutically sponsored studies are uniformly positive for the funding company.

However, clinicians who have not engaged in research know little of this process. To them, it might seem easiest to ignore all these studies. Yet there are many good studies, with important data, either funded by pharmaceutical companies or in some way assisted by those companies. And such clinicians usually are woefully unaware of these important, scientifically sound studies.

There is no easy answer here. It is simply ignorant to reject pharmaceutically sponsored studies as biased. It is also naive to accept them all, since the process is influenced by economic considerations of the private marketplace. Clinicians, and patients, need to become somewhat educated about research and statistics, just as they know they need to be educated about clinical signs and symptoms. Empirical psychiatry is not ideal, but it has its strengths. It cannot be ignored, or devalued, simply because it is complex.

CHAPTER 20

A Climate of Opinion

What Remains of Psychoanalysis

> There is no doubt that the main task of therapy of the neuroses will be dealt with by means which new discoveries in the area of inner secretions will provide. I hear the steps of endocrinology behind us and it will catch up with us and overtake us. But even then psychoanalysis will be very useful. Endocrinology will then be a giant who is blind and does not know where to go, and psychoanalysis will be the dwarf who leads him to the right places. —SIGMUND FREUD

In the public mind, psychiatry is still identified with Sigmund Freud. It might appear surprising, then, that I have avoided a lengthy discussion of Freud's work until now. This is because, in my opinion, what is useful in Freud needs to be placed in the context of the previous chapters.

W. H. Auden famously concluded that Freudianism was not simply a theory but had become a climate of opinion. I would suggest that though this may still be the case to some extent in the larger culture, it is no longer so in psychiatry proper. Yet it is also not the case that psychoanalysis has simply been dismissed as irrelevant, replaced by neuroscience. Many ideas derived from Freud continue to be central in psychiatry, but not in the ways originally envisaged by him. In this chapter I will assess what is living and what is dead in Freud's opus, from the perspective of clinical psychiatry.

1.

What is dead in Freudianism? Infantile sexuality, the interpretation of dreams, the Oedipus complex, the Electra complex, object cathexes, catharsis, Eros, the death instinct, the cultural effects of the incest taboo, the neurosis of religion, the genesis of psychiatric illness in most cases as a result of childhood familial problems, and the myriad machinations of id, ego, and superego as they struggle for the soul of man. In other words, most of the great man's most creative speculations—brilliant notions when born, mere dogmas in the hands of disciples—have basically been shown to be wrong, or worse, irrelevant.

What is living in Freudianism? Transference, countertransference, defense mechanisms, the concept of unconscious mental states, the irrational nature of much human behavior, the importance of sexual desire in human life, the utility of listening without judgment, the likely importance of childhood trauma in some psychiatric disorders.[1]

It can be seen by this list that psychiatry today is finally coming to a nuanced assessment of Freud's ideas. No longer is his word holy writ, nor are his ideas simply wrong.

2.

Let's look at some of his more useful concepts. Transference is a good place to start. By *transference* Freud meant to describe the special emotional relations that occur between a psychotherapist and a patient. For Freud, this relationship consisted of unconscious emotional connections made to one's parents. In other words, the patient unconsciously sees the therapist as her parents, and she feels emotions toward the therapist that derive from emotions toward her parents. These emotions, usually sexual or aggressive (or both), are expressed in the psychotherapy. Freud taught therapists to be ready for and make use of these transference emotions. Although he initially saw these unusual emotional reactions in his patients as problems, he later made use of them as a means to move the psychoanalysis forward. In fact, he came to believe that the transference relationship was the key to successful treatment. This is because of the problem of *resistance,* that is, the patient's unwillingness to accept the therapist's interpretations. Freud long struggled with this problem. Sometimes it would seem clear to him that a patient's associations and unconscious emotions were explainable by a particular interpretation. But when Freud would express such interpretations, either patients would expressly reject them, or, even worse, patients would accept them and yet continue to have the same symptoms or problems that brought them to treatment. Thus, it seemed that a purely cognitive, or rational, acceptance of a psychoanalytic interpretation did not have sufficient force to remove emotional symptoms or change behavioral problems. Freud concluded that he needed to recruit more emotional forces from the patient's psyche. He ultimately called upon the transference relationship to do this. Under the influence of transference emotions, patients could understand and experience psychoanalytic interpretations at the appropriate times and in the appropriate manner during a course of psychotherapy. Only then would the interpretations be effective.

This is how Freud came to see transference. The specific views he held regarding the role of transference in promoting psychotherapeutic change are less relevant here than the general concept itself. It seems clinically useful and accurate to note that patients often seem to have unconscious feelings toward their psychotherapists or doctors. These feelings often seem sexual or aggressive in nature, and recognizing these transference feelings for what they are— reflections of the patient's habits and wishes—is an important part of psychiatric treatment. When such feelings are not recognized appropriately, doctors and therapists can misinterpret transference feelings for mature feelings. This may explain some cases of psychiatric abuse of patients for sexual purposes, as well as many cases of failed treatment owing to psychological conflict between patient and doctor.

This brings us to another useful psychoanalytic notion: *countertransference.* Freud only briefly touched on this concept, but later psychoanalysts shed helpful light on it. Just as the patient brings unconscious feelings to the treatment relationship, so does the therapist. Countertransference describes the unconscious emotions the therapist experiences, based on the therapist's own past relationships but directed at the patient. These feelings, too, are frequently sexual or aggressive. The psychoanalyst Otto Kernberg (1975, 1976) highlighted the presence of "countertransference hate" in the treatment of patients with borderline personality disorder. In other words, doctors and therapists frequently dislike those patients, or even have aggressive feelings toward them. I recall having these feelings myself, in the course of my training as a psychiatric resident. I remember initially feeling quite guilty: how could I dislike this patient? I knew she had suffered in the past in various ways; I was supposed to help her, I was being trained to help her, I was being paid to help her. Yet I did not want to. Often, these countertransference feelings were preceded by similar transference feelings: when I had barely met a patient, she seemed to already hate me. This all was quite a shock at first, but I found that understanding transference and countertransference helped me make sense of these confused feelings.

3.

One of the most difficult aspects of psychoanalysis has been the problem of empirically validating psychoanalytic theories. A good example of empirical research related to psychoanalytic ideas is the work on defense mechanisms by the psychiatrist George Vaillant (Vaillant, Bond, and Vaillant 1986). Vaillant showed that the more "developed" mechanisms, like altruism and sublimation, were associated with markers of "success" in life. Success was operationalized as having a stable long-term marriage that was reported to be satisfying to both partners and having a conventionally productive career. The work of Vaillant and his associates is one of the few large, prospective, empirical outcome studies of psychoanalytic ideas. In daily clinical practice, psychotherapists frequently find Freud's concept of defense mechanisms helpful. For instance, patients sometimes do not seem to be aware of patterns of behavior that are completely obvious to others, suggesting the defense mechanism of denial. Other patients ascribe to others feelings that they themselves possess, making the defense mechanism of projection seem relevant.

Behind the notion of defense mechanisms lies the concept of unconscious mental processes. One does not need to accept the entirety of Freud's theories about mental states to recognize the applicability of the concept of unconscious mental life. One also does not need to accept Freud's views regarding the exact nature of unconscious mental life to recognize that such unconscious feelings may exist. The minimum fact one might say that modern psychiatry accepts from Freud is that not all feelings and thoughts are conscious. That is, much of one's mental activities exist at a level below that of superficial awareness. Some individuals have doubted the existence of unconscious mental processes, since they are difficult to establish empirically, but one can turn to research in neuropsychology for such empirical backing. Those studies show that memory and other mental activities frequently occur without conscious awareness (Kandel 1999). This neuropsychological evidence does not exactly support Freudian ideas about the content of unconscious processes, since Freud held that those underlying unconscious aspects of mental life had a specifically sexual character. Empirical studies in neuropsychology do not show that this is the case, nor do they disprove it. However, that there are mental processes below the level of conscious awareness—that is, unconscious mental processes—seems almost indubitable. And Freud can be commended for clearly arguing for this fact.

Another aspect of Freud's theories that is taken for granted today is the idea that much of human life does not function at the level of reason alone. That is, the irrational aspects of humanity make up a good part of our psychology, culture, and history. The proposition that much of human mental life does not follow the rules of reason was revolutionary in Freud's day. Even other approaches to psychology, such as cognitive behavioral ideas, no longer completely deny the relevance of irrationality to understanding the mind. Unlike the early behaviorists, such as B. F. Skinner, many modern cognitive behavioral psychologists are quite willing to admit that many of the problems in human behavior have to do with the effects of irrational mental processing. These persons may not accept Freudian ideas about what constitutes those irrational ideas, but Freud deserves credit in retrospect for convincing the field of the relevance of irrational thoughts and feelings.

Although Freud can be justly criticized for overemphasizing the importance of sexuality in human life, one must recall that in the Victorian age he deserved credit for addressing this topic at all. Clearly, sexuality has relevance to human psychology, although Freudians certainly appear to overdo it when they reduce every aspect of psychopathology to a sexual complex of one kind or another.

The issue of childhood trauma has generated the most controversy recently in relationship to Freud (Forrester 1997).[2] There are those who think that Freud intentionally ignored the scope of sexual trauma in Victorian Vienna. Others believe that Freud altogether mistakenly introduced the notion of sexual trauma into psychiatry. Some hold that almost all psychiatric problems are due to sexual trauma, whether this trauma is consciously known or unconsciously buried in the depths of one's memory. Others believe that almost no psychiatric problems are related to sexual trauma and that so-called memories of childhood sexual trauma are cultural fallacies, based on trendy notions passed around in the confines of a psychotherapist's office. This controversy is large, and I will not attempt to judge it. I will merely contend that mainstream psychiatry is taking a middle road on this issue. Most psychiatrists believe that some psychiatric problems are due to childhood sexual trauma but not that all psychopathology can be traced to a sexual source. Specifically, personality disorders, including borderline personality disorder, are thought to be related to childhood sexual trauma; there is empirical research of some rigor to support this connection. Similarly, many clinicians, including child psychiatrists, have come across cases of sexual trauma that are real and supported by medical and forensic evidence. Yet many of us have also seen cases of individuals who seem to have had memories of childhood sexual trauma that later turned out to be false or unlikely. Again, I think that Freud deserves credit both for opening the eyes of his medical colleagues and the culture at large to this problem and for recognizing the limits of the sexual trauma explanation for psychiatric conditions.

Many nonpsychiatrists identify Freud with his theories, rather than his methods. Yet I feel that his methods are much more relevant today than his theories. As described earlier, one of Freud's major contributions to psychiatry was to introduce the method of free association. Freud taught psychiatrists to listen. And he taught them to listen without making judgments or spinning theories. Freud's theories themselves were concepts he devised *after* seeing his patients. Freud emphasized the need, during the treatment sessions, to listen attentively to people; thinking about ideas interfered with this ability to listen. One of Freud's patients once remarked that the aspect of the man that stood out most for him was how he felt listened to. You can't imagine how it felt to be *listened to* like that, Freud's former patient noted.[3]

4.

Freud's contributions are not minor, nor is he the sole fount of psychiatric wisdom. Psychiatry is finally coming to a more balanced perspective on Freud and his ideas.

Since psychoanalysis is no longer as powerful as it once was, the role of psychotherapy in general, as part of psychiatry, has been put into question. Another form of psychotherapy, long overshadowed by psychoanalysis, that may have new relevance today is existential therapy, which I will discuss next.

CHAPTER 21

Being There

Existential Psychotherapy

Always the rule of rules is to treat the individual who is sick, not an abstract disease. —HENRY MAUDSLEY

1.

The "existential" school of psychiatry has three main branches, based on different aspects of its philosophical fathers. The first, based on Edmund Husserl, emphasizes the phenomenological reduction; Karl Jaspers worked in this tradition, which formed the mainstream of Continental psychiatry for decades. The second, resting on the early Martin Heidegger, emphasizes the existential structure of each individual's world; here Ludwig Binswanger made his mark. The third, building on the late Heidegger, centered itself on the importance of authenticity for the understanding of persons; Jean-Paul Sartre was associated with this approach, along with assorted others such as R. D. Laing and Erich Fromm.[1]

The existential psychiatry that was much in vogue three decades ago is largely ignored today. It has become identified with extreme views, such as those of Thomas Szasz and Laing, and mainstream psychiatry has distanced itself from it. Yet the tradition in existential psychiatry developed through interpretations of the work of Martin Heidegger by the Swiss psychiatrist Ludwig Binswanger, which focuses on the methods of phenomenology, should be useful to contemporary psychiatrists. Binswanger is the source of the ideas presented here, since he wrote extensively, as a psychiatrist grounded in clinical work, on how to relate Heidegger's existential ideas to psychiatry. Contrary to his own protestations in his main philosophical text, *Being and Time* ([1927] 1962), Heidegger took a keen interest in pursuing the psychiatric implications of his ideas. For more than sixteen years, Heidegger persistently tried to teach his ideas to medical students and young doctors in the Zurich clinic of his student Medard Boss. Boss has provided a painfully truthful transcript, which includes long delays (with Boss's own exclamation points [e.g., "seven minutes delay!"]) following profound Heideggerian questions that were met with complete silence on the part of the young medical personnel (Binswanger 1963a). Binswanger tried to make Heidegger's ideas clinically relevant.

In this chapter I will discuss some of Heidegger's philosophical ideas, then present two of Binswanger's cases applying those ideas.

2.

For Binswanger, Heidegger's ideas, mainly as described in section 1 of *Being and Time,* provided an understanding of normal human psychology. One could not fully understand psychopathology, he thought, unless one first understood normal psychology. Freud failed to fulfill this role for Binswanger; he was too averse to explicit philosophizing. When *Being and Time* was published in 1927, Binswanger found a theory that fit his needs better.

Binswanger identified two aspects of Heidegger's thought that were particularly important for psychiatry. First, he felt that Heidegger could lead psychiatry beyond the mind-body problem and thus provide psychiatry with a tolerant overarching theory that could allow an integration of its different approaches, ranging from the biological to the psychoanalytic. Second, he believed that Heidegger's analysis of human existence as "Being-in-the-World" served as a lodestar in reference to which abnormalities in mental illness could be understood. Binswanger felt that abnormal "existential structures," or ways of Being-in-the-World, were the primary pathologies of mental illnesses and provided the key to understanding their origins and treatment.

3.

Binswanger saw the mind-body problem as an artifact of most philosophical traditions before Heidegger, and he attributed the crisis of modern psychiatry to the ill effects of this philosophical heritage. Heidegger held that one could get beyond traditional problems in philosophy by engaging in analysis of being rather than logical arguments about knowing. In traditional philosophy, the problems of epistemology are central: how a subject can have knowledge about an object is a core feature of traditional philosophy. The ontology that follows from this approach leads in the direction of common metaphysical controversies in the history of philosophy, for example, arguments regarding subjective versus objective realms of existence.

Heidegger sought to supersede this philosophical path by asking a different primary question. Instead of asking "How do we know?" he asked "What is the nature of Being?" or, more precisely, "What is the nature of our Being?" He wished to proceed by "concrete demonstrations" of the character of Being, rather than logical argument about the nature of knowledge. Thus, instead of emphasizing logical analysis, his philosophical method emphasized finding new words or definitions to describe the character of Being as *Dasein*. This term in Heidegger referred loosely to the being of humans or, more precisely, anything that exists and "takes a stand" on its existence. In other words, *Dasein* asserts something about itself when it exists, such as the fact that it has this or that capability or engages in this or that activity. It is "being there," something that is present outside of itself ("there") in a way that allows it to recognize itself (Gelven 1989; Dreyfus 1994).[2]

Heidegger's aim was to delineate the "pretheoretical" nature of the being of *Dasein*—what its characteristics are, what it depends on, before any cognitive appraisals it makes about itself or other things. This method was his attempt to start at a different beginning point than that of traditional philosophy.

In his description of the being of *Dasein,* Heidegger discussed what *Dasein* finds in the world around it. *Dasein* does things; it acts in relationship to other things in the world. This is a primary characteristic of *Dasein*. Intentionality represents this characteristic of the "comportment" of *Dasein*. It is involved with other things and beings around it. These other objects are either "available" for *Dasein,* or they are "unavailable." They are available if *Dasein* makes use of them, "manipulates" them, in its activity; and when it does so, *Dasein* is not aware of its use of the objects; it is "absorbed" in the world. When, for some reason, the objects fail to perform the use *Dasein* makes of them, due to some "obstacle," they become unavailable, and then *Dasein* becomes aware of their independent existence outside of *Dasein*. Then *Dasein* faces them in the traditional subject-object relationship. *Dasein* "decontextualizes" them in order to understand what went wrong in its use of them. If *Dasein,* engaged in science, "recontextualizes" them in some model or theory, then the objects are "occurrent." If *Dasein* does not recontextualize them, and merely "stares" at them in curiosity, then the objects are "purely occurrent" and *Dasein* faces them in the extreme stand of "traditional philosophy of mind": the isolated subject beholding the isolated object.

Heidegger holds that the primary relationship between *Dasein* and other objects is an "ontic transparency," where *Dasein* manipulates objects as "equipment" instead of thinking about them as independent objects. Thus this primary relationship is ontological and not one consisting of mental states. In other words, the primary problem in epistemology and philosophy of mind, the relationship between subject and object, is preempted by an even more primary condition of existence, in which there is no distinction between *Dasein* and the world in which it is absorbed.

Binswanger felt that this approach, by bypassing the subject-object distinction altogether, also bypassed the mind-body problem (1963b). For psychiatry, this might mean that Heidegger could provide a theoretical scope that can reveal why differing schools of thought only understand a part of the patient's experience and only partake of partial, rather than absolute, knowledge.

4.

Heidegger's second major contribution to psychiatry, as interpreted by Binswanger, was the concept of Being-in-the-World as a means of understanding the existential structure of each individual. For persons with mental illness, Binswanger argued, these existential structures differ from the ones that persons without mental illness have (and even among persons without mental illness, all sorts of variation exists). It is these differences in existential structure that underlie the most primary differences of mental illness; everything else—symptoms and signs, biological changes, psychosocial aspects—follow from and are secondary to the changes in existential structure.

Binswanger interpreted Heidegger's conception of *Dasein* as Being-in-the-World as an "existential a priori," in a way, whose job it was to ground an individual in the characteristics of his life and his world of relationships and roles.[3] If this structure of one's existence was in some way altered, owing to biological or psychological reasons, then it could lay the basis for varied manifestations of mental illnesses. Heidegger nowhere makes such explicitly clinical use of the concept of Being-in-the-World, but this aspect of his thought is central to his contribution to Binswanger's theory and practice, as Jacob Needleman (1963) stresses in his introduction to Binswanger's writings. This core concept is most clearly described by Binswanger in his classic case studies.

It is interesting that Binswanger's adaptation of Heidegger avoids certain of Heidegger's ideas that would seem to have a direct relationship to psychology.

For instance, Heidegger describes three attitudes that *Dasein* can take toward its own being: (1) it can "fail to take a stand" on its being, so that it allows itself to be formed by "public interpretation," (2) it can "disown" its being, "actively identifying" with public social roles as a way of "fleeing its unsettledness," or (3) it can "own up" to its own being, where social roles never become one's identity but merely ways of expressing *Dasein*'s "understanding of the groundlessness of its existence" (Dreyfus 1994, 236). Binswanger nowhere takes up these notions directly in his description of the theoretical contribution of Heidegger to psychiatry.

Neither does Binswanger make use of certain aspects of Heidegger's thought in section 2 of *Being and Time* that seem more readily applicable to psychology, such as *dread of death* and *authenticity*. Instead, Binswanger sticks to a more limited reading of Heidegger's description in section 1 of the ontic realities that *Dasein* faces and of the ontological underpinnings of *Dasein*'s experiences in the world.

5.

Binswanger's best work is in his published clinical cases, all discussed in his translated papers (Binswanger 1963a; May, Angel, and Ellenberger 1958), where his allusions to theory are forced to face the concrete demands of patients. I will limit myself to two of those cases here.

Ilse was a thirty-nine-year-old woman who, after watching *Hamlet*, decided to force her father to treat her mother more kindly (Binswanger 1958b). She one day hit upon her method: as her father reproved her mother, she placed her arm into a hot oven and then exclaimed: "Look, this is to show you how much I love you!" (215). Over the next few months, she was "vigorous, agile, energetic," and began to experience delusions of reference and, upon hospitalization, erotomania, with the belief that her doctors were in love with her. In the course of her thirteen-month institutionalization, Ilse "passed through severe states of excitation with suicidal tendencies" and ultimately was discharged "completely cured of her acute psychosis" (216). Today we might have reason to doubt whether it was her doctors who "cured" her or nature, in what seems to be the duration of a rather typical manic-depressive episode. To analyze this case of what might today be called bipolar disorder, Binswanger appears to rely on the notion of the existential a priori. His first comment is: "Much as war is described as a continuation of politics by different means, so in our case we could interpret Ilse's delusions as a continuation of her sacrifice, but by different means" (218). His method again seems to be a Heideggerian take on Kant's transcendental method: given Ilse's delusions, what existential structure must exist in her that would allow such delusions to exist? Binswanger's specific interpretation of Ilse's case is, to me, not particularly convincing: he discusses different stages in her life and interprets her actions and beliefs from her perspective of what was going on in these life stages.

What is most interesting to me is Binswanger's *method,* rather than the content of his interpretations. His method, it seems to me, is an altogether original version of an *empathic* approach to psychosis. Binswanger is explicit about this. He emphasizes the need to live in the world of *Mitsein*, the world of "being-with," where one becomes an equal, so to speak, of the person one is analyzing (224). Standing shoulder to shoulder with the patient in the *mitsein*, the patient's world becomes intelligible as a series of "modes of being-together" *(Mitseinandersein)* (226); one would be tempted to call these modes of being-together the world of interpersonal relationships, but it may mean more; Binswanger is not overly clear about what he means here.

What he says next, though, implies that he wishes to contrast this "being-together" approach to traditional types of empathy, such as in Karl Jaspers's work. Jaspers famously defined psychosis, in his *General Psychopathology,* as happening when empathy with the patient breaks down. That point, where the patient's world becomes unintelligible to the doctor, is the phenomenological boundary of psychosis, he asserts. Binswanger challenges this idea, without directly referring to Jaspers, and implies that it is an overly intellectualized approach to empathy. Empathy is not a matter of understanding ideas; it involves "being-together," that is, understanding the existential structures that function in the *Mitsein* world of the psychotic person. Binswanger seems to proceed from this point in his discussion of the case to a direct extension of his criticism of Jaspers's approach, an approach that is similar to what is considered to be the mainstream "medical model" of "biological psychiatry" today. The psychiatrist, Binswanger says, is not too different in his approach from the "layman": "He *judges* Ilse's sacrifice" (228). The italics are Binswanger's, not mine, and he goes on to emphasize the evaluative, as opposed to the avowed descriptive, nature of the approach in traditional psychiatry:

> He [the psychiatrist] sees the complex and dramatic life-historical *phenomenon* of the sacrifice as an individual *event* "in time" and "in" a human being, he places it

in the category of bizarre, absurd, or "eccentric" acts . . . and lists the latter as a symptom of schizophrenia. . . . But now we have to ask ourselves: what has happened here? . . . If we judge abnormal social behavior—a cultural fact—psychiatrically as a pathological phenomenon, we have left the area of purely biological judgment and entered the area of judgment of biological *purpose*. . . . Health and illness are value concepts . . . based on biological purpose. (228–29)

The modern reader may hear echoes of Thomas Szasz in Binswanger's emphasis on the origin of psychiatric diagnosis in abnormal social behavior and in his implication that the movement from there to biological etiology may not be warranted. Further, he betrays a philosophy of medicine that is at odds with today's mainstream approach in psychiatry; instead of basing medicine on science, that is, the empirical facts of normal and abnormal functioning, he bases medicine on ethics, on the value judgments we make about our biological purpose. Binswanger goes on to assert that when a biological basis for a psychiatric symptom is asserted, nothing more is done than to "name" the "hidden," but "its being [*Sein*] or essence" is not revealed (230).

So, it is worth noting, Binswanger advances an essentialism obviously at odds with the type of rigorous empiricism with which mainstream psychiatry identifies itself. But Binswanger seeks to build a bridge to the mainstream approach. Although he denies that Ilse's specific delusions can, one by one, be identified with brain phenomena, he does allow that "the total form in which the life-historical theme is treated, the form of solution to the task which is posed by the theme, can be pathological and thus dependent on disturbances in the central organ . . . for it is not the 'brain' that thinks and treats a life-historical theme, but the 'man' [*der Mensch*]" (230–31). He seems to be saying that the altered existential structure, in a way, may be linked with brain pathology; Ilse's interpretation of the world as a place of sacrifices and love, as an existential theme, may be driven by some brain phenomena; but the details of her beliefs about this world are the product of her thinking self, not of stereotypic or static brain abnormalities.

Binswanger concludes that Ilse's illness needs to be understood both as a disease and as a life-historical phenomenon. He refuses to take sides on this conflict between Wilhelm Dilthey's famously conflicting approaches of the natural sciences and the humanities *(Geisteswissenschaften)*, because, he thinks, the unity of mind and body precludes such divisions. This is where he uses Heidegger's approach to the mind-body problem clinically. Since the separation of mind and body is an artifact of science, the philosophical approach need not accept it, and existential analysis is based on this "philosophical insight" (232–33).

So Binswanger, in his characteristically eclectic fashion, uses the case of Ilse to describe how a traditional biological approach to "schizophrenia" could be combined with an existential approach that perceives the "life-historical phenomenon" at work in the patient's life. Allowing for the diagnostic inaccuracy of what I think was probably a case of bipolar disorder, one would have to say that Binswanger's claim in this case is not as radical as those of many later existential writers, such as Szasz and Laing.[4]

6.

Except for the fact that the unfortunate Ellen West committed suicide, her story might be the most compelling case history in the history of psychiatry (Binswanger 1958a). Ellen West was a walking test case of different psychiatric theories. She underwent two periods of psychoanalysis, was treated as an inpatient in a psychiatric hospital by Binswanger, and was consulted upon by the doyens of biological psychiatry Emil Kraepelin and Eugen Bleuler. Perhaps so much expertise expended upon one person was bound to be dangerous.

Briefly, she was born of Jewish parents, with a strong family history of completed suicide, probable depression, and manic-depressive psychosis, according to Binswanger. From her childhood she often seemed unhappy, with "days when everything seemed empty to her" (238). Binswanger noted that at age 18, based on diary notes, she wanted "to gain fame—great, undying fame; after hundreds of years her name should still ring out on the lips of mankind" (240). At age 20 she was extremely happy; "from her poems stream radiant joy of life—indeed wild ecstasy of life" (241). She then falls into a deep depression, from which she never completely recovers until her death at age 33. Apparently at the same time, around age 21, she develops the other main pathology that never leaves her, "a dread of getting fat" (242). This is around the same time as the end of a romantic relationship.

Over the years, she alternates between bingeing on food and starving herself; she takes long walks to burn her weight off; she abuses thyroid pills and laxatives to control her weight. She falls in love with her cousin and marries him at age 25. He remains supportive throughout her life. But she is obsessed with being thin, and, at the same time, she is distressed by this obsessive idea and wishes that she could eat food normally.

Today, she would be diagnosed with bulimia nervosa, with possibly a brief period of anorexia as well, and her psychopathology would be discussed mainly in terms of the obsessive-compulsive phenomenology of those eating disorders. In Binswanger's day, "obsessive neurosis" indeed was her initial diagnosis, apparently provided by her first psychoanalyst, who saw her for six months at age 32. She stopped this analysis because she felt it was "useless" but started another one with a more "orthodox" Freudian, according to Binswanger, who apparently saw her for about a year (249). He seemed to be an imperious man, ignoring a period of one month when she made at least four serious suicide attempts by overdosing twice, trying to throw herself in front of a car, and even attempting to throw herself out of her analyst's office. She then began to see an internist with common sense who felt she should be treated in a hospital. Her analyst disagreed.

A consultation was arranged with the most famed clinician of the day, Emil Kraepelin, who diagnosed "melancholia" and recommended rest and treatment in a hospital. The analyst "considered this diagnosis incorrect" and continued outpatient psychoanalysis. Ellen's diary describes her frustrations in the analysis despite an apparently sincere motivation to engage in it: "I wanted to get to know the unknown urges which were stronger than my reason and which forced me to shape my entire life in accordance with a guiding point of view . . . to be thin. The analysis was a disappointment. I analyzed with my mind, and everything remained theory. The wish to be thin remained unchanged in the center of my thinking" (257). At one point, she apparently developed an erotic transference to the analyst, jumping on his lap and kissing him. Ultimately, her internist prevailed upon her to be hospitalized and she ended the analysis after about one year. She remained very ill with her (probable) bulimic and depressive symptoms.

Enter Binswanger, who treated her for a two-month-long hospitalization at age 33. During the hospitalization, Binswanger essentially got nowhere. Attempts to reform Ellen's eating habits produced few results, and she became more and more suicidal. Surprisingly, however, Binswanger tellingly observed that she did not seem deeply despondent as in typical severe depression. "One has less the impression that she suffers under a genuine depressive affect than that she feels herself physically empty and dead, completely hollow, and suffers precisely from the fact that she cannot achieve affect" (262). This perceptive comment is typical of what would today be called a characteristic dysphoric affect of borderline personality disorder or other personality disorders.

Since she was held in an unlocked unit but was becoming more and more suicidal, Binswanger recommended transfer to a locked unit. Ellen and her husband insisted on evidence that she would improve before agreeing to the transfer. Binswanger, who had diagnosed "a progressive schizophrenic psychosis"
(266), could only offer a poor prognosis.

One final consultation was made, with Eugen Bleuler and "a foreign psychiatrist" (perhaps an American?) "whose views were not too close to the Krae-
pelin-Bleuler theory of schizophrenia." Not surprisingly, Bleuler felt that "the
presence of schizophrenia [was] indubitable." The other psychiatrist opined
(probably rightly) that her great concern with her weight did not represent a
delusion (and thus did not represent a symptom of schizophrenia) but rather
an "overvalent idea," or what today we would call an overvalued idea (one step
short of an obsession); her symptoms were part of a "psychopathic constitu-
tion" (i.e., a personality disorder), he surmised (266). Neither held out any
hope for a good prognosis. With that final word, she was discharged, and three
days later, after one day of "a positively festive mood" and an uncharacteristi-
cally healthy appetite, she killed herself with poison (267).

Binswanger made a great effort to understand Ellen West's Being-in-the-
World using his new existential techniques. He began a discussion of her *Eigenwelt*, the "own world" of her subjective purely personal experience, compared
with her *Mitwelt*, the "with world" of interpersonal relationships, and her
Umwelt, the "in world" of natural objects, including our bodies, existing inde-
pendently of us (269–73). He held that Ellen West's mode of existence was
marked by a withdrawal during childhood into her *Eigenwelt* from her *Umwelt*
and her *Mitwelt*. "The *Eigenwelt* does not go trustingly over into the *Umwelt* and
Mitwelt, to let itself be carried, nourished, and fulfilled by it, but separates itself sharply from it" (270). She met a few failures in love and work as a young
adult; Binswanger mentions these apparently in passing, leaving the impression that they were common and unavoidable, part of Shakespeare's ubiquitous "slings and arrows of outrageous fortune."

Yet, as a result of these expected setbacks, her interest in others in the
Mitwelt began to shrink more and more. Soon her interest in her existence in
terms of her future fell away, and her existence became more and more identified by her past, an unchanging remembrance of failures and unfulfilled
wishes. "Her failure to realize 'the old plans and hopes' transforms the world
into boundless desolation, soundless stillness, and icy cold, in which the Eigenwelt shrivels to an infinitely tiny point. Her soul is weary, the bells of death in

her heart cannot be silenced" (276). Thus her existence, spatially conceived, moved from being a line pointing toward the future to a circle imprisoned in the past.

By her early twenties her existence was held up in this "vicious circle" (354), which she would never break until the end of her life. At the age of 21, her existential development had ended, just as her psychopathological symptoms would begin.

> The dread of becoming fat . . . with which the true illness in the psychiatric sense manifests itself, has thus to be seen anthropologically not as a beginning but as an end. It is the end of the encirclement process of the entire existence, so that it is no longer open for its existential possibilities. . . . Existence now gets hemmed in more and more, confined to a steadily diminishing circle of narrowly defined possibilities, for which the wish to be thin and the dread of getting fat represent merely the definitive [psychophysical] garb. The way of the life-history is now unmistakably prescribed: it no longer runs into the expanse of the future but moves in a circle. The preponderance of the future is now replaced by supremacy of the past. All that remains are the fruitless attempts at escaping from this circle. (281)

The fundamental existential structure of her life was set, and her future was preordained by it. The onset of her bulimic symptoms was merely an expression of her constricted circular mode of existence. The irrelevance of the *Mitwelt* and the *Umwelt* was symbolized by her fixation on her "bodily eigenwelt" (352) of her eating habits. Her particular symptoms were an expression of her existential pathology. "The dread of becoming fat has revealed itself as a concretization of a severe existential dread, the dread of the 'degenerating life,' of withering, drying up, moldering, rotting, becoming a husk, eroding, being buried alive, whereby the world of the self becomes a tomb, a mere hole" (349).

As she focused more and more on food, the existential structure of her life developed into a process of being-in-a-hole, the hole of her unfulfilled need for food, rather than a process of being-for-others in the *Mitwelt* and being-for-herself in an authentic *Eigenwelt*.

Ultimately, she had her one moment of authentic existence when, paradoxically, she ended her physical existence. For when she died of her own volition, she broke the circle of existence that imprisoned her for the first (and last) time. Binswanger seemed to approve rather explicitly of her suicide in this way. She had already been dead, he asserted, existentially dead, since her early twenties when her Being-in-the-World was distorted into that vicious circle. The rest of her life was a mere waiting for her physical death. Like a chronologically old person, who looks upon death as a welcome deliverance after becoming gradually more and more detached from "the needs of life," the "young . . . Ellen West had already become old." She had aged existentially very rapidly and was "ripe for death," and finally she hastened herself what nature would not speed up. "The suicide is the necessary-voluntary consequence of this existential state of things" (295). In that moment, she reconciled herself with her mode of existence; since it took death for her to reach such harmony of life, her story was a tragedy. "The festival of death was the festival of the birth of her existence. But where the existence can exist only by relinquishing life, there the existence is a tragic existence" (298).

Binswanger refused to pass judgment on her or to assume that continued life would have been better or more right for her (although he speculated that she possibly might have recovered somewhat had electroconvulsive therapy been available at that time). He wished to understand her way of Being-in-the-World, and he did so by recognizing her death as in some way necessary. "Life and death are not opposites . . . death too must be lived . . . life is 'encompassed' by death" (294).

7.

Binswanger deserves a number of distinctions for his contributions. He was the first to systematically apply Heidegger's ideas to clinical psychopathology. He was original and independent-minded, not allowing himself to be bound by the niceties of the orthodox interpretation of the philosopher. He was adept with psychoanalysis and descriptive clinical approaches to his cases as well. In his cases he was at his most brilliant, providing rich material in which he tried to concretize the application of existentialist ideas to human psychology. His biggest weakness, it seems to me, was a certain intellectual sloppiness, marked by his overly eclectic use of different ideas that, in retrospect, seem little related. Most typical of this failing is his painful distortion of Ellen West into a Bleulerian schizophrenic, and that after a masterful understanding of the meaning of her suicide and the existential basis of her bulimia.

There are crimes of passion and crimes of logic, Camus once wrote, and the border between the two is not always clear. Although Binswanger may have committed misdemeanors of logic, he committed no crimes. If anything, he was too wary of commitments of any kind to expose himself to such criticism. Binswanger was passionate about understanding something more about persons with psychiatric symptoms than most orthodoxies would admit. Contemporary psychiatry would likely benefit from reexamining some of his ideas.

CHAPTER 22

Beyond Eclecticism

Integrating Psychotherapy and Psychopharmacology

> Because each [school of thought] represents a significant attitude toward
> life and people and is strongly attractive to certain temperaments, the
> person who means to master psychiatry has to withstand strong exclusive
> pulls in one direction or another. Further the psychiatrist or psychologist
> does not want to be merely eclectic, that is, borrowing whatever pleases
> him from various sources. He wants to be *pluralistic,* able to use all the
> methods. —LESTON HAVENS, 1973

1.

In psychiatric education, eclecticism is a popular professed approach, implying theoretical lack of bias and an evenhanded biopsychosocial approach.
However, with the economic pressures of managed care and the influence of
advances in empirical research, some observers have noted a drift in psychiatric teaching programs toward biological approaches, with a concomitant decline in psychotherapy training. A professed adherence to eclecticism has failed
to halt this shift.

An alternative is the pluralist approach, which holds that *specific* theoretical approaches are best applied to *specific* disorders; it supports an integrationist
approach to treatment, wherein each psychotherapy technique is used with
appropriate psychopharmacological treatments when most applicable to each
relevant psychiatric disorder. In contrast, the eclectic approach, in practice, applies both psychotherapy and psychopharmacology treatments to practically
all disorders. This distinction will be clarified below.

Also, psychiatric education programs have taught psychotherapy through
individual supervision separate from the psychopharmacological training received in clinics or on inpatient wards. Although this approach undoubtedly
will remain in place, I suggest here that psychotherapy teaching can be

strengthened by including supplementary psychotherapy education as an integral part of psychopharmacological training. This approach to psychiatric education, though in many ways simplistic, may help clarify the roles of psychotherapy and psychopharmacology in modern psychiatric theory and practice for the next generation of students and residents.

2.

Words are the main tools psychotherapy possesses. One perspective, derived from Havens, is that psychotherapeutic techniques involve different ways in which words can be used. Havens divides psychotherapy techniques into four major schools, based, in one descriptive sense, on their methods of using words: the psychoanalytic school uses words for interpretations of hidden meaning; the existential school uses words to create a process of empathy with the patient's meaning; the objective-descriptive school (which includes the supportive types of psychotherapy) uses words to show sympathy for the patient; and the interpersonal school uses words to undo the patient's distortions of meaning (as will be discussed shortly).

Good bedside manner in the physician suggests psychotherapeutic skill with words, and it is practiced spontaneously and unconsciously. The psychopharmacologist, however, needs to begin where the intuitive physician leaves off, since treating psychiatric disorders involves a need to directly address the patient's emotional concerns in a way that may not allow for the influence of bedside manner. Thus, the use of psychotherapeutic approaches needs to be more explicit in psychopharmacology than in general medicine.

I will provide examples of different types of psychotherapy geared to specific psychiatric disorders that are treated with medications as well. While reading them, one should keep in mind the main suggestion of this chapter: by teaching psychotherapies that are specific to certain disorders at the same time as teaching the relevant psychopharmacology, the amount of psychotherapy teaching possible in the typical contemporary residency program is expanded.

3.

In patients with mild psychiatric disorders, such as mild forms of anxiety or affective disorders, supportive psychotherapeutic techniques involve a straightforward discussion of the risks and benefits of treatment and a clear-cut professional relationship based on the doctor's competence to treat and the patient's commitment to honestly cooperate. From one, albeit simplified, perspective, the psychotherapeutic relationship here is not different from most relationships in life, where words are spoken with little deliberation or intended meaning beyond the superficial. They are simply aimed at bolstering the patient's sense of self in the face of troubling but not overwhelming symptoms and providing information for autonomous decision-making. The doctor's goal with this method is to tell the truth and to set the patient's mind at ease.

4.

In moderate depression, an essential psychotherapeutic aspect of psychiatric treatment involves empathy. Depressed patients suffer from deadening worldviews. They are unable to see beyond these worldviews, and the recognition of the need for medication may lie beyond the horizon of a depressive worldview. Depressed patients also feel a need for the doctor to be in touch with the content of their depressive experiences. It then becomes the psychopharmacologist's task, by utilizing empathy, to delve into their worldviews, gain their trust, and slowly pull them out far enough so that they can see the need for treatment with medications. This task can be achieved by the use of our own existential despair, which should be immediately available to all human beings on reflection, as a tool to contact patients ensconced in depressive worldviews. The goal is to initiate a connection with patients; all treatment follows that initial contact.

In mild to moderate personality disorders (especially of the borderline and narcissistic types) and mild to moderate affective disorders, another psychotherapeutic technique, probably the most popular technique in general, is interpretation. Empathy may initiate the process whereby patients feel understood, but they may need insightful interpretations of their thoughts and feelings in order to feel better understood.

5.

In severe psychiatric illnesses, such as severe personality disorders, schizophrenia, and severe affective disorders (psychotic depression and bipolar disorder), the psychotherapeutic aspects of psychiatric treatment need to become at once simpler and more complex than in traditional psychotherapy. They need to be simpler because the severely ill patient is most in need of the basic ego-bolstering activity of supportive psychotherapy. Since complete cure is rare in severe illness, relapse and persistently poor functioning are constant dilemmas. Supportive psychotherapy works here by encouraging the patient to focus on the positive aspects of recovery, where they exist, rather than the negative aspects of continuing disability. Also, like traditional medical bedside manner, the plain sympathy of supportive psychotherapy can diminish the sense of aloneness and impotence of the suffering patient.

Psychotherapeutic techniques in the psychopharmacological management of severe illness also need to be rather sophisticated, sometimes as complex as those employed in the most intensive formal psychotherapy treatments. A special psychotherapeutic sensitivity is needed here because paranoia, the antithesis of the trusting therapeutic alliance, is rife in severe psychiatric illness. In severe personality disorders, it may take the form of projective identification and rage directed toward the doctor. In severe psychotic disorders, it may be directly reflected in paranoid delusions and hallucinations. And in severe affective disorders (especially psychotic depression), it may be expressed in a distrustful rejection of the empathic approaches of the doctor.

Where sympathy, empathy, and interpretation fail, counterprojective techniques may work. In other words, it is in severe psychotic, affective, and personality disorders that counterprojective psychotherapeutic techniques become useful.

Counterprojection is an idea developed by Harry Stack Sullivan (1954). In its simplest form, as described by Havens (1983), it involves the following logical process: The patient says "You are Jack," which is a projection of his own feeling about an internal object-representation of a man named Jack. The doctor, when counterprojecting, needs to convince the patient of the following proposition: "No, I am not Jack. I'm Jim. Jack is out there." Jack is out there in the world, not in the doctor (where the projection places him), nor in the patient's mind (where he truly resides). At this point in treatment, the severely ill patient is unable to tolerate the idea that Jack resides within him or her as an internal object-representation. Only through repeated counterprojection can the doctor begin to convince the patient that the doctor, at least, is not Jack. If the patient can accept that fact, then psychopharmacological treatment can begin. Only then can the patient divert the paranoia that lives with the concept of Jack away from the doctor and toward all those Jacks in the external world. Colluding against those other Jacks, the doctor and the patient are free to form some kind of therapeutic alliance. This alliance is to some extent superficial, but in the context of psychopharmacological treatment, it may create just enough of a wedge in the patient's paranoid worldview to allow a pill to enter. With the acceptance of medication treatment, the paranoid worldview might be biologically shattered, thus making counterprojection no longer necessary and allowing further psychotherapeutic work to proceed.

6.

Today's student of psychiatry often is confused by psychiatry's schools of thought, especially the different approaches of psychotherapies and psychopharmacology. These two different treatment approaches tend to be taught separately, but, as mentioned above, I suggest teaching them together, in an integrated manner. Havens's theoretical framework may be a useful starting point. Its main use here is that it allows the recognition of the utility of *specific* psychotherapeutic techniques derived from *specific* psychiatric schools of thought, along with medication, in different psychiatric disorders. Thus, these different approaches each are given a definite, albeit limited, validity. This *pluralism* is both theoretically more detailed than the traditional eclectic approach and, in my experience, more clarifying for new students of psychiatry.

The practitioner and advanced teacher may object that this approach seems quite oversimplified; certainly psychiatric theory and practice are more complex than suggested here. No doubt the application of particular psychotherapeutic techniques to specific psychopathological entities has its limitations. Often, techniques need to be combined, and the specific conditions for their utilization depend on the particular circumstances of treatment for each patient. I seek here only to provide a broad outline toward integrating psychotherapeutic methods into the psychopharmacology setting. In actual practice, undoubtedly, this integration will be more complex than what for the sake of clarity I present here. But this integrated approach to teaching psychotherapy and psychopharmacology to new students is meant to serve as an introduction toward getting some theoretical grounding in this complicated field. Being simplified, it has the virtue of comprehensibility, and it is amenable to being deepened and made less rigid with further experience. In my experience, students react positively to this kind of structured introduction to the field, which helps clear away the initially daunting confusion many face when encountering complicated clinical and historical aspects of psychiatry.

Part III / After Eclecticism

CHAPTER 23

Bridging the Biology-Psychology Dichotomy

The Hopes of Integrationism

1.

In chapter 2, where I discussed current philosophies of mind, the basic dichotomy that I described was the split between dualism and monism. Until the twentieth century, dualism was commonly accepted, the basic idea being that mind and brain are separate and generally unrelated entities. Contemporary philosophy is greatly influenced by the advances of science, however, and most philosophers would likely accept the proposition that the mind is dependent on the brain. That is, without the brain there would be no mind. Almost all scientists also take this view, as do most physicians.

Yet, though dead in theory, dualism is alive in practice. This is because many laypersons still adhere to an essentially dualistic theory of mind. And I am not implying here that laypersons are wrong simply because scientists and many philosophers are no longer dualists. I happen to believe that dualism is misconceived, but it would be elitist to argue against it simply based on the current consensus of philosophers and scientists. Dualism does seem to have been dealt serious blows by the advances of science. First Darwin, then Einstein, showed that many beliefs based on another realm of existence (the divine) could be explained within the realm of the natural world. Neuroscience has gradually extended the same explanations to the brain.

Dualism in practice remains a problem, however, not only because many persons are dualists in theory (though frequently almost unconsciously), but also because straightforward monism also has received a great deal of philosophical criticism. This kind of materialism would hold that the mind simply *is* (rather than is dependent on) the brain. This approach would *reduce* the mind to brain. Hence, this view is a reductionist materialism. A number of philosophical criticisms have been directed at this way of thinking, such as the qualia problem and other topics discussed in chapter 2. Furthermore, neuroscience has not yet progressed to the point where the actual translation of mental to brain phenomena is obvious.

As a result, there have been a number of attempts at avoiding dualism and reductionist materialism, such as emergence and some types of functionalism. These are examples of *nonreductive materialism*. According to this view, although mind is dependent on brain, mental phenomena are not reduced to brain states. I think that nonreductive materialism makes the most sense in philosophy of mind, given our current state of knowledge. In psychiatry, I suggest that a pluralist approach works best, and the pluralism I propose could be linked with either emergence or some kinds of functionalism as its underlying philosophy of mind. I have reviewed the utility of a pluralist approach to many clinical phenomena in psychiatry in earlier chapters.

There is at least one other viable perspective in current psychiatry that is also nonreductionist and antidualist. I call this the *integrationist* perspective, and it is intuitively more appealing than pluralism to many persons. In the next chapter, I will discuss why pluralism, when considered carefully, is not attractive to everyone. The attractions of integrationism, in contrast, are many. A recent proponent of this view is Eric Kandel, a prominent neuroscientist and psychiatrist. In this chapter, I will assess the strengths and limits of the integrationist view and spell out some of its claims and implications.

2.

A major attraction of integrationism is that it promises to be one large explanatory theory for psychiatry. Clinicians and patients are always looking for a final explanation for everything. The dogmatisms of psychoanalysis (which relies on a dualistic mind-brain theory) and biological reductionism have failed. Integrationism promises a potentially coherent alternative.

Another benefit of integrationism is that it sounds good. Just as eclecticism and pluralism seem innocuously benign, no one would seem to want to be opposed to the pleasant sound of *integration*. But as with eclecticism and pluralism, once one asks what the word means, many opportunities for disagreement exist.

Also, for those who want to be as materialist as possible, integrationism has the potential for avoiding too much talk of non-brain-related phenomena. This contrasts with pluralism, which requires a willingness to allow for phenomena or aspects of mental phenomena that are best understood quite separately from the underlying neurophysiology.

For these reasons and more, integrationism has its attractions. But what does it really entail?

3.

I discussed the basic concepts of integrationism in chapter 1. Here I will examine these ideas in the context of the work of Eric Kandel. And then I will expand on the implications of this approach as a general theory of psychiatry, focusing as well on its limitations.

Kandel expressed his mature views in a 1998 paper entitled "A New Intellectual Framework for Psychiatry," based on a speech given at the New York State Psychiatric Institute. This paper was followed by another, also published prominently in the *American Journal of Psychiatry* (as was the first), entitled "Biology and the Future of Psychoanalysis" (1999), which represented his response to a number of critiques of the first paper. Since Kandel received the Nobel Prize in 2000, his views have gained even more prominence and deserve careful attention.

In his primary paper, Kandel (1998) reviews his psychiatric training at the Massachusetts Mental Health Center in Boston in the 1960s with a mixture of nostalgia and regret. Kandel clearly has nostalgia for the days when psychoanalysis was more creative and influential, but he also suffered from the indifference of his psychoanalytic teachers toward empiricism, science, and research. Kandel went his own way, obtaining experience at the National Institutes of Health in basic science research and then developing his own career in neuroscience. Yet his research was influenced by his early exposure to psychoanalysis, resulting in his focus on the mechanisms of memory and learning. In retrospect, Kandel rather clearly indicts the leaders of psychoanalysis for ignoring scientific method, to their own detriment as well as to that of the field of psychiatry as a whole. This critique led to many responses, which Kandel addressed in his second paper.

But before I assess Kandel's view of psychoanalysis further, I want to review Kandel's own stated principles for his new intellectual framework, which I consider to be basic tenets of integrationism. Kandel lays them out as five principles:

This framework can be summarized in five principles that constitute, in simplified form, the current thinking of biologists about the relationship of mind to brain.

Principle 1. All mental processes, even the most complex psychological processes, derive from the brain. . . . As a corollary, behavioral disorders that characterize psychiatric illness are disturbances of brain function, even in those cases where the causes of the disturbances are clearly environmental in origin. . . .

Principle 2. Genes . . . are important determinants of the pattern of interconnections between neurons. . . . As a corollary, one component contributing to the development of major mental illnesses is genetic. . . .

Principle 3. . . . Just as combinations of genes contribute to behavior . . . so can behavior and social factors exert actions on the brain by feeding back upon it to modify the expression of genes and thus the function of nerve cells. Learning . . . produces alterations in gene expression. Thus all of "nurture" is ultimately expressed as "nature."

Principle 4. Alterations in gene expression induced by learning give rise to changes in patterns of neuronal connections. These changes not only contribute to the biological basis of individuality but presumably are responsible for initiating and maintaining abnormalities of behavior that are induced by social contingencies.

Principle 5. Insofar as psychotherapy or counseling is effective and produces long-term changes in behavior, it presumably does so through learning, by producing changes in gene expression that alter the strength of synaptic connections and structural changes that alter the anatomic pattern of interconnections between nerve cells of the brain. As the resolution of brain imaging increases, it should eventually permit quantitative evaluation of the outcome of psychotherapy. (1998, 460)

This, in a nutshell, is Kandel's integrationist model of psychiatry. The first principle is simply nonreductive materialism: the mind is dependent on the brain. The second and third principles are, at one level, statements of the fact that genes and environment contribute to the formation of the brain. Thus, if one connects all three principles, the following logical argument develops:

1. Mind is dependent on brain.
2. Brain is partly dependent on genes.
2a. Therefore, mind is partly dependent on genes.
2b. Therefore, abnormal mental phenomena are partly dependent on genes.
3. Brain is partly dependent on social environment.

3a. Therefore, mind is partly dependent on social environment.

3b. Therefore, abnormal mental phenomena are partly dependent on social environment.

Thus far, this summary, though correct, is not very original. The originality of Kandel's proposal lies in the tail end of principle 3, as well as principles 4 and 5, all of which are variations on one general theme: that the environment influences the brain directly, through neuronal changes, as suggested by the concept of neuroplasticity. Kandel's own neuroscientific work on learning and memory has focused on this concept, and he has been a trailblazer in establishing the relevance and importance of neuroplasticity. Kandel has also long had an interest in the association between psychotherapy and changes in the brain produced via neuroplasticity (earliest expressed in a 1979 article called "Psychotherapy and the Single Synapse"). Hence, we can add a fourth premise to Kandel's proposal:

4. Social environment influences abnormal mental phenomena by means of the brain.

4a. Psychiatric treatments, whether biological or psychological, ultimately act through the mechanism of changes in the brain.

The integrationist steps are premises 3 and 4. If we accept that the brain is influenced by social environment and that mental illness is partly influenced by social environment, then the brain is the link between the social environment and mental illness. The integration occurs at that link between brain and social environment.

4.

Kandel admits that the details of this connection between the environment and the brain are not well understood. But he thinks it is only a matter of time and effort before this connection is clarified. He provides two examples in his 1998 paper.

The first example comes from his own work with the snail *Aplysia*. He described his findings this way: "Animals subjected to controlled learning that gave rise to long-term memory had twice as many presynaptic terminals as untrained animals. Some forms of learning, such as long-term habituation, produce the opposite changes; they lead to a regression and pruning of synaptic connections. These morphological changes seem to be a signature of the long-term memory process. They do not occur with short-term memory" (1998, 464).

In other words, as one remembers something, the brain is changing. If one remembers something for a long time, the brain changes in a different way than if one remembers something for a short time. The environment is changing the brain, structurally, in its very anatomy! This certainly would seem to argue for an integration between mind and brain, emphasizing that this integration is a two-way street.

Kandel's other example involves a study with monkeys: "Adult monkeys were encouraged to use three middle fingers at the expense of two other fingers of the hand to obtain food. After several thousand trials, the area of cortex devoted to the three fingers was greatly expanded at the expense of the area normally devoted to the other fingers. Practice alone, therefore, may not only strengthen the effectiveness of existing patterns of connections, but also change cortical connections to accommodate new patterns of actions" (1998, 465). Practice, another form of learning, can actually make part of the brain grow in size!

All this adds up to the brain being a plastic organ, highly responsive to the environment. It is a short step from this observation to the conclusion of Edward Hundert, described in chapter 3. Hundert uses these findings to argue that the external world literally shapes the brain, ensuring that our brain accurately represents the external world. Hundert thereby seeks to reach the same conclusion as Hegel reached three hundred years ago, this time based on the idea of integration of mind and brain.

Kandel and Hundert do not lay out the details of exactly how mental phenomena are brain phenomena other than in these examples. But what these examples suggest, I think, is that, *in principle,* mental phenomena and brain phenomena might translate into each other. I suggested a way of thinking about this issue in figure 1.2 in chapter 1.

The idea here (which again is not explicit in the work of Kandel and Hundert, but which I think logically follows from their work) is that, *at some level,* mental phenomena and brain phenomena translate into each other. The question is, What is that level? It is not the level of general mental phenomena (e.g., what it feels like to see the color red). At such general levels of mental phenomena, the idea of emergence seems valid, and mental phenomena are not directly linked to brain phenomena. However, at a fine-grain level of analysis, such mental phenomena can be broken down into very simple cognitive structures and principles. This is the work of cognitive neuroscience. Hence, in the snail *Aplysia,* experimenters can examine conditioned learning (a simple cognitive principle) of a very basic behavior (a simple cognitive structure in a simple invertebrate). Researchers can show that this conditioned learning of a simple behavior leads to specific changes in the structure of the brain (synaptic growth or pruning). Where that behavior is present, the brain changes are present. Where the brain changes are present, that behavior is present. One cannot occur without the other. One is directly linked to the other. One translates into the other.

Notice three issues. I did not say one is *reduced* to the other. But it seems clear that a mental phenomenon, the learning of a behavior, is inextricably linked to a brain phenomenon, such as synaptic pruning of a certain region of the brain of *Aplysia*. Without the brain changes, the mental phenomena would not occur. But the mental phenomena are still not exactly the same as the brain changes. One does not say that synaptic pruning of this part of the brain *is the same as* learning this kind of behavior. However, one might be able to say that such synaptic pruning *causes,* or leads to, learning this kind of behavior. Yet, this translation is two-sided. So one might just as easily say that learning this kind of behavior causes, or leads to, such synaptic pruning in this part of the brain. Translation is not the same thing as reduction. Hence, integrationism remains a nonreductive materialism. To that extent, the arguments of dualists and others against reductive materialism are not refuted by integrationism, nor do they affect the central argument of integrationism.

Second, whereas we needed very fine-grained cognitive analysis to allow a translation into brain phenomena, we need a very large view of neuronal structure to allow such a translation. Fine-grain brain phenomena, such as alterations in neurotransmitters and cellular proteins, are too complex and redundant to be directly linked to specific cognitive events.

Third, the examples in *Aplysia* occur in a very simple invertebrate by design. Kandel found that the mechanisms of memory were too complex to study with much success in complex vertebrates or mammals. To be able to make the mind-brain connection he was seeking, he had to go to a simple invertebrate with a very simple neuronal structure as well as a very simple behavioral repertoire. However, what Kandel is doing is establishing that, in principle, a mind-brain translation can happen. Once established in principle, the relevance to human beings becomes one of complexity, rather than one of possibility. In other words, we now have a biological example of mind-brain integration. The possibility that the same process happens in humans is no longer simply a metaphysical or theoretical one; it is biologically possible.

5.

Is integrationism valid? Is it a better approach than pluralism?

It is too early to answer these questions definitively. Integrationism, especially as proposed by Kandel, has a potential for providing a useful general theory that, at certain levels, will provide a kind of glue between mental and brain sciences, between psychiatry and neuroscience. Yet, at least in the interpretation of integrationism I have offered here, it would still be nonreductive. Many psychological phenomena would still autonomously function in social sciences and psychiatry, and many neuroscientific phenomena would still autonomously be studied in molecular biology. The change is in the use of the word *many* rather than the word *all*. Hence, to some extent, pluralism and integrationism are not at odds. An integrationist would still need to be a pluralist in psychiatry, recognizing the need for and limits of strictly psychological approaches as well as strictly biological approaches, even if, at some level, the integrationist believes that the two approaches can translate into each other. Furthermore, for those phenomena which can be translated, the integrationist may indeed move back and forth from biological to psychological language, without reducing one to the other. So little is known about mind-brain integration in humans that, even if one accepts the idea in principle, *in practice* integrationists would have to be pluralists (unless they wanted to accept either of the other alternatives of dogmatism or eclecticism).

But it is not easy to be a pluralist.

CHAPTER 24

Why It Is Hard to Be Pluralist

Man is a larger whole than any single method. —HENRY MAUDSLEY

The object of psychiatry is man. What sets man apart from all things in
the world is the fact that he as a whole can no more become an object
than the world as a whole. When we know him, we know something
about him, rather than himself. —KARL JASPERS

1.

The danger of advocating pluralism is the "So what?" problem. Readers
might be inclined to ask that question when I suggest the benefits of pluralism. Especially when pluralism is set against the term *dogmatism,* most persons
would not want to identify themselves with the latter. But I use the word *dogmatism* as shorthand: in reality it is always dogmatism about something. Thus,
in politics, one might be a conservative, or a socialist, or a liberal and hold his
views dogmatically. Such a person is a dogmatist, and such dogmatists have
much more in common than one might expect, despite differing ideologies.
One could be a nondogmatic conservative, or socialist, or liberal, and such persons would have much more in common with each other than with dogmatists of their own ideology.[1] Similarly, in psychiatry, the content of the ideology can be psychoanalysis or it can be neuroscience, but dogmatism reflects
the attitude taken by the adherent. And it is this attitude that is important,
more than the content. By dogmatism, then, I mean the dogmatic attitude.
Dogmatists do not, as a rule, revel in their dogmatism, and thus it is not up to
them to accept or deny this label. They are dogmatists whether they like it or
not. And there are many of them practicing in the mental health professions
today.

Besides not wanting to accept the label of dogmatism, many might think of
pluralism as a "So what?" option because they identify it with eclecticism. By

now it should be clear that nothing could be further from the truth. Eclecticism, enshrined in the biopsychosocial model, is the status quo in psychiatry. Pluralism is the ignored pretender to the throne. Distant cousins, they have almost nothing in common besides an opposition to dogmatism. I hope that readers of previous chapters will now see that pluralism simply is not eclecticism, and thus it cannot be easily accepted in the same way that eclecticism can be accepted. A "pox on all the schools" attitude is the high road to eclecticism; that is easy. Pluralism is hard.

In fact, the alternative closest to pluralism is integrationism, and the two are not incompatible. Both are hard.

Why is it hard to be a pluralist? What is so bad about the biopsychosocial model? I will explain in this chapter that most clinicians today are dogmatists in practice and eclectics in theory, and I will lay the fault of this state of affairs at the feet of the biopsychosocial model. I will also argue that accepting pluralism means fighting dogmatism in all the nooks and crannies of psychiatry into which it has seeped, a guerilla war that will be never-ending.

2.

In 1995, psychiatrists J. Alexander Bodkin, Harrison G. Pope Jr., and Robert Klitzman conducted a fascinating study that proves that most clinicians are dogmatists in practice (Bodkin, Klitzman, and Pope 1995). They sent a questionnaire to 435 academic psychiatrists to assess whether they were primarily biologically oriented or primarily psychotherapeutically oriented, or whether they demonstrated evidence of mixing both approaches. Most clinicians claim to be open to both approaches and to mix them, consistent with the biopsychosocial model. The researchers found that they could classify 27 percent of practitioners as biological and 37 percent as psychotherapeutic. These practitioners spent more than three-fourths of their time solely working in their approach. Hence 64 percent of practitioners limit their practice to one approach or the other, and their perspectives on psychiatry usually follow their approach. Sixty-four percent of psychiatrists are dogmatists. Thirty-six percent are "eclectic" practitioners who spend almost equal time practicing in both approaches. These are the biopsychosocialists.

These numbers may seem surprising to some readers. The psychotherapeutically oriented dogmatists were greater in number than the biological dogmatists in 1995. This largely reflects the fact that psychiatry was so dominated by psychoanalytic dogmatism for so many decades. It will take decades for these practitioners to leave the field and be replaced by newly minted clinicians without older biases. Further, the 36 percent eclectic group may seem small. But I think this finding highlights how psychiatrists do not practice what they proclaim. Bodkin and colleagues did not ask their respondents to describe their own philosophies of psychiatry, but it is my experience that most psychiatrists claim to be biopsychosocial eclectics. Yet in practice, only one-third are in fact eclectics. Most clinicians are eclectics only in theory; they are dogmatists in practice.

Is this an unwholesome fact? Proponents of the biopsychosocial view think so, and Glen Gabbard and Jerald Kay recently published a prominent article to that effect. Gabbard and Kay's argument neatly summarizes the faults of the biopsychosocial school, so I will review it here and then explain again why and how pluralism is so different and so difficult.

3.

In their paper "The Fate of Integrated Treatment: Whatever Happened to the Biopsychosocial Psychiatrist?" Gabbard and Kay (2001) begin by assuming the validity of eclecticism and blaming its decline on others: "Almost all psychiatrists, and certainly those who are leaders in our field, endorse the notion that psychiatrists are distinct from all other mental health professionals in that their training and expertise allow them to be the ultimate integrators of the biological and psychosocial perspectives underlying diagnostic understanding and treatment. However, the biopsychosocial model made famous by Engel has been relegated to political lip service in our managed care era" (1956). The first sentence of this influential article demonstrates that it is hard to be a pluralist. Gabbard and Kay assume, right at the start, that "almost all" psychiatrists would wish to "integrate" biological and psychological approaches. Readers should realize that this use of the word *integrate* has no relation to what I describe as integrationism. Rather, it reflects the eclectic mixing of the biopsychosocial model. I, for one, am a psychiatrist who does not want to integrate biological and psychological approaches in a manner such as that proposed by the biopsychosocial model. A pluralist would have to be opposed to this assumption. Clearly, then, pluralism is not simply the easy task of accepting the common assumption above that "almost all" psychiatrists make.

Gabbard and Kay then note that some data suggest that most patients receive psychotherapy along with medication treatment and that combined treatment is thus the standard of care in psychiatry. However, increasingly, this treatment has evolved from the previous paradigm of being provided by one psychiatrist to the current paradigm of being divided between two or more clinicians, usually a psychiatrist (or general practitioner or nurse practitioner) for pharmacology and a psychologist or social worker for psychotherapy. They approvingly quote the work of the anthropologist Tanya Luhrman about how managed care has worsened the polarity between biological and psychological approaches in psychiatry: "These approaches are presented in different lectures, taught by different teachers, associated with different patients, learned in different settings. The new policies have sharply enhanced that separation and severely truncated the psychotherapeutic side" (1956). Gabbard and Kay then state their thesis, which they oppose to biological reductionism: "In this communication, we wish to emphasize that combined treatment in many respects is the essence of psychiatric practice and the most obvious exemplar of the biopsychosocial foundation on which treatment decisions are ideally based" (1957).

I will argue below that combined treatment is the essence of an eclectic approach to psychiatry, but if one gives up on eclecticism and replaces it with pluralism, then a separate treater approach becomes more central to psychiatry. But first, let me point out a few issues on which I agree with Gabbard and Kay as they proceed in their line of argument. They describe studies, especially in depression, where combined treatment with medication and psychotherapy was more effective than medication alone. They then appear poised to draw the classic mistaken eclectic conclusion: Therefore, combined treatment with medication and psychotherapy is the preferred treatment in psychiatry. The problem with this conclusion is that it generalizes from specific research studies for specific conditions, like depression, *to the entire field of psychiatry.* This would be like saying since treatment X works for urinary tract infections, it should be used for all infectious diseases. This is obviously an egregious logical error of generalization, yet it is amazing how frequently I hear proponents of the biopsychosocial model make it. To their credit, Gabbard and Kay do not fall into this common mistake. They state that these studies are specific to specific conditions, such as depression, and even in those conditions can be limited to only certain subgroups (more severely ill depressed patients appear to benefit from combined therapy more than mildly ill depressed patients). Gabbard and Kay also make the same point I made in chapter 22 regarding the utility of psychotherapeutic techniques in psychopharmacologic practice: "Psychotherapeutic principles should optimally be employed in every interaction with the patient, including the 15 minute medication management format. Successful treatment depends on a solid therapeutic alliance, and psychotherapy techniques enhance the formation of that alliance" (1958). I could not agree more, as I suggested in chapter 16 in my comments on the therapeutic alliance as a mood stabilizer for bipolar disorder. I would go further and argue that good psychopharmacology, which must include use of psychotherapeutic techniques, cannot be conducted during fifteen-minute "med checks." A minimum of twenty minutes, and preferably thirty minutes, is required for a beneficial psychopharmacology visit. Gabbard and Kay go on to emphasize the importance of medication compliance (or "adherence"), which they relate to the importance of psychotherapeutic methods in psychopharmacology. Again, I agree.

But these practical points do not argue for the necessity of formal psychotherapy and psychopharmacology treatment, either by one person or two. They do argue for the need for psychopharmacology that is not simply "med checks," that is, a psychopharmacology that is informed by psychotherapeutic methods.

Where Gabbard and Kay make their strongest claim is also where they make their mistake. They proceed to claim that the presence of separate treaters for one patient reflects Cartesian dualism and that combined treatment reflects mind-brain identity:

> Beyond issues of cost-effectiveness, however, there is a conceptual price to pay for dividing treatment between a psychiatrist-prescriber and a nonpsychiatrist psychotherapist. Such an arrangement often has the symbolic meaning to all parties of a tacit endorsement of Cartesian dualism that potentially fragments the patient into a "brain" and a "mind." By contrast, the one-person treatment model implicitly endorses an integration of mind and brain in both the psychiatrist's and the patient's perspective. The dichotomization of mind and brain has long been associated with a view in psychiatry that psychotherapy is a treatment for "psychologically-based" disorders, while "brain-based" disorders should be treated with medication. What we commonly refer to as "mind" can be understood as the activity of the brain. Psychotherapy must work by its impact on the brain. Kandel has elaborated on how these processes might work at the synaptic and intracellular levels. . . .

To say that mind is dependent on brain, of course, is not to say that mental states are easily reducible to neural states. As contemporary mind/brain philosophers have stressed, the irreducible subjectivity of consciousness defies description in nonmental terms. . . . Hence the language of psychology and the language of biology involve two different levels of discourse when working with a patient. The biopsychosocial psychiatrist must be conceptually bilingual.

The one-person treatment model demands that the psychiatrist must think both in terms of a dysfunctional brain and a psychologically distressed human being. . . . While this balancing act is challenging, it is also the essence of good medical and psychiatric practice and epitomizes Engel's biopsychosocial model. The psychiatrist, like any other good physician, treats the whole person.

Many psychiatrists find this integration daunting. It is easy to scapegoat managed care policy as the sole culprit responsible for the demise of integrated treatment. However, biological reductionism may appeal to all of us when immersing ourselves in human suffering is too much to bear. (2001, 1959)

In this section, Gabbard and Kay make their major philosophical claim, the limitations of which readers of previous chapters will recognize.[2] It is worthwhile teasing apart these claims one by one. First, they wrap themselves in the cloak of Kandel's integrationism, rejecting dualism. This is something of a feat, since the psychoanalytic tradition, as it has developed, has tended to be quite dualistic. As Kandel made quite clear in his paper and the subsequent follow-up article, his psychoanalytic colleagues were completely uninterested in the brain. Not only did the analysts treat the brain like a black box; they also denigrated research in neuroscience. For psychoanalysis, the psychological realm was more than enough. Nothing could be more dualistic. Now Gabbard and Kay seek to defend psychotherapy, especially the psychoanalytic version, from an antidualistic stance. This is quite a change, and the fact that it is happening may suggest a welcome recognition on the part of psychotherapeutically oriented psychiatrists of the importance of the biological approach.

Gabbard and Kay essentially then defend psychotherapy using the language of emergence, the mind being dependent on the brain but mental phenomena not being identical to brain phenomena. With this I can only agree. I would go even further, though: the clinician needs to be multilingual, not just bilingual. This is where Gabbard and Kay's lack of pluralism is evident. By clinging to the biopsychosocial model as they interpret it, they divide psychiatry up into two approaches, biological and psychosocial. But that is at best a minimal

division. There are more, along Jaspers's epistemological lines (causal explanation and meaningful understanding), or Havens's methodological schools
(objective-descriptive, existential, interpersonal, and psychoanalytic), or
McHugh and Slavney's perspectives (disease, dimension, behavior, life story).
Clinicians would do well to be familiar with most if not all of these approaches
to the mind. We can all agree that unilingualism (dogmatism) is misplaced.
Gabbard and Kay's version of bilingualism is little better, though. The pluralism of psychiatry requires us all to be multilingual. And this multiplicity of approaches cannot be easily translated into the superiority of psychotherapy and
medication provided by a single clinician.

Indeed, what this pluralism asks of clinicians is much more daunting than
the bilingualism of Gabbard and Kay. It is harder to be a biopsychosocial psychiatrist, as Gabbard and Kay rightly assert, than to be a dogmatist (they focus
on biological reductionism while downplaying the equally deplorable effects
of psychoanalytic reductionism). It is harder still to be a pluralist. Pluralism is
the toughest of all approaches to psychiatry. It asks much of us and gives little
in return. But what it gives is gold compared to the dross of biopsychosocial
eclecticism.

4.

Let me clearly state that by rejecting the biopsychosocial model, I am not
thereby turning to a biological reductionist approach. I am seeking an even
more rigorous openness, a pluralism that asks us to give up on the eclectic me-
anderings of the past. Pluralism argues for an even closer cooperation of psychiatrists, psychologists, and social workers. It does so despite arguing against
dearly held shibboleths. But my social-work and psychology colleagues should
know that they have better friends among pluralists than among eclectics.

This is because there is a subtle but important medical bias to the biopsychosocial claims of some psychoanalytically oriented psychiatrists. For instance, in summarizing the limits of the two-treater approach, Gabbard and
Kay conclude: "Finally, the psychiatrist is often assumed to have overall primary responsibility for the patient and all treatment decisions, even though a
poorly trained professional providing psychotherapy may have made a major
decision about the patient's treatment without consulting the psychiatrist"
(2001, 1960).

Nonpsychiatrists will rightfully wince at this statement. The underlying assumption of the biopsychosocial psychiatrists' approach is that nonpsychiatrists often provide shabby psychotherapy. They argue that for many reasons (knowledge of biology, medical experience, frequency of contact, transference, therapeutic alliance) the psychiatrist can provide the best overall treatment for a patient (namely, psychotherapy plus medication). They conclude that the psychotherapy provided in this setting is better than psychotherapy provided by a second non-M.D. treater (psychologist or social worker). One cannot ignore the economic aspects of this debate. The economic livelihood of psychotherapists who are psychiatrists depends on having a rationale for doing psychotherapy. The one-treater biopsychosocial psychiatry argument provides this rationale. The biopsychosocial model is, for these psychiatrists, a convenient justification for what they do.

In arguing for pluralism, I am asking all clinicians, whether psychiatrists or social workers or psychologists, to forget about trying to justify what they do. I am asking them to think about why they do what they do. If they agree that pluralism is the best alternative, I am asking them to alter what they do consistent with what a pluralist approach would suggest.

What does this mean in practice?

First, there is absolutely no general reason why one treater would be better than two, three, or four. There is absolutely no general reason why a psychiatrist would provide better psychotherapy treatment than a psychologist or social worker. For that matter, there is no reason to assume that a psychiatrist would provide better psychopharmacology treatment than a highly skilled and experienced nurse practitioner. It all comes down to knowledge, experience, and conceptual clarity.

The best treatment is provided by the most expert treater. On the whole, no single clinician can be extremely expert at more than one approach or method in psychiatry. Since there are many methods (Havens's schools, McHugh and Slavney's perspectives, psychopharmacology of specific conditions, psychotherapeutic approaches), there are many experts. The specific combination of treatment depends on the patient and the condition. A patient with bipolar disorder, for instance, would benefit the most from a highly expert psychopharmacologist who specializes in bipolar disorder. A good general psychopharmacologist would not be optimal. Someone who specializes in bipolar disorder is preferable. That patient may also benefit from a highly expert psychotherapist. This person might be a social worker, or a psychologist, or a psychiatrist. He or she might practice cognitive behavioral psychotherapy, or family therapy, or interpersonal therapy, or psychoeducational therapy, but the psychotherapist ideally should be expert at the specific therapy that is being provided. And that therapy should have empirical evidence of being effective in bipolar disorder. That patient may also benefit from vocational rehabilitation with a specialist in that field, or occupational therapy from a specialist in that field, or substance abuse therapy with a specialist in that field. There is just no way that one person would do an excellent job. One person might do an adequate job, or perhaps a poor job. But the best outcome will arise from multiple treaters, each of whom is expert in what she or he does.

Now this does not mean that we should all become closed-minded specialists. I specialize in psychopharmacology of bipolar disorder, for instance, but I think I am an able psychopharmacologist for unipolar depression, most anxiety disorders, and most psychotic disorders. However, as a pluralist, I will admit that I am not as good a psychopharmacologist for schizophrenia as a colleague who is expert in that area. Similarly, I have some experience and background in existential psychotherapy, but almost none in cognitive-behaviorally oriented psychotherapy. Thus, although I will treat a patient with psychotherapy in certain conditions, I will carefully select that circumstance where I think the patient would benefit from my particular skills. I frequently refer patients either to other psychopharmacologists who specialize in other relevant conditions that I think the patient has or might have and to other psychotherapists (mostly social workers and master's level colleagues) who are highly experienced in specific methods or conditions that I or the patient, or both, think might be useful. For instance, one of my colleagues is a man with a master's degree in counseling (who also has bipolar disorder). He has a great deal to offer patients with bipolar disorder in terms of existential and supportive psychotherapy. Furthermore, it is very important for psychotherapists to be highly familiar with bipolar disorder if they are to treat these patients. It is important to be able to distinguish symptoms of mood episodes from emotions unrelated to mood episodes; it is relevant to be able to pick up on potential early signs of relapse, especially as weekly therapy allows more frequent contact than what occurs in monthly psychopharmacology sessions; and it is useful to understand the rationale for and be a partner in assessing the effects of medication changes. For all these reasons, I think my colleague is a much more expert psychotherapist for most of my patients with bipolar disorder than a psychoanalytically trained biopsychosocial psychiatrist who might have little experience with bipolar disorder.

5.

The pluralist must be exceedingly humble. For him there are no finished systems. There are no ideologies to which he can cling. He sees the mind as complex, yet he still seeks to be clear in his attempts to explain and understand it. He cannot claim to know anything for certain. Yet he must reject all relativism. He is the eternal skeptic, yet he is also always open to belief. Belief for him is not an ideology, though; it is faith in James's definition: the need to make choices because the decisions are momentous, even in the absence of sufficient evidence. Which takes us back to the need for humility.

These questions for the clinician will determine whether he or she can be a pluralist and, for the mental health professions, will determine whether we are to progress beyond the stalemate of dogmatism and eclecticism:

— Can you accept the absence of a single overarching theory in psychiatry, yet also reject relativism and eclecticism?

— Despite the absence of a single theory, can you accept the need to be conceptually clear about what we do?

— Do you recognize that in certain conditions and certain circumstances, a single method is more appropriate than any other?

— Do you recognize the strengths and limitations of the many methods of psychiatry?

— Do you accept that each method has its role?

— Do you accept your own limitations in terms of what your skills can be? Can you accept the strengths of others in terms of what their skills are? Will you fit the treatment to the individual condition and the individual patient's circumstances?

— Can you do all this while never being completely certain?

We are far from being pluralists in psychiatry today.

Afterword

It is in the nature of our subject that every thoughtful psychiatrist can
choose only between having his philosophic standpoint explicit or leaving it implicit; a philosophic standpoint of some sort he must have.
—AUBREY LEWIS, 1967

Psychiatry rests on philosophical questions and assumptions.

The main purpose of this book has been to raise questions and discuss concepts, rather than to provide answers. No single theoretical framework has
been suggested that will satisfy those who seek a single ideology. Philosophers
may find this a weakness, but it is only so if one accepts that such is the purpose of philosophy: system-building. That is not a purpose I accept.

I have tried to do something along the lines of Socrates' tradition: I have
sought to clarify the concepts of psychiatry by asking questions, by providing
insights, by using ideas from different sources. In so doing, I have applied ideas
from Karl Jaspers, Freud, existentialists, and others.

I have sought to show that research and practice in psychiatry rely on certain concepts—hidden, confused, and vague as they may be. And the discussion of concepts is what philosophy is all about. Those who might deny having any conceptual assumptions suffer from a myopia of not recognizing that
they too have philosophical ideas, which they impose on their psychiatric research or practice without realizing it. The purpose of this book has been to
make the discussion of these philosophies overt, to bring them to the surface,
follow their outlines, and delineate their implications. For psychiatrists, this
should help us to choose and apply our philosophies in psychiatry more ra-
tionally. For patients and the lay public, this book hopefully provides an ex-
plication of what psychiatry is all about and helps demystify the field.

Psychiatry, as a field of theory and practice, is committed to certain views
regarding what there is (mind-brain theories), how we know about psychiatric
realities (epistemology), and what we value (ethics). Which view one espouses
on these matters has important practical consequences.

The purpose of this type of investigation is to promote conceptual clarity
about one's assumptions and values. This in turn leads us to the general

theoretical framework of pluralism, which entails open-mindedness toward diverse ideas, flexibility in using different methods in psychiatry, and a commitment to finding and applying the best method for a specific circumstance. Emil Kraepelin wrote in 1917, when surveying the previous one hundred years of psychiatric practice: "Our satisfaction over the progress already made is tinged with regret. . . . We must openly admit that the vast majority of the patients placed in our institutions are according to what we know forever lost, that even the best of care can never restore them to perfect health. . . . Even under the most favorable conditions, the fruits of scientific labor generally ripen very slowly, and in our field, quick, dazzling results are unthinkable" ([1917] 1962, 152, 154). As the end of a second hundred years of psychiatric research and practice approaches, I think it is not implausible to have expected more progress than we have achieved, given the tireless work of so many brilliant psychiatric clinicians and researchers. Yet, much progress was stymied by fruitless conflict and inflexible beliefs. If psychiatric theory and practice can achieve and sustain a pluralistic, pragmatic attitude, the profession might be able to better serve the purposes of scientific progress and its ultimate goal of healing those suffering from these all-too-human afflictions.

Notes

ONE: The Status Quo

1. Emil Kraepelin is not anywhere nearly as famous as Freud among nonpsychiatrists. Even in psychiatry, at least in the United States, he was, until the 1970s, considered a dusty old German ideologue whose views were hopelessly old-fashioned. Kraepelin was largely ignored because Freud was so popular, and because Freud's methods and theories were so different. In American psychiatry, the influence of Adolf Meyer also led to a downgrading of Kraepelin's ideas, since Meyer was more interested in psychosocial factors related to behavioral problems than in a strictly medical approach to psychiatric diagnosis as exemplified by Kraepelin. The 1970s saw a rebirth of a consciously neo-Kraepelinian school in psychiatry, which led to DSM-III and the radical restructuring of psychiatric nosology. Today, references to Kraepelin are quite frequent in psychiatric articles in the standard nonpsychoanalytic journals, whereas those to Freud are few and far between. This does not mean that history has passed its judgment on these two fathers of psychiatry; the seesaw between the two men seems to go on indefinitely.

2. One might include Thomas Szasz (1970) and some other scholars in this school of thought. One of the limitations of individuals such as Szasz and Laing is that they appear to take a dogmatic approach to psychiatry. The existential approach is but one approach to psychiatry, with many limitations as well as some strengths. (According to one of my themes in this book, the same is true of any single approach.) Because in many persons, life situations can be misinterpreted as mental illness, Szasz and Laing conclude that in no instance is any psychological symptom reflective of a mental illness. This is simply a type of extremism that differs in no way, in terms of form, from the strictest psychoanalytic orthodoxy or from blind biological reductionism. Reality is much more complex, the wishes of true believers to the contrary notwithstanding.

3. Obviously the content of the works of these individuals differs, but they all share the method of applying interpersonal and social methods to psychiatry. Havens focuses most on the contributions of Sullivan.

4. My colleague David Brendel has emphasized this point to me.

5. Kandel was co-awarded the prize along with Arvid Carlsson and Paul Greengard, but of the three, Kandel was the only one with an M.D. who had trained in a clinical psychiatry residency program.

6. Paul Roazen has pointed out to me that this retrospective criticism of Wagner-Jaurregg may not do justice to his skills and dedication. He apparently was a careful, dedicated clinician and researcher of high caliber.

7. I am indebted here to the work of Jillian Craigie and Ian Gold (2002), presented at a recent conference. They describe the concept of *fractionation,* the attempt to break

down cognitive properties to simple terms and then to link these simple cognitive terms to complex neural terms. Their idea is that each level of description explains the level above it, owing to shared properties. There is an isomorphism, in that one thing is explained in two different languages. Although, in the presentation I attended, Craigie did not make the direct link to the type of integrationism espoused by Kandel, I think a link could indeed be made. Another well-known effort along similar lines, more indebted to evolutionary theory, is that of Gerald Edelman (1988).

TWO: What There Is

1. Jackson's example of Mary the color scientist is the classic thought experiment used to illustrate the problem of qualia.

2. The pain thought experiment is an old one, well described by Flanagan. This text is, in my opinion, the most comprehensive and comprehensible summary of modern philosophy of mind.

3. Dennett's views are best laid out in *Consciousness Explained*. His recent work (1995) has expanded into attempting to find a basis in evolutionary theory for his views.

4. Aviel Goodman (1991) has tried to bring some of the philosophical concepts of emergence into psychiatry, while linking them to the *Erklaren-Verstehen* distinction. Goodman links the emergence concept to mind-body dualism and to the biopsychosocial theory of Engel. Although this is not illogical, emergence does not need to be linked only with the biopsychosocial theory.

5. Cobb was a unique figure in modern psychiatry. He was fully trained in neurology and neuropathology, and he also completed his psychiatry residency with Adolf Meyer at Johns Hopkins during World War I. He ran the neurology service at Harvard's Boston City Hospital for about a decade in the 1920s until moving to found the first psychiatry department at Massachusetts General Hospital in 1934. He ran that service until his retirement in 1955, and he remained a spiritual advisor to trainees and faculty there until his death in 1967. Cobb was essentially a Meyerian and roughly eclectic in his overall view of psychiatry. He continued to use Meyerian life charts to understand psychiatric cases throughout his career. However, he was also sensitive to the limitations of dogmatism and the need for a pluralism similar to that defined in this book. For instance, when offering his perspective on psychiatric nosology, in a passage in which he suggests four basic categories, he writes: "There is nothing magic about four; five, ten, or twenty may be more true. I only insist on being pluralistic and practical" (Cobb 1943, 21). In the 1940s and onward, as the psychoanalytic trend began to take hold in the United States, Cobb, who had been one of the first to welcome psychoanalysis as another perspective on psychiatry, appears to have become somewhat disenchanted with it as the resurgence of another form of dogmatism. Ultimately, I think, he was a psychiatric William James, tolerant and open-minded above all, but lacking, somewhat like James, the ability to provide a conceptual framework for his pluralism. Peirce and Jaspers serve as important figures precisely because they are more conceptually rigorous.

6. See Goodman 1991 and Cobb 1943. A good philosophical source is Kim 1993.

7. These ideas are based on the writings of Paul Churchland (1988, 1989) and Patricia Churchland (1986), who have become known for holding a view called *eliminative materialism*. This theory states that beliefs, such as folk psychological concepts, are eliminated with time as scientific empirical knowledge regarding them increases.

8. No doubt Penfield was God's gift to neurosurgery. It is somewhat striking, as my father (also a neurosurgeon) always pointed out to me, that this gifted neurosurgeon ended his autobiography by asserting a dualist commitment to the existence of a divine reality beyond the natural world. His ground-breaking work argues much more strongly for a more materialistic interpretation of human spirituality. The great British neurologist Sir Charles Symonds (1970) took a materialistic view of the matter.

9. Since Goodman's 1991 paper, the *American Journal of Psychiatry* did not publish a special article on philosophy of mind until a recent wonderful contribution by Kenneth Kendler (2001).

10. I cannot emphasize enough how one chapter cannot do sufficient justice to the labyrinthine world of philosophy of mind. This chapter is by no means complete or particularly original, nor is it meant to be an original contribution to philosophy of mind. Since this book is not primarily about philosophy, but rather about concepts in psychiatry, I can only discuss the topic of philosophy of mind in such a way as to bring up the relevant issues for psychiatry and suggest some connections to topics that would be helpful to those philosophers interested in psychiatry. I understand all too well that philosophers will find this material limited, but I really intend this chapter to be more of an introduction to these topics for nonphilosophers, hopefully providing an impetus for intensive examination of these issues in primary sources and the larger philosophical literature.

THREE: How We Know

1. Much of the following discussion attempts to offer a general understanding of Jaspers's philosophy, which is best summarized in this collection of his works, with annotations by academic experts in his philosophy.

2. If someone could choose only one text of psychiatry to best understand the field, this would be it, even almost a century after it was first written.

3. Apparently, a chronic lung disease (L. Ehrlich, personal communication, 2001).

FOUR: What Is Scientific Method?

1. James's essential insights have been taken up by the statistical discipline of decision analysis (Hunink et al. 2001). James would likely be proud that this approach is taken so seriously, but at the same time he might cringe at its being made a science, with numbers to multiple decimal places identifying the probable outcomes of forced momentous decisions.

FIVE: Reading Karl Jaspers's *General Psychopathology*

1. Except as noted, all quotations from Jaspers's *GP* are from the recent Hopkins edition ([1913] 1997), with page numbers provided in the text.

2. Shepherd was an unusual figure in psychiatry. In the late 1960s, he was quite skeptical about the evidence regarding the efficacy of lithium in manic-depressive illness; it proved to be effective despite Shepherd's skepticism. Later, Shepherd (1995) turned on the rehabilitated figure of Emil Kraepelin, accusing Kraepelin of Nazi sympathies. Jaspers appears to be one of the few figures toward whom Shepherd was sympathetic.

SIX: **What Is Scientific Method in Psychiatry?**

1. A view in the tradition of Jaspers has been espoused by these authors, who argue that there is a science of meaning that is, on the one hand, science and, on the other, deals with meanings rather than simple empirical facts.

2. I am greatly indebted to these verbal and written contributions of Professor Ehrlich in response to an earlier presentation of some of these ideas that I gave to the Karl Jaspers Society.

3. Jaspers expanded his discussion of philosophy of science in future works, which have been expertly interpreted by Professor George Pepper (1988).

SEVEN: **Darwin's Dangerous Method**

1. Dennett deserves a great deal of credit for putting Darwin back on the intellectual map in a thorough, engaging, broad-ranging manner in his recent book. Dennett's specific description of Darwin's dangerous idea is the concept that "the fruits of evolution can be explained as the products of an algorithmic process" (1995, 60). By this he means that Darwin's theory of natural selection explains evolution using chance, mindless variations, thus removing the influence of a Creator or of some special spiritual realm on biological existence. This approach can be expanded to philosophy, psychology, and other fields, argues Dennett, with great explanatory power and providing a basically materialist explanation for many matters on which we are often inclined to take religious, spiritual, or nonmaterialistic perspectives. I would tend to agree with him that Darwinian ideas are quite useful, though I focus on Darwin's anti-essentialist method, rather than his algorithmic method. The two are not exclusive of each other, and Dennett does take the approach I support throughout this book of focusing on methods used rather than on the content of theories.

2. Ernst Mayr (1991) emphasizes this point.

3. I refer here to Charles Sanders Peirce, William James, Chauncey Wright, and, later, John Dewey. Louis Menand fleshes out this intellectual history in his recent book (2001).

4. The critiques of these figures in no sense argue for the unreality of mental illness, just as Marx's critique of capitalism does not prove the value of communism. These critics recognize the chinks in the armor of simplistic essentialism and positivism as applied to psychiatry. This calls for more sophisticated perspectives on scientific method and psychiatry, which is part of the goal of this book.

EIGHT: **What We Value**

1. The source for this famous reference is unclear. In asking various Freud scholars, I have heard that it may derive from Sandor Ferenczi, to whom Freud mentioned it in a conversation. At the very least, it appears that Freud has not left us a carefully thought-out written discussion about the relationship of psychoanalysis to ethics.

2. The following discussion represents a brief summary of standard modern moral philosophy. Two good general sources have been written by Norman (1983) and Thomas (1993), and a good reference is Singer's text (1993).

3. Franklin's autobiography remains a treasure trove of moral philosophy and psy-

chotherapeutic thinking mingled together. If read from this perspective, I think it has great relevance to psychiatry. Another wonderful source is Rogers's recent collection (1990).

4. Psychiatrists would also profit from some familiarity with MacIntyre's work. I once heard him give a lecture at the Harvard Divinity School, in which he was asked what aspects of a person's upbringing best inculcated virtue. He replied that one's profession was quite important, since one spends so much time in training and working in one's occupation. Specifically, he felt that some professions, like medicine, promoted the acquisition of virtues, while others, like law (at least in the United States), generally impeded this process. I have been struck by how little thought physicians in general, and psychiatrists in particular, give to this line of thinking.

5. The work by Havens that most clearly addresses these issues is *Coming to Life* (1993). Jaspers discusses these matters in the psychotherapy sections of the *General Psychopathology* ([1913] 1997, 790–822).

NINE: Desire and Self

1. This discussion is greatly indebted to the work of Martha Nussbaum (1994) and largely rests on her sources and interpretations.

2. This adaptation is taken from the wonderful work of the American poet Coleman Barks. The original parable does not translate smoothly into English. Barks has adapted it somewhat so that it is much more effective in English, while capturing all important details of the text and the underlying meaning. The story did not originate with Rumi but had also been told by earlier poets such as Sanai and Ghazali, though with some minor differences, for example that the wise men might be blind rather than in a dark room. Ghazali, who was an important medieval Islamic philosopher, even drew rather straightforwardly pluralistic conclusions from the story: "Every one of these persons spoke the truth in a way, since he described the qualities of the elephant so far as his knowledge of it reached; yet the whole party failed to comprehend the real form of the elephant. Now consider this parable carefully, for it illustrates the nature of our controversies" (Nicholson 1989, 34). The controversies to which Ghazali refers are the religious and philosophical conflicts between the rationalist/empiricist philosophers in the Islamic world, as described in the text of this chapter, and mystically oriented Sufi thinkers as well as orthodox religious leaders. Unfortunately, Ghazali did not follow up his pluralistic interpretation of this parable with an open-minded tolerance of the opposition, but rather joined in the attack on and ultimate extermination of the rationalist/empiricist school.

3. I have modified this section and translated it from the original Persian.

4. A good source that reviews this material is Nasr 1976.

5. Dr. Hairi Yazdi, who was a friend to my family, was a Renaissance man hidden in a modern theological state. He can justly claim to be one of certainly not more than a handful of individuals who have received formal training in Shiite Islamic theology in Iranian religious seminaries as well as formal Ph.D. training in philosophy at Western universities. For some time, he served on the faculty of Georgetown University, where, as a child, I had the privilege of meeting him. His father was also a revered Ayatollah. In later years, Hairi taught theology in Iran and published this work. He died a few years ago.

6. To me this is an amazing example of Plato's dictum that all knowledge is remembrance.

7. Readers may be justifiably confused about the similarities and differences between Sufism and illuminationism. There is some overlap, in that some writers are identified with both approaches in different aspects of their writings. Rumi is an excellent example, since he writes frequently on Sufi themes, as discussed above, but he also frequently refers to illuminationist themes about divine light. In Arabic, there is a distinction between Sufism and Irfan that parallels the distinctions I am making here between Sufism and illuminationism. Sufism is an approach to the practice of life; it does not intend to be a philosophy in the academic sense or to compete with rational or empiricist theories. Irfan is an attempt to engage with rational and empiricist philosophies, essentially defending the Sufi position, but attempting to do so to some extent by rational or even potentially empiricist means. In some way, then, one might see Irfan as a mediation between Sufism and rational-empiricist philosophies. This may be what Hairi meant by defining Irfan as the "linguistic methodology of introspective knowledge." Some, like Hussein Nasr (1976), use the word *gnosis* to denote Irfan, as opposed to *mysticism* to denote Sufism. This distinction in English is close to capturing the Arabic meaning, if gnosis is viewed as a means of trying to explain mysticism in nonmystical terms.

8. Hairi represented such a figure.

TEN: On the Nature of Mental Illness

1. All quotations by Lewis in this chapter are from this source. The original article was titled "Health as a Social Concept."

2. It is important to recognize the differences that exist between mental and physical action failures. In most cases, physical action failures are recognized by the patient, who suffers or experiences pain (thus the root of the word *disease*). Yet in many mental action failures, the problem is not apparent to the person who is failing in his activities, but rather to others (the vexing problem of insight, discussed in chapter 17).

ELEVEN: Order out of Chaos?

1. It is notable that in this book, Menninger's prime text on psychiatry, Menninger felt that Kraepelin only merited comment in an appendix.

2. Gerald Klerman was perhaps the main intellectual source behind the changes in American nosology with DSM-III. In practice, I believe he was a pluralist, and in some of his historical writings he describes schools of psychiatry in a manner similar to Havens's. His work was much more empirical and clinical than that of Havens or McHugh and Slavney, but I conceive Klerman's work to have been conducted with a similar pluralistic mind-set. As an active researcher and political leader in psychiatry, Klerman had a great deal of real influence, for the better, toward a pluralistic psychiatry. However, he and his disciples did not sufficiently express and explain the conceptual rationale for this approach (Hirschfeld 1994).

3. All quotations from this debate in this chapter derive from this source. Subsequent quotations are identified by page number.

4. Full disclosure requires that I inform the reader that Kendler and Eaves were my first teachers in psychiatric research. They introduced me to the wonders and potential of psychiatric research, and I have ever since been thankful for the luck of being exposed to them so early in my medical career.

5. John Sadler (personal communication, 2002), also has suggested a similar analogy, with DSM-IV compared to a gardener's terminology for flowers and plants, as opposed to the nomenclature of botany, which is more detailed and more useful for scientific purposes, though less useful for the practical needs of gardeners. This analogy is not meant, I wish to emphasize, to degrade the utility of DSM-IV, conceived as a folk nosology, but rather, in a pluralistic spirit, to highlight its strengths and weaknesses.

TWELVE: A Theory of DSM-IV

1. A good source, especially for German sources on ideal types, is Pepper 1963. Much has been written about the ideal-type concept, and many other sources exist. Original work by Weber includes Weber 1949 and 1993. Jaspers discusses ideal types in the *General Psychopathology* ([1913] 1997, 1:434–35).

2. A closer study of Dilthey is indispensable to these topics. Unfortunately, his original works, like those of his compatriot Hegel, are dense and difficult. A very useful reading companion is Makkreel 1992. Dilthey, like Hegel, is one of those thinkers who must be read slowly over a long period of time with the careful assistance of knowledgeable commentators. A great deal in Jaspers's work, as well as that of Weber, stands or falls with the epistemological validity of Dilthey's *Erklaren-Verstehen* distinction.

3. Some have suggested that this work should be seen as the twentieth century's answer to Marx's *Capital*. Together, the two works provide a comprehensive view of human history and sociology. For psychiatry, they supply sources for many of the assumptions that clinicians and researchers bring into our field.

4. Like so many ideas in psychiatry, this view that ideal types are central to psychiatric diagnosis was first expressed by Karl Jaspers in *General Psychopathology*. More recently, Wiggins and Schwartz (1991) reminded the field of the relevance of this perspective. Working in experimental psychology, apparently unaware of Jaspers's views, other researchers have produced theories that border on the ideal-type concept, such as the view that diagnosis often proceeds by analogy to "prototypes" of certain illnesses, rather than by specific enumeration and elicitation of signs and symptoms (Rosch and Mervis 1975; Zachar 2001). I am not justifying this prototype or ideal-type approach as clinically accurate. I think clinicians do practice this way but that conscious probing of signs and symptoms is also required to counteract the subjective biases of clinicians.

THIRTEEN: Dimensions versus Categories

1. In the following comments, I am greatly indebted to the groundbreaking work of Frederick Goodwin on this topic (Goodwin and Jamison 1990), as well as the recent research of Ross Baldessarini (2002).

2. Hagop Akiskal clearly deserves priority for arguing for over two decades now for a broad definition of the bipolar spectrum.

3. I borrow the term *Cade's disease* from Terrence Ketter (personal communication, 2002).

4. It is striking how many psychiatrists, like many scientists in general, profess a Popperian view of science but practice according to the Peircean paradigm. In fact, Popper's perspective has gained an intellectual dominance that is somewhat surprising (see chapter 4).

5. An excellent source on Bernard is Olmsted and Olmsted 1961. The development of diagnostic theory and pathology in medicine is relatively well-known (Porter 1997). The beginning of this trend in modern medicine is generally attributed to Thomas Sydenham (Sydenham and Dewhurst 1966).

6. This article was a seminal point in the evolution of psychiatric nosology toward the DSM-III culmination. This basic approach of having multiple sources for nosological validation (in the absence of a gold standard) is very similar to the general concept of pluralist psychiatry derived from Jaspers. Epidemiological circles have generally accepted this methodology, though I have not noticed much in the way of conceptual writings in psychiatric epidemiology in its justification. Perhaps the best overall source is Goodwin and Guze 1989, which is probably the single best summary of modern psychiatric nosology, ascetically conducted in the framework of the neo-Kraepelinian school.

7. The history of the concept of borderline personality is long and tortuous. A succinct, readable clinical text on the topic was written by John Gunderson (1984). The two classic psychoanalytic approaches are found in texts by Otto Kernberg (1975, 1976) and Heinz Kohut (1971).

8. I cannot do justice to the large field of personality disorders here. I am trying to briefly summarize some potential interpretations of this field so as to situate my comments in the larger discussion regarding dimensional versus categorical nosology. No claim is made that my brief interpretation of personality disorders is comprehensive or that it is supported sufficiently with references.

FIFTEEN: The Slings and Arrows of Outrageous Fortune

1. Joshua Shenk (2003) has investigated Lincoln's melancholia in careful detail.

2. Paul Roazen (1969) has examined how Freud was driven to write this paper apparently in response to the work of one of his disciples, Viktor Tausk. Tausk, who had a recurrent mood illness (probably bipolar disorder, in my opinion), was one of the first in Freud's circle to be interested in applying Freudian ideas to major psychiatric conditions like depression and psychosis. Freud was driven, mostly against his inclinations, to comment on melancholia in response to Tausk's activities. Freud was quite ambivalent, though, as witnessed by the fact that he avoided further comment of significance in later years. Freud's testy relationship with Tausk, which led to the disciple's suicide, is a blemish in the psychoanalytic world that was covered up until Roazen's courageous rediscovery and publication of it.

3. The psychiatrist Hermann van Praag (1993b) has emphasized this issue in regard to controversies in psychiatric nosology.

SIXTEEN: Life's Roller Coaster

1. Goodwin and Jamison 1990, now a classic text, is undoubtedly the most comprehensive work on mania, where past theories are reviewed. A second edition is in press for 2004.

2. I borrow this concept from Ronald Pies (personal communication, 2002), and I modify it in existential terms.

SEVENTEEN: Being Self-Aware

1. This phenomenon is nicely discussed in its philosophical implications by Flanagan (1991).

EIGHTEEN: Psychopharmacology

1. Almost any 1960s book will do. One source that I think captures the temper of the times in unique detail is Solomon 1966.

2. Despite the fact that these writers, particularly Marcuse, have fallen out of favor, partly as a result of an intellectual backlash in the United States against 1960s-era theories, their relevance to contemporary society (minus, in the case of Marcuse, some remnants of Marxist ideology) seems as clear as ever, in my opinion.

3. I think the basic observation made by Peter Kramer relates to the effect of serotonin reuptake inhibitors (like Prozac) on personality, beyond their simple effects on depressive syndromes.

NINETEEN: Truth and Statistics

1. I review this topic in greater detail in my book *Polypharmacy in Psychiatry* (Ghaemi 2002). This quote got Holmes into a great deal of controversy with many of his colleagues, who felt it could too easily be transformed into an extreme attack on any pharmacology. The controversy even made it to the front page of the New York newspapers of his day.

2. Osler emphasized the need to move from a focus on treating symptoms to a focus on diagnosing diseases. He felt that once the pathology of disease states was understood well enough, prevention and treatment solutions would soon follow. This has largely been the course of scientific medicine in the twentieth century. See Ghaemi 2002.

3. This is a key issue, rarely understood in psychiatry. A good reference is a series of papers outlining the relevance of Bayesian methods to medical research and practice (Goodman 1999a, 1999b). These comments are equally applicable to psychiatry.

TWENTY: A Climate of Opinion

1. Undoubtedly, pro- and anti-Freudians will object to this list based on their own preferences. It may be notable that many of the aspects of psychoanalytic thought, such as countertransference and the defense mechanisms, were not ideas put forward by Freud himself but rather developments beyond Freud's own views, deriving from his followers in the "ego psychology" school of psychoanalysis, especially Anna Freud, and the somewhat less orthodox "object relations" school of thinking, especially Melanie Klein, D. W. Winnicott, and Otto Kernberg. When I use the word *Freudian*, I use it to mean the entire broad development of psychoanalysis, rather than Freud's own specific views, and I do this because I believe that the term has come to have this meaning in the general population and among nonspecialist academics.

2. Frankly, these issues have been more salient in nonpsychiatric academic and lay circles. They are much more commonly and heatedly discussed in the *New York Review*

of Books than in the *American Journal of Psychiatry*. Within psychiatry, it should be said, there has been a loud minority, which in the 1970s and 1980s exerted much more influence, that believes early childhood (usually sexual) trauma is the holy grail of the field. These individuals would likely view much of this book as completely off the mark, since I have not focused on this issue. The same group also views biological psychiatry as dangerously wrong and perhaps simply a politically sinister force. The vagaries of this type of extremism are exemplified by Pam and Ross 1995. This dogmatic approach to psychiatry is simply one more sect, no different from all the rest of the past century. If nothing else, a pluralistic approach, as promoted in this book, provides an exhaustive and, I hope, convincing answer to this smug sectarianism.

3. Paul Roazen (1995) provides the case histories that concretize Freud the clinician.

TWENTY-ONE: Being There

1. There are, according to my reading, no comprehensive accounts of existential psychiatry. Perhaps the single best source is May, Angel, and Ellenberger 1958. Another highly readable resource is found in the works of Leston Havens ([1973] 1987). Alfred Marguelis (1989) has also written an excellent modern clinical application. A fascinating source on Heidegger's attempt to teach his views to psychiatrists has been preserved by his student Medard Boss (1988). The single best source on Binswanger is Binswanger 1963a.

2. Heidegger's ideas are an important source for many views in modern philosophy and psychiatry, ranging from existentialism to postmodernism. These two sources are excellent and popular approaches to his complex work. Personally, I am quite put off by Heidegger's attachment to Nazism, and I feel that Jaspers's philosophical work includes most of what is also useful in Heidegger, without the relativistic, postmodernistic, and frankly totalitarian threads that run through much of Heidegger's work. Nonetheless, Binswanger's interpretation of Heidegger is creatively useful.

3. The concept of a priori mental structures derives from Kant (see chapter 3).

4. When an earlier version of this chapter was published in an academic journal, I heard from strong partisans of Szasz about how immensely correct he was in his views. It is indeed a major drawback for existential approaches in psychiatry (much like psychoanalytic views) that many of those interested in these methods become extremist true believers. It should be obvious to the reader who has made it to this note that the whole thrust of this book is to resist and refute such extremism.

TWENTY-FOUR: Why It Is Hard to Be Pluralist

1. Hans Eysenck (1954) identified the relevance of such personality traits to political ideology; thus communists and fascists are similar, despite opposite contents to their extremist ideologies. William James ([1890] 1950) probably first made the basic distinction between "tough-minded" and "tender-minded" dispositions, which James believed formed the basis for difference among philosophers' opinions. I think the same effects occur in differing beliefs about mental illness and psychiatry.

2. Scott Waterman brought the essential misunderstanding of mind-brain issues in this paper to my attention (personal communication, 2002).

References

Akiskal, H. S. 1996. The prevalent clinical spectrum of bipolar disorders: Beyond DSM-IV. *Journal of Clinical Psychopharmacology* 16 (suppl. 1): 4S–14S.

Ali ibn Abú Talib. 1984. *Nahjul Balagha: Peak of eloquence: Sermons, letters, and sayings of Imam Ali ibn Abu Talib.* New York: Tahrike Tarsile Quran.

Alloy, L. B., and L. Y. Abramson. 1988. Depressive realism: Four theoretical perspectives. In *Cognitive processes in depression,* ed. L. B. Alloy, 223–65. New York: Guilford Press.

Amador, X. F., D. H. Strauss, S. A. Yale, et al. 1991. Awareness of illness in schizophrenia. *Schizophrenia Bulletin* 17:113–32.

Ambrose, W. E. 1967. William T. Sherman: A personality profile. *American History Illustrated,* January 11, 5–11.

Andreasen, N. C., S. Paradiso, and D. S. O'Leary. 1998. "Cognitive dysmetria" as an integrative theory of schizophrenia: A dysfunction in cortical-subcortical-cerebellar circuitry? *Schizophrenia Bulletin* 24 (2): 203–18.

Angst, J. 1998. The emerging epidemiology of hypomania and bipolar II disorder. *Journal of Affective Disorders* 50:143–51.

Baer, L. 1996. Behavior therapy: Endogenous serotonin therapy? *Journal of Clinical Psychiatry (supplement)* 57 (suppl. 6): 33–35.

Baldessarini, R. J. 2000a. American biological psychiatry and psychopharmacology, 1944–1994. In *American psychiatry after World War II,* ed. R. W. Menninger and J. C. Nemiah, 371–412. Washington, DC: American Psychiatric Press.

———. 2000b. A plea for the integrity of the bipolar concept. *Bipolar Disorders* 2:3–7.

———. 2002. Historical evolution of Kraepelin's *Manic-Depressive Illness* concept. Paper presented at the Boston chapter of the Association for the Advancement of Philosophy and Psychiatry, June 6.

Binswanger, L. 1958a. The case of Ellen West. In *Existence,* ed. R. May, E. Angel, and H. Ellenberger, 237–364. New York: Simon & Schuster.

———. 1958b. Insanity as a life-historical phenomenon: The case of Ilse. In *Existence,* ed. R. May, E. Angel, and H. Ellenberger, 214–36. New York: Simon & Schuster.

———. 1963a. *Being-in-the-world.* New York: Basic Books.

———. 1963b. Heidegger's analytic of existence and its meaning for psychiatry. In *Being-in-the-world,* by L. Binswanger, 206–21. New York: Basic Books.

Bodkin, J. A., R. Klitzman, and H. G. Pope. 1995. Treatment orientation and associated characteristics of North American academic psychiatrists. *Journal of Nervous and Mental Disease* 183:729–35.

Boss, M. 1988. Martin Heidegger's Zollikon seminars. In *Heidegger and psychology,* vol. 16, ed. K. Hoeller, 7–21. Seattle: Review of Existential Psychiatry and Psychology.

Brown, E. S., A. J. Rush, and B. S. McEwen. 1999. Hippocampal remodeling and damage by corticosteroids: Implications for mood disorders. *Neuropsychopharmacology* 21 (4): 474–84.

Brown, T. M. 2000. The growth of George Engel's biopsychosocial model. *Free Associations,* www.human-nature.com/free-associations.

Churchland, P. 1986. *Neurophilosophy: Toward a unified science of the mind/brain.* Cambridge, MA: MIT Press.

Churchland, P. M. 1988. *Matter and consciousness.* Cambridge, MA: MIT Press.

———. 1989. *A neurocomputational perspective: The nature of mind and the structure of science.* Cambridge, MA: MIT Press.

Cloninger, C. R. 1999. A new conceptual paradigm from genetics and psychobiology for the science of mental health. *Australia and New Zealand Journal of Psychiatry* 33 (2): 174–86.

Cloninger, C. R., D. Svrakic, and T. Przybeck. 1993. A psychobiological model of temperament and character. *Archives of General Psychiatry* 50:975–90.

Cobb, S. 1943. *Borderlands of psychiatry.* Cambridge, MA: Harvard University Press.

Craigie, J., and I. Gold. 2002. *Unification in psychiatry.* Paper presented at the 14th annual meeting of the Association for the Advancement of Philosophy and Psychiatry, Philadelphia, May 18–19.

Crow, T. J. 1990. Nature of the genetic contribution to psychotic illness—a continuum viewpoint. *Acta Psychiatrica Scandinavica* 81:401–8.

———. 1998. From Kraepelin to Kretschmer leavened by Schneider: The transition from categories of psychosis to dimensions of variation intrinsic to homo sapiens. *Archives of General Psychiatry* 55:502–5.

Daniels, N. 1985. *Just Health Care.* Cambridge: Cambridge University Press.

Darwin, C. [1859] 1998. *The origin of species.* New York: Gramercy.

David, A. S. 1990. Insight and psychosis. *British Journal of Psychiatry* 156:798–808.

Dennett, D. 1991. *Consciousness Explained.* Boston: Little, Brown.

———. 1995. *Darwin's dangerous idea.* New York: Simon & Schuster.

Dreyfus, H. L. 1994. *Being-in-the-world: A commentary on Heidegger's* Being and Time. Cambridge, MA: MIT Press.

Eaves, L., J. Eysenck, and H. Martin. 1989. *Genes, culture, and personality: An empirical approach.* London: Academic Press.

Edelman, G. 1988. *Neural Darwinism: The theory of neuronal group selection.* New York: Basic Books.

Ehrlich, E., L. Ehrlich, and G. Pepper, eds. 1994. *Karl Jaspers: Basic philosophical writings.* Atlantic Highlands, NJ: Humanities Press.

Ehrlich, L. 1999. *Commentary on SN Ghaemi: Karl Jaspers and scientific method in psychiatry.* Paper presented at the annual meeting of the American Philosophical Association, Boston.

Einstein, A., and S. Freud. [1933] 1978. *Why war? The correspondence between Albert Einstein and Sigmund Freud.* Chicago: Chicago Institute for Psychoanalysis.

Engel, G. L. 1980. The clinical application of the biopsychosocial model. *American Journal of Psychiatry* 137:535–44.

Eysenck, H. J. 1953. *The structure of human personality.* London: Methuen.

———. 1954. *The psychology of politics.* New York: Praeger.

Farber, S., and R. Wilson, eds. 1961. *Man and civilization: Control of the mind.* New York: McGraw-Hill.

Flanagan, O. 1991. *The science of the mind.* Cambridge, MA: Bradford Press.

Flexner, J. T. 1974. *Washington: The indispensable man.* New York: Mentor Books.

Forrester, J. 1997. *Dispatches from the Freud wars: Psychoanalysis and its passions.* Cambridge, MA: Harvard University Press.

Foucault, M. 1994. *The birth of the clinic: An archaeology of medical perception.* New York: Vintage Books.

Franklin, B. 1996. *Autobiography.* New York: Dover Books.

Freud, S. [1910] 1963. Observations of "wild" psychoanalysis. In *Sigmund Freud: Therapy and technique,* ed. Philip Rieff, 89–96. New York: Collier.

———. 1917. *Mourning and melancholia.* London: Hogarth.

———. [1927] 1953–74. *The future of an illusion.* In *Standard edition of the complete psychological works,* vol. 21. London: Hogarth.

———. [1937] 1953–74. Analysis terminable and interminable. In *Standard edition of the complete psychological works,* vol. 16, pp. 59–99. London: Hogarth.

Fulford, K. W. M. 1989. *Moral theory and medical practice.* Cambridge: Cambridge University Press.

Gabbard, G., and J. Kay. 2001. The fate of integrated treatment: Whatever happened to the biopsychosocial psychiatrist? *American Journal of Psychiatry* 158:1956–63.

Galbraith, J. K. 1958. *The affluent society.* Boston: Houghton Mifflin.

———. 1973. *Economics and the public purpose.* New York: New American Library.

Gelven, M. 1989. *A commentary on Heidegger's Being and Time.* Rev. ed. DeKalb, IL: Northern Illinois University Press.

Gerth, H., and C. Mills, eds. 1978. *From Max Weber: Essays in sociology.* New York: Oxford University Press.

Ghaemi, S. N. 1997. Insight and psychiatric disorders: A review of the literature, with a focus on its clinical relevance for bipolar disorder. *Psychiatric Annals* 27:782–90.

———, ed. 2002. *Polypharmacy in psychiatry.* New York: Marcel Dekker.

Ghaemi, S. N., J. Y. Ko, and F. K. Goodwin. 2002. "Cade's disease" and beyond: Misdiagnosis, antidepressant use, and a proposed definition for bipolar spectrum disorder. *Canadian Journal of Psychiatry* 47 (2): 125–34.

Glantz, K., and J. K. Pearce. 1989. *Exiles from Eden: Psychotherapy from an evolutionary perspective.* New York: Norton.

Goodman, A. 1991. Organic unity theory: The mind-body problem revisited. *American Journal of Psychiatry* 148:553–63.

Goodman, S. N. 1999a. Toward evidence-based medical statistics 1: The P value fallacy. *Annals of Internal Medicine* 130:995–1004.

———. 1999b. Toward evidence-based medical statistics 2: The Bayes factor. *Annals of Internal Medicine* 130:1005–21.

Goodwin, D., and S. Guze. [1974] 1989. *Psychiatric diagnosis.* New York: Oxford University Press.

Goodwin, F. K., and K. R. Jamison. 1990. *Manic depressive illness.* New York: Oxford University Press.

Gould, S. J. 1989. Sociobiology and the theory of natural selection. In *Philosophy of biology,* ed. M. Ruse, 253–80. London: Macmillan.

Gunderson, J. 1984. *Borderline personality disorder.* Washington, DC: American Psychiatric Press.

Hairi Yazdi, M. 1992. *The principles of epistemology in Islamic philosophy: Knowledge by presence.* Albany: State University of New York Press.

Harris, J. R. 1998. *The nurture assumption.* New York: Free Press.

Harrison, P. 1991. *General psychopathology:* Karl Jaspers: A trainee's view. *British Journal of Psychiatry* 159:300–302.

Havens, L. L. [1973] 1987. *Approaches to the mind: Movement of the psychiatric schools from sects toward science.* Cambridge, MA: Harvard University Press.

———. 1983. *Participant observation: The psychotherapy schools in action.* Northvale, NJ: Jason Aronson.

———. 1984. The need for tests of normal functioning in the psychiatric interview. *American Journal of Psychiatry* 141 (10): 1208–11.

———. 1986. *Making contact: Uses of language in psychotherapy.* Cambridge, MA: Harvard University Press.

———. 1989. *A safe place.* New York: Ballantine.

———. 1993. *Coming to life.* Cambridge, MA: Harvard University Press.

———. 1994. *Learning to be human.* Reading, MA: Addison-Wesley.

Healy, D. 1998. *The antidepressant era.* Cambridge, MA: Harvard University Press.

Heidegger, M. [1927] 1962. *Being and time.* New York: Harper & Row.

Heilman, K. M., E. Valenstein, and R. T. Watson. 1985. The neglect syndrome. In *Handbook of Clinical Neurology,* vol. 1, ed. J. A. M. Frederiks, 153–83. New York: Elsevier.

Hirschfeld, Robert M. A. 1994. Diagnosis and classification in psychiatry: Gerald Klerman's contribution. *Harvard Review of Psychiatry* 1:306–9.

Holmes, O. W. [1860] 1911. Currents and counter-currents in medical science. In *Medical Essays (1842–1892),* 173–208. Boston: Houghton Mifflin.

Huesmann, L. R. 1978. *Learned helplessness as a model of depression.* Washington, DC: American Psychological Association.

Hume, D. [1777] 1988. *An enquiry concerning human understanding.* La Salle, IL: Open Court.

Hundert, E. H. 1989. *Philosophy, psychiatry, and neuroscience: Three approaches to the mind.* Oxford: Clarendon Press.

Hunink, M., P. Glasziou, J. Siegel, J. Weeks, J. Pliskin, A. Elstein, and M. C. Weinstein. 2001. *Decision-making in health and medicine.* Cambridge: Cambridge University Press.

Irvine, W. 1959. *Apes, angels, and Victorians: Darwin, Huxley, and evolution.* New York: Meridian Books.

Jablensky, A. 1999. The nature of psychiatric classification: Issues beyond ICD-10 and DSM-IV. *Australia and New Zealand Journal of Psychiatry* 33 (2): 137–44.

Jackson, F. 1982. Epiphenomenal qualia. *Philosophical Quarterly* 32:127–36.

Jackson, J. H. 1958. *Selected writings of John Hughlings Jackson.* New York: Basic Books.

James, W. [1890] 1950. *The principles of psychology.* 2 vols. New York: Dover.

———. [1897] 1956. *The will to believe and other essays in popular philosophy.* New York: Dover.

———. [1901] 1958. *The varieties of religious experience.* New York: Mentor Books.

Janowsky, D. S., M. Leff, and R. S. Epstein. 1970. Playing the manic game: Interpersonal maneuvers of the acutely manic patient. *Archives of General Psychiatry* 22 (3): 252–61.

Jaspers, K. [1913] 1997. *General psychopathology.* 2 vols. Trans. J. Hoenig and M. W. Hamilton. Baltimore: Johns Hopkins University Press.

———. [1957] 1986. An autobiographical account. In *Karl Jaspers: Basic philosophical writ-*

ings, ed. Ehrlich, E. L. Ehrlich, and G. B. Pepper, 4–7. Atlantic Highlands, NJ: Humanities Press.

Kandel, E. R. 1979. Psychotherapy and the single synapse: The impact of psychiatric thought on neurobiologic research. *New England Journal of Medicine* 301 (19): 1028–37.

———. 1998. A new intellectual framework for psychiatry. *American Journal of Psychiatry* 155:457–69.

———. 1999. Biology and the future of psychoanalysis. *American Journal of Psychiatry* 156:505–24.

———. 2000. Autobiography. *www.nobel.se.*

Kant, I. [1781] 1998. *Critique of pure reason.* Cambridge: Cambridge University Press.

Kasanin, J. J. [1933] 1994. The acute schizoaffective psychoses. *American Journal of Psychiatry* 151 (suppl. 6): 144–54.

Kendell, R. E. 1989. Clinical validity. *Psychological Medicine* 19 (1): 45–55.

Kendell, R. E., and I. F. Brockington. 1980. The identification of disease entities and the relationship between schizophrenic and affective psychoses. *British Journal of Psychiatry* 137:324–31.

Kendell, R. E., J. E. Cooper, A. J. Gourlay, et al. 1971. Diagnostic criteria of American and British psychiatrists. *Archives of General Psychiatry* 25 (2): 123–30.

Kendler, K. S. 1990. Toward a scientific psychiatric nosology: Strengths and limitations. *Archives of General Psychiatry* 47 (10): 969–73.

———. 2001. A psychiatric dialogue on the mind-body problem. *American Journal of Psychiatry* 158 (7): 989–1000.

Kendler, K. S., W. M. Glazer, and H. Morgenstern. 1983. Dimensions of delusional experience. *American Journal of Psychiatry* 140:466–69.

Kendler, K. S., and D. Walsh. 1998. The structure of psychosis: Syndromes and dimensions. *Archives of General Psychiatry* 55:508–9.

Kernberg, O. F. 1975. *Borderline conditions and pathological narcissism.* New York: J. Aronson.

———. 1976. *Object-relations theory and clinical psychoanalysis.* New York: J. Aronson.

Kety, S. S. 1960. A biologist examines the mind and behavior. *Science* 132:1861–70.

Kim, J. 1993. *Supervenience and mind: Selected philosophical essays.* New York: Cambridge University Press.

Kirby, J., J. Chu, and D. Dill. 1993. Correlates of dissociative symptomatology in patients with physical and sexual abuse histories. *Comprehensive Psychiatry* 34:258–63.

Kleinman, A. 1988. *Rethinking psychiatry: From cultural category to personal experience.* New York: Free Press.

Klerman, G. 1986. Historical perspectives on contemporary schools of psychopathology. In *Contemporary directions in psychopathology: Toward the DSM-IV,* ed. T. Millon and G. Klerman, 3–28. New York: Guilford Press.

Klerman, G., G. Vaillant, R. Spitzer, et al. 1984. A debate on DSM-III. *American Journal of Psychiatry* 141:539–53.

Kohlberg, L. 1981. *The philosophy of moral development: Moral stages and the idea of justice.* San Francisco: Harper & Row.

Kohut, H. 1971. *The analysis of the self: A systematic approach to the psychoanalytic treatment of narcissistic personality disorders.* New York: International Universities Press.

Kraepelin, E. [1917] 1962. *One hundred years of psychiatry.* New York: Citadel Press.

———. 1921. *Manic-depressive insanity and paranoia.* Ed. G. M. Robertson. Edinburgh: E & S Livingstone.

Kramer, P. D. 1993. *Listening to Prozac.* New York: Viking.

Kripke, S. 1972. *Naming and necessity.* Cambridge, MA: Harvard University Press.

Kuhn, T. S. 1962. *The structure of scientific revolutions.* Chicago: University of Chicago Press.

Laing, R. D. 1969. *The divided self.* Baltimore: Pelican.

Leber, P. 2000. Clinical trials and the regulation of drugs. In *Oxford Textbook of Psychiatry,* ed. M. G. Gelder, J. J. Lopez-Ibor Jr., and N. C. Andreasen, 2:1247–52. Oxford: Oxford University Press.

Lee, R. E., G. Bradford, W. T. Thom, et al. 1988. *Recollections and letters of General Robert E. Lee.* Wilmington, NC: Broadfoot.

Lewis, A. 1934. The psychopathology of insight. *Journal of Nervous and Mental Disease* 14:332–48.

———. 1967. *The state of psychiatry: Essays and addresses.* New York: Science House.

Luhrmann, T. M. 2000. *Of two minds: The growing disorder in American psychiatry.* New York: Knopf.

MacIntyre, A. C. 1984. *After virtue: A study in moral theory.* 2d ed. Notre Dame, IN: University of Notre Dame Press.

Maher, B. A. 1990. The irrelevance of rationality to adaptive behavior. In *Philosophy and Psychopathology,* ed. M. Spitzer and B. A. Maher, 73–85. New York: Springer-Verlag.

Makkreel, R. 1992. *Dilthey: Philosopher of the human studies.* Princeton, NJ: Princeton University Press.

Marcuse, H. 1968. *One-dimensional man.* Boston: Beacon Press.

Marguelis, A. M. 1989. *The empathic imagination.* New York: Norton.

Martin, M. 1999. Depression: Illness, insight, and identity. *Philosophy, Psychiatry, Psychology* 6:271–98.

May, R., E. Angel, and H. F. Ellenberger, eds. 1958. *Existence.* New York: Simon & Schuster.

Mayr, E. 1991. *One long argument: Charles Darwin and the genesis of modern evolutionary thought.* Cambridge, MA: Harvard University Press.

McGinn, C. 1990. *The problem of consciousness.* Oxford: Blackwell.

McHugh, P. R. 1997. Foreword to *General psychopathology,* by Karl Jaspers, v–xii. Baltimore: Johns Hopkins University Press.

McHugh, P. R., and P. R. Slavney. 1998. *The perspectives of psychiatry.* 2d ed. Baltimore: Johns Hopkins University Press. Originally published in 1983.

McLaren, N. 1998. A critical review of the biopsychosocial model. *Australia and New Zealand Journal of Psychiatry* 32:86–92.

Menand, L. 2001. *The metaphysical club: A story of ideas in America.* New York: Farrar, Straus & Giroux.

Menninger, K. 1967. *The vital balance.* New York: Viking Press.

Meyer, A. 1948. *The commonsense psychiatry of Dr. Adolf Meyer.* New York: McGraw-Hill.

Nagel, T. 1974. What is it like to be a bat? *Philosophical Review* 83:435–50.

———. 1986. *The view from nowhere.* Oxford: Oxford University Press.

Nasr, S. H. 1976. *Three Muslim sages: Avicenna, Suhrawardi, Ibn Arabi.* Delmar, NY: Caravan Books.

Needleman, J. 1963. *Being-in-the-World.* New York: Basic Books.

Nicholson, R. A. 1989. *The Mathnawi of Jalaluddin Rumi. Books III–IV Commentary.* Lahore, Pakistan: Islamic Book Service.

Nierenberg, A. A., S. N. Ghaemi, K. Clancy-Colecchi, et al. 1996. Cynicism, hostility, and suicidal ideation in depressed outpatients. *Journal of Nervous and Mental Disease* 184:607–10.

Norman, R. 1983. *The moral philosophers: An introduction to ethics.* Oxford: Clarendon Press.

Nussbaum, M. C. 1994. *The therapy of desire: Theory and practice in Hellenistic ethics.* Princeton, NJ: Princeton University Press.

Olmsted, J., and E. Olmsted. 1961. *Claude Bernard and the experimental method in medicine.* New York: Collier Books.

Osler, W. [1889] 1948. *Aequanimitas.* Philadelphia: Blakiston Co.

Pam, A., and C. A. Ross, eds. 1995. *Pseudoscience in biological psychiatry.* New York: Wiley & Sons.

Partington, A., ed. 1994. *The concise Oxford dictionary of quotations.* Oxford: Oxford University Press.

Peirce, C. [1905] 1958. What pragmatism is. In *Selected Writings,* ed. P. Weiner, 180–202. New York: Dover.

———. 1958. *Selected writings.* Ed. P. Weiner. New York: Dover.

Pellegrino, E. D., and D. C. Thomasma. 1981. *A philosophical basis of medical practice.* New York: Oxford University Press.

Penfield, W. 1958. *The excitable cortex in conscious man.* Springfield, IL: C. C. Thomas.

———. 1975. *The mystery of the mind: A critical study of consciousness and the human brain.* Princeton, NJ: Princeton University Press.

———. 1977. *No man alone: A neurosurgeon's life.* Boston: Little, Brown.

Penfield, W., and H. H. Jasper. 1954. *Epilepsy and the functional anatomy of the human brain.* Boston: Little, Brown.

Pepper, G. 1963. A re-examination of the ideal type concept. *American Catholic Sociological Review* 24:185–201.

———. 1988. Karl Jaspers on the sciences: In retrospect. In *Karl Jaspers today: Philosophy at the threshold of the future,* ed. L. Ehrlich and R. Wisser, 153–78. Washington, DC: Center for Advanced Research in Phenomenology and University Press of America.

Perris, C. 1966. A study of bipolar (manic-depressive) and unipolar recurrent depressive psychoses. *Acta Psychiatrica Scandinavica* 42 (suppl. 194): 15–152.

Pinel, P. [1806] 1983. *A treatise on insanity.* Trans. D. D. Davis. Birmingham, AL: Classics of Medicine Library.

Popper, K. 1959. *The logic of scientific discovery.* New York: Basic Books.

Porter, R. 1997. *The greatest benefit to mankind: A medical history of humanity.* New York: Norton.

Ramachandran, V. S., and S. Blakeslee. 1998. *Phantoms in the brain: Probing the mysteries of the human mind.* New York: William Morrow.

Reik, T. 1956. *The search within: The inner experiences of a psychoanalyst.* New York: Farrar, Straus & Cudahy.

Roazen, P. 1969. *Brother animal: The story of Freud and Tausk.* New York: Knopf.

———. 1995. *How Freud worked: First-hand accounts of patients.* Northvale, NJ: J. Aronson.

Robins, E., and S. B. Guze. 1970. Establishment of diagnostic validity in psychiatric illness: Its application to schizophrenia. *American Journal of Psychiatry* 126:983–87.

Rogers, G., ed. 1990. *Benjamin Franklin's The art of virtue.* Eden Prairie, MN: Acorn Publishers.

Rosch, E., and C. Mervis. 1975. Family resemblances: Studies in the internal structure of categories. *Cognitive Psychology* 7:573–605.

Rumi, Jalaludin. 1995. *The essential Rumi.* Trans. Coleman Barks, with John Mayne, A. J. Arberry, and Reynold Nicholson. San Francisco: Harper San Francisco.

Sadler, J., ed. 2002. *Descriptions and prescriptions: Values, mental disorders, and the DSMs.* Baltimore: Johns Hopkins University Press.

Sadler, J., O. Wiggins, and M. Schwartz, eds. 1994. *Philosophical perspectives on psychiatric diagnostic classification.* Baltimore: Johns Hopkins University Press.

Sadock, B., and V. Sadock, eds. 2000. *Kaplan and Sadock's comprehensive textbook of psychiatry.* 7th ed. Philadelphia: Lippincott, Williams & Wilkins.

Schweitzer, A. 1969. *Reverence for life.* New York: Harper & Row.

Shafii, M. 1998. *Freedom from the self: Sufism, meditation, and psychotherapy.* New York: Human Sciences Press.

Shenk, J. In press. *The melancholy of Abraham Lincoln.* New York: Viking Press.

Shepherd, M. 1982. Review of *General Psychopathology,* by Karl Jaspers. *British Journal of Psychiatry* 141:310–12.

———. 1995. Two faces of Emil Kraepelin. *British Journal of Psychiatry* 167 (2): 174–83.

Shweder, R. A. 2001. A polytheistic conception of the sciences and the virtues of deep variety. In *Unity of knowledge: The convergence of natural and human science,* vol. 935, ed. A. Damasio, A. Harrington, J. Kagan, et al., 217–32. New York: New York Academy of Sciences.

Sims, A. 1988. *Symptoms in the mind: An introduction to descriptive psychopathology.* London: Balliere Tindall.

Singer, P. 1993. *A companion to ethics.* Oxford: Blackwell Reference.

Smart, J. J. C. [1959] 1991. Sensations and brain processes. *Philosophical Review* 68:141–56.

Solomon, P., ed. 1966. *Psychiatric drugs: Proceedings of a research conference held in Boston.* New York: Grune & Stratton.

Spitzer, M. 1990. On defining delusions. *Comprehensive Psychiatry* 31:377–97.

———. 1994. The basis of psychiatric diagnosis. In *Philosophical perspectives on psychiatric diagnostic classification,* ed. J. Sadler, O. Wiggins, and M. Schwartz, 163–77. Baltimore: Johns Hopkins University Press.

Starkstein, S. E., S. Vazquez, R. Migliorelli, et al. 1995. A single-photon emission computed tomographic study of anosognosia in Alzheimer's disease. *Archives of Neurology* 52:415–20.

Stevens, A., and J. Price. 2000. *Evolutionary psychiatry.* 2d ed. London: Routledge.

Sullivan, H. S. [1940] 1953. *Conceptions of modern psychiatry.* New York: Norton.

———. 1954. *The psychiatric interview.* New York: Norton.

Sulloway, F. J. 1996. *Born to rebel: Birth order, family dynamics, and creative lives.* New York: Pantheon Books.

Swann, A., J. Bjork, F. Moeller, et al. 2002. Two models of impulsivity: Relationship to personality traits and psychopathology. *Biological Psychiatry* 51:988–94.

Sydenham, T., and K. Dewhurst. 1966. *Dr. Thomas Sydenham (1624–1689): His life and original writings.* Ed. K. Dewhurst. Berkeley: University of California Press.

Symonds, C. 1970. *Studies in neurology.* London: Oxford University Press.

Szasz, T. S. 1970. *Ideology and insanity.* New York: Doubleday.

———. 1974. *The myth of mental illness: Foundations of a theory of personal conduct.* Rev. ed. New York: Harper & Row.

Tannen, D. 1990. *You just don't understand: Women and men in conversation.* New York: Morrow.

Thomas, G. 1993. *An introduction to ethics: Five central problems of moral judgment*. London: Gerald Duckworth.

Tsuang, M., S. Faraone, and M. Lyons. 1993. Identification of the phenotype in psychiatric genetics. *European Archives of Psychiatry and Clinical Neuroscience* 243:131–42.

Vaillant, G. E., M. Bond, and C. O. Vaillant. 1986. An empirically validated hierarchy of defense mechanisms. *Archives of General Psychiatry* 43:786–94.

Valenstein, E. S. 1986. *Great and desperate cures: The rise and decline of psychosurgery and other radical treatments for mental illness*. New York: Basic Books.

Van Praag, H. M. 1990. Two-tier diagnosing in psychiatry. *Psychiatry Research* 34 (1): 1–11.

———. 1992. Reconquest of the subjective: Against the waning of psychiatric diagnosing. *British Journal of Psychiatry* 160:266–71.

———. 1993a. Diagnosis, the rate-limiting factor of biological depression research. *Neuropsychobiology* 28 (4): 197–206.

———. 1993b. *"Make-believes" in psychiatry; or, The perils of progress*. New York: Brunner/Mazel.

———. 1996. Comorbidity (psycho)analysed. *British Journal of Psychiatry* 168 (suppl. 30): 129–34.

———. 1997. Over the mainstream: Diagnostic requirements for biological psychiatric research. *Psychiatry Research* 72 (3): 201–12.

———. 1999. Nosologomania: A disorder in psychiatry. *Tijdschrift voor Psychiatrie* 41:703–12.

Weber, M. 1949. *The methodology of the social sciences*. Trans. E. A. Shils and H. A. Finch. Glencoe, IL: Free Press.

———. [1904] 1993. *The Protestant ethic and the spirit of capitalism*. London: Routledge.

Wiggins, O. P., and M. A. Schwartz. 1991. Is there a science of meaning? *Integrative Psychiatry* 7:48–53.

Williams, T. H. 1962. *McClellan, Sherman, and Grant*. New Brunswick, NJ: Rutgers University Press.

Winnicott, D. W. 1958. *Collected papers: Through paediatrics to psycho-analysis*. New York: Basic Books.

Yolles, S. 1966. The government's stake in psychiatric drug research. In *Psychiatric drugs: Proceedings of a research conference held in Boston*, ed. P. Solomon, 121. New York: Grune & Stratton.

Zachar, P. 2000. *Psychological concepts and biological psychiatry: A philosophical analysis*. Amsterdam: J. Benjamins.

———. 2001. Psychiatric disorders are not natural kinds. *Philosophy, Psychiatry, and Psychology* 7:167–94.

Index

About the Author

S. Nassir Ghaemi is an assistant professor of psychiatry at Harvard Medical School and director of the bipolar disorder research program at Cambridge Hospital. He holds a B.A. degree in history from George Mason University, an M.D. from the Medical College of Virginia, and an M.A. in philosophy from Tufts University. He completed his psychiatric residency training at McLean Hospital, Belmont, Massachusetts.